AF803875

Signals and Communication Technology

Series Editors

Emre Celebi, Department of Computer Science, University of Central Arkansas, Conway, AR, USA

Jingdong Chen, Northwestern Polytechnical University, Xi'an, China

E. S. Gopi, Department of Electronics and Communication Engineering, National Institute of Technology, Tiruchirappalli, Tamil Nadu, India

Amy Neustein, Linguistic Technology Systems, Fort Lee, NJ, USA

Antonio Liotta, University of Bolzano, Bolzano, Italy

Mario Di Mauro, University of Salerno, Salerno, Italy

This series is devoted to fundamentals and applications of modern methods of signal processing and cutting-edge communication technologies. The main topics are information and signal theory, acoustical signal processing, image processing and multimedia systems, mobile and wireless communications, and computer and communication networks. Volumes in the series address researchers in academia and industrial R&D departments. The series is application-oriented. The level of presentation of each individual volume, however, depends on the subject and can range from practical to scientific.

Indexing: All books in "Signals and Communication Technology" are indexed by Scopus and zbMATH

For general information about this book series, comments or suggestions, please contact Mary James at mary.james@springer.com or Ramesh Nath Premnath at ramesh.premnath@springer.com.

Athina Bourdena •
Constandinos X. Mavromoustakis •
Evangelos K. Markakis • George Mastorakis •
Evangelos Pallis
Editors

Intelligent Technologies for Healthcare Business Applications

Springer

Editors
Athina Bourdena
Department of Business Administration & Tourism
Hellenic Mediterranean University
Heraklion, Iraklion, Greece

Constandinos X. Mavromoustakis
Department of Computer Science
University of Nicosia and University of Nicosia Research Foundation
Nicosia, Cyprus

Evangelos K. Markakis
Department of Electrical and Computer Engineering
Hellenic Mediterranean University
Heraklion, Crete, Greece

George Mastorakis
Department of Management Science and Technology
Hellenic Mediterranean University
Agios Nikolaos, Crete, Greece

Evangelos Pallis
Department of Industrial Design and Production Engineering
School of Engineering University of West Attica
Athens, Greece

ISSN 1860-4862 ISSN 1860-4870 (electronic)
Signals and Communication Technology
ISBN 978-3-031-58526-5 ISBN 978-3-031-58527-2 (eBook)
https://doi.org/10.1007/978-3-031-58527-2

© The Editor(s) (if applicable) and The Author(s), under exclusive license to Springer Nature Switzerland AG 2024

This work is subject to copyright. All rights are solely and exclusively licensed by the Publisher, whether the whole or part of the material is concerned, specifically the rights of translation, reprinting, reuse of illustrations, recitation, broadcasting, reproduction on microfilms or in any other physical way, and transmission or information storage and retrieval, electronic adaptation, computer software, or by similar or dissimilar methodology now known or hereafter developed.
The use of general descriptive names, registered names, trademarks, service marks, etc. in this publication does not imply, even in the absence of a specific statement, that such names are exempt from the relevant protective laws and regulations and therefore free for general use.
The publisher, the authors and the editors are safe to assume that the advice and information in this book are believed to be true and accurate at the date of publication. Neither the publisher nor the authors or the editors give a warranty, expressed or implied, with respect to the material contained herein or for any errors or omissions that may have been made. The publisher remains neutral with regard to jurisdictional claims in published maps and institutional affiliations.

This Springer imprint is published by the registered company Springer Nature Switzerland AG
The registered company address is: Gewerbestrasse 11, 6330 Cham, Switzerland

If disposing of this product, please recycle the paper.

Preface

The healthcare industry has consistently been a leader in innovation and technological advancement. As the world moves toward an increasingly digital future, the integration of intelligent technologies in healthcare offers transformative potential. These advancements promise to revolutionize healthcare business operations, enhance patient outcomes, and streamline administrative processes, bringing a myriad of benefits to the industry. It is against this backdrop that we present "Intelligent Technologies for Healthcare Business Applications," a comprehensive exploration of the most promising technologies and their applications within the healthcare sector. This book is a collaborative effort by experts from various fields, aiming to provide a holistic view of how intelligent technologies can reshape healthcare. From predictive analytics and telehealth to administrative efficiencies and personalized medicine, this volume covers a wide range of topics crucial for understanding the current and future landscape of healthcare innovation.

Predictive analytics stands out as one of the most promising areas of intelligent technology in healthcare. By utilizing data mining, machine learning, and other advanced analytics techniques, predictive analytics can identify patterns and relationships within large datasets. This capability allows healthcare providers to anticipate and prevent health problems before they occur, ultimately leading to improved patient outcomes. For instance, predictive analytics can help identify patients at high risk of developing specific diseases, enabling targeted interventions that can prevent or mitigate these conditions. Telehealth, or telemedicine, represents another significant advancement facilitated by intelligent technologies. Through video conferencing, remote monitoring devices, and other telecommunication technologies, telehealth enables healthcare professionals to provide remote care to patients. This approach is particularly beneficial for those in rural or remote areas, offering them improved access to healthcare services. Additionally, telehealth can help reduce healthcare costs by minimizing the need for in-person visits. Machine learning and natural language processing further enhance telehealth by analyzing patient data from remote visits and providing personalized care recommendations. Administrative efficiency in healthcare can also be significantly improved through the application of intelligent technologies. Machine learning algorithms can optimize scheduling and resource allocation by analyzing patient data to identify patterns. Similarly, natural language processing can automate the processing of medical records and other administrative documents, freeing up healthcare professionals to focus on patient care. These advancements not only streamline operations but also enhance the overall efficiency and effectiveness of healthcare delivery. Personalized medicine is yet another exciting area where intelligent technologies are making a substantial impact. By leveraging data analytics and other advanced technologies, healthcare providers can tailor treatment plans to the unique characteristics of individual patients. Genetic data, for example, can identify patients at high risk for certain diseases, allowing for personalized interventions that can prevent or effectively treat these conditions.

Despite the numerous benefits, the integration of intelligent technologies in healthcare also presents challenges and concerns. Data privacy and security are paramount, as healthcare businesses must ensure that patient data is kept secure and confidential. Furthermore, it is crucial to train employees to use these technologies safely and ethically, understanding both their potential and limitations. "Intelligent Technologies for Healthcare Business Applications" is a small yet significant step toward exploring recent advances, disseminating state-of-the-art techniques, and deploying novel technologies in intelligent healthcare services and applications. We extend our gratitude to the contributors and experts whose efforts have made this book possible. We also thank our readers for their interest in this vital field. Together, we can unlock the full potential of intelligent technologies in healthcare, paving the way for a healthier and more efficient future.

Heraklion, Greece — Athina Bourdena
Nicosia, Cyprus — Constandinos X. Mavromoustakis
Heraklion, Greece — Evangelos K. Markakis
Agios Nikolaos, Greece — George Mastorakis
Athens, Greece — Evangelos Pallis

Contents

Chapter 1
An Introductory Perspective on Machine Learning for Health Care

Reinaldo Padilha França, Ana Carolina Borges Monteiro, Rangel Arthur, and Rodrigo Bonacin

1.1 Introduction

In essence, machine learning is the study of pattern recognition and computational learning in artificial intelligence (Fig. 1.1), basically considering two types of approaches featuring supervised and unsupervised learning; and two types of algorithms: classification and regression. This technology allows machines to work in digital "learning" mode so that they can process data independently and, considering that there are several uses for this type of data-oriented technology, including predictive analysis with historical information, description of patients via habits, detection of diseases by patient profile, among others [1].

Machine Learning in Health has the potential to work with data analysis and machine learning techniques in medicine, ranging from the reduction of operating costs and individual health expenses to the possibility of people enjoying longer, healthier, and more productive lives. In general, health applications are supervised learning techniques for classification algorithms. This means that, through a database of several patients containing the list of their symptoms and diagnoses, one seeks to find patterns of symptoms for each disease. In this way, the application can

R. P. França (✉) · R. Bonacin
Renato Archer Information Technology Center (ITC), Campinas, SP, Brazil

A. C. B. Monteiro (✉)
School of Electrical and Computer Engineering (FEEC), University of Campinas (UNICAMP), Campinas, SP, Brazil
e-mail: monteiro@decom.fee.unicamp.br

R. Arthur
School of Technology (FT), University of Campinas (UNICAMP), Limeira, SP, Brazil
e-mail: rangel@ft.unicamp.br

© The Author(s), under exclusive license to Springer Nature Switzerland AG 2024

A. Bourdena et al. (eds.), *Intelligent Technologies for Healthcare Business Applications*, Signals and Communication Technology,
https://doi.org/10.1007/978-3-031-58527-2_1

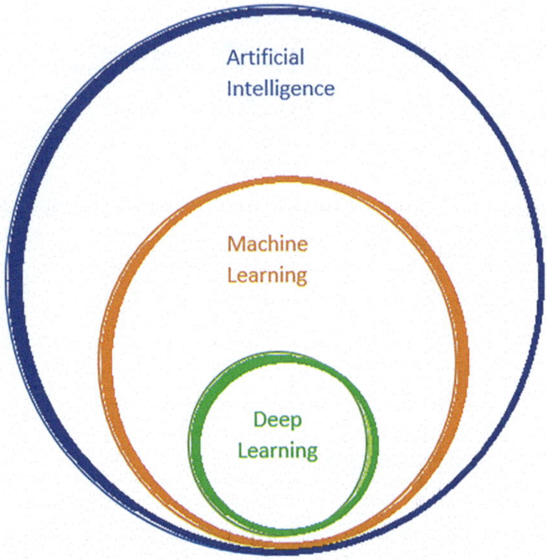

Fig. 1.1 Artificial intelligence concept illustration

inform whether the patient has a certain disease or not, according to the symptoms they present [2, 3].

With regard to the COVID-19 pandemic, this has been seen as the main accelerating element of digital transformation in different sectors of society, and in the area of health, machine-learning techniques have been applied in various research related to the development of vaccines and evaluation of medicines. In addition, it is used for the purposes of early diagnosis, supported by blood and imaging tests, and to prevent the clinical condition of patients. Machine learning addresses one of the concerns arising from the new coronavirus regarding the isolation of symptomatic people to reduce the contagion and spread of the disease, considering intelligent processes capable of relating symptoms presented with the disease, resulting in a more agile targeting of those infected [4, 5].

Considering that COVID-19 symptoms are very similar to flu symptoms, machine-learning models serve as true allies to find patterns combining large masses of data of different natures, relating to the need to adopt analytical technologies in health processes. It became vital to evolve hospital processes and implement specialized dynamics of mass data collection, including the structuring of different types of data, evaluation of research fronts, and constant training of models and validation by health professionals [4, 5].

Machine learning is a powerful tool in the diagnosis of cancer in that it analyzes the characteristics of a nodule on the magnetic resonance image, according to a database that has already been defined, making it possible to classify the nodule as malignant or benign, or even making it possible to estimate the probability that the nodule belongs to each of the classifications, to then define the patient's diagnosis and the next steps of treatment. Considering that the development of a database large enough to cover as much information as possible for the machine-learning model, considering that diseases behave and evolve differently in each organism, in this respect, the model must be able to absorb these differences, evaluating a wide set of variables [6–8].

The use of machine learning in health may also not be as specific, indicating not only one but all the possible illnesses that the patient may have according to the symptoms they present. Being a great tool during the screening of a patient when they arrive at the emergency room, given the symptoms presented and with the help of data already pre-defined in the system, the patient is referred to the most appropriate specialist [9].

It is also worth highlighting several types of recent research bringing machine-learning methodologies as a perspective for interpreting large databases, focusing on various specialties such as supporting the diagnosis and treatment of diseases, facilitating laboratory tests, and developing and prescribing medications, to name a few. These studies describe the view of the machine-learning model on the importance of risk factors, which can be compared with other studies with the same analysis, but statistically [9].

Establishing a machine-learning process in a health institution requires a series of specific analyses; after all, each institution has its particularities, as it is up to management to know how to identify them, using an investigative approach, and we seek to understand exactly where it is and what are the opportunities to implement solutions based on machine learning to deliver maximum usability and value, tailored to the specificities of each health institution. This makes it possible to reduce costs and improve the quality of health services. Investing in machine-learning technology is a way to maximize results. Some challenges, however, are inherent to the reality of health institutions [9, 10].

The benefits of machine learning in health are reducing the time of diagnosis; optimizing virus genetic sequencing processes in the research and developing treatments and drugs; reducing examination costs, indicating the most decisive for obtaining each diagnosis; improving diagnostic and prevention models; reducing the operational team necessary to meet the demand, as a doctor will be able to define the diagnosis more accurately and in a shorter consultation time, being able to attend more patients; and even applying remote service predictive processes, with periodic programming for staff reevaluation [9–11].

In this sense, the convergence of several technological trends, such as the disruptive technology of machine learning and the growing accumulation of data, have been accelerating the progress of technological development in health; the obstacle, however, lies in extracting value from this universe of available data. Given the technological panacea, knowing which technology is best to be implemented to help a medical decision, such as which machine-learning approach to employ, can be decisive in a patient's life. And institutions need tools capable of transforming data into information that allows for more assertive decision-making [10–12].

Therefore, this chapter demonstrates a landscape view of the applied aspect, as well as the key concerns and challenges, aiming to provide an updated overview of machine learning for health care and technologies, with a concise bibliographic background featuring their potential, showing the fundamentals of this disruptive technology.

The novelty in work concerning the discussion of machine learning for health care and technologies has as motivation focused on conceding a major scientific contribution. It is also worth mentioning that this manuscript differs from the existing contributions of various previous works [13–21], as it offers a new perspective on an element missing in the literature, a scientific collection around the topic addressed, whereas a survey or review [13–21] describing and explaining the theoretical aspects is often employed in science documenting how each discovery is aggregated to the store of knowledge, fitting into a theoretical model. Therefore, this type of research work gives examples of the most recent research, applications, and technological developments, which are scarce in the literature. This chapter deals with tools and approaches focusing on an updated discussion summarizing scientific techniques.

1.2 Literature Review on Machine-Learning Fundamentals

Artificial intelligence encompasses several methods, techniques, and algorithms that convert software into an intelligent system, having several applications that can even be seen in distinct fields of society. Currently, these systems can perform more specific tasks, in many cases, more efficiently and accurately than humans themselves [22].

Machine learning has behavior autonomously based on its own experience, i.e., it is a system that can modify its training as we discussed earlier, as human interference here is minimal, capable of analyzing a large amount of data using specific statistical methods. Basically, in the establishment of logical rules, i.e., the rules are generated based on the recognition of patterns within the analyzed data, in addition to using a variety of algorithms to find patterns in the database, considering that based on these patterns, it can make determinations or predictions, which are aimed at improving the performance of a task or, depending on the application, making the most appropriate decision for the context [23].

Its main characteristic, however, is that it does not have to have routines implanted manually because the machine-learning system performs tasks with ever greater precision and can learn from data analysis. An example is the spam filter of emails, without the need for configuration, improving itself automatically, and, with time, it becomes more and more efficient at blocking unwanted messages from the inbox [23].

In supervised mode, when trying to predict a dependent variable from a list of independent variables, the algorithm learns by receiving data that contain the right answer; there is a relationship between input and output used to train the algorithm, considering that the information entering the system is already labeled as positive or negative. The basic characteristic of supervised learning is that the data used to train them contain the desired response; that is, the data are annotated with the responses or classes to be predicted, i.e., it contains the dependent variable resulting from the observed independent variables [24].

In the case of the unsupervised mode, the data received do not carry labels; that is, the effects of the variables are not predicted. It is desired to find a more informative representation of the data available. With this, the results are related to the patterns found in the data, as well, according to certain variables, improving as the system meets new selected standards. Generally, this more informative representation is also simpler; this is a method that extracts references from datasets consisting of input data with no marked responses, condensing the information into more relevant points, used as a process to find a meaningful structure, generative characteristics, underlying explanatory processes, and groupings inherent in a set of examples [24, 25].

Reinforcement learning depending on the circumstances in which this action will be performed is what the machine tries to learn, i.e., what is the best action to take. It is a way of teaching the computer which action to prioritize given a certain situation; it is still possible to link rewards and punishments for possible outcomes and, weighing them in the right way, teach the priority level of each goal [24–26].

Machine learning techniques usually use various statistical methods to improve their performance. Among the main ones most frequently used is regression, which is used in supervised learning algorithms, in which the input variables are mapped, determining their characteristics, and is used when the value that is being predicted differs from a "yes or no." It follows a continuous spectrum, thus predicting the output results [24–27].

The classification used in supervised learning is the method in which the answer can have two or more variables; it is the process of taking some type of input and assigning a label to it. Using this method, the results can be grouped into variables of a certain size that is below a certain value and the group of those that are above that. This is generally used when the forecasts are of a different nature, that is, a simple "yes or no" [24–27].

Clustering is used in an unsupervised learning algorithm based on a database in which it is not possible to perceive the effects of variables, performing grouping or segmentation or separation into similar characteristics through an algorithm that can be k-means, principal component analysis, or even hierarchical. This method finds patterns and the data are grouped according to the relationships found between the variables. It is basically a collection of objects based on their similarity and dissimilarity; this is the task of dividing the population or the data points into several groups. So, in the same group and different from the data points in other groups, the data points in the same groups are more similar to other data points [24–27].

Using an machine-learning algorithm and the method appropriate to the objectives, it is possible to obtain good predictions; considering the learning flow, the machine is capable of learning only once. In other words, machine learning is only possible when the program improves performance and accuracy by increasing experience. For this reason, when faced with new data, it is necessary to add algorithms that will act on the existing models when additional data are inserted [24–27].

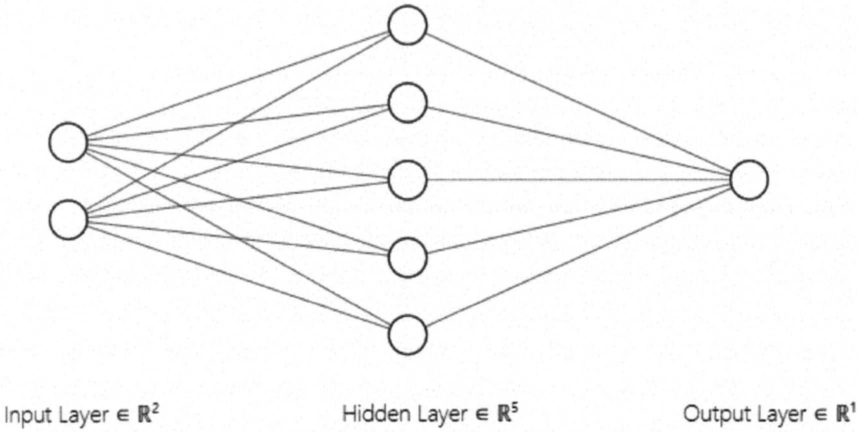

Fig. 1.2 Neural networks

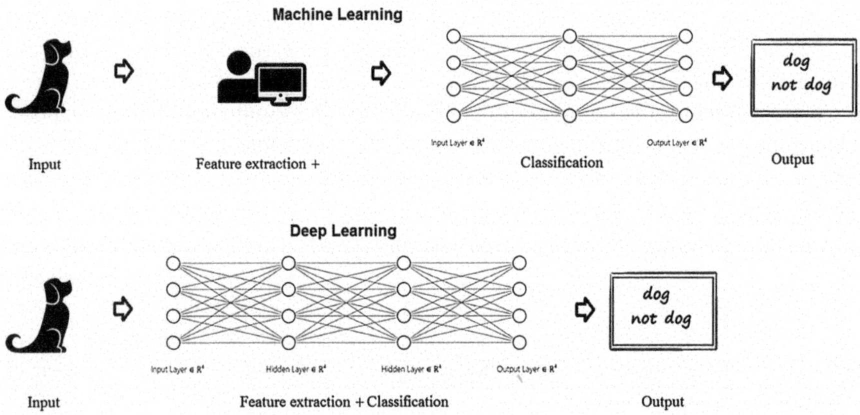

Fig. 1.3 Machine learning × deep learning

Artificial neural networks (Fig. 1.2) are one of the methods used in machine learning, seeking to simulate the way in which the human brain works; that is, it mimics the connections between neurons (synapses). This means that the inputs travel through the neural network of a system, where the data are processed and produce some outputs in response. A neural network is the essential building block of an artificial neural network, whereas the basic unit of the brain is the neuron, and these are then connected to a large mesh network. A perceptron performs simple signal processing, allowing the computer to learn by incorporating new data. The larger the mesh, the more "intelligent" the machine is and the more the machine can learn [24–27].

Instead of organizing the data to be executed through predefined equations, which is also one of the techniques used by machine learning, deep learning (Fig. 1.3) trains the computer to learn on its own, configuring basic parameters about the data and recognizing patterns in various layers of processing. For example, it manages to perform image recognition, differentiating a photo of a person from an animal, It is possible that a layer of a neuron has prior knowledge about the dog's nose and ears, whereas another layer has information about the texture of the dog's hair, eyes, and teeth, and a third layer is known as the paws and tail. This technique is a class of machine-learning algorithms that employs multiple layers to progressively extract top-level resources from raw input; it can also be used to recognize the voice and natural language as well [26–28].

1.3 Applications, Issues, and Challenges

A machine-learning algorithm is able to identify movement patterns and reconstruct the digital image as if the patient were immobile. An example is machine-learning technology applied to imaging equipment for patients with Parkinson's. This type of technological solution is an alternative to sedation, because of a certain difficulty in performing imaging tests relative to tremors, which impairs the formation of medical imaging, i.e., improves access to these tests for this population [28–30].

Another application is based on an machine-learning-oriented algorithm that makes it possible to find incidental findings in chest examinations for pulmonary nodules, the premise of which is to diagnose early problems that may intensify the symptoms of pneumonia or even COVID-19. Other AI-oriented solutions suggest better results than dermatologists or radiologists, for example, in the identification of cancerous lesions on the skin or in the diagnosis of pneumonia through the analysis of radiographic examinations. After all, technology has already changed the way in which patients and doctors communicate, and AI is changing the way in which health care is perceived [30–32].

Another application uses AI and machine learning for digital emotional detection to detect emotions in the human face and help the physician at a distance, via telemedicine, to interpret this nonverbal language, and even the use of machine learning in the ICU remotely, collecting information about the prognosis and using algorithms for decision making. Both examples of applications in real contexts are aimed at bringing the patient and the specialist doctor closer and making the medical decision as accurate as possible [33].

Telemedicine, especially teleconsultation, has experienced and continues to experience growth since the advent of COVID-19, even though there was a great cultural prejudice that delayed its implementation until society was forced to take advantage of digital services, not only to ask for meals but also to have work and family meetings and, finally, to carry out medical consultations online. Telemedicine is one of the areas that has advanced using AI resources. New technologies have enabled the intensive use of data as well as added speed and quality to the exchange of information and the acquisition of knowledge. By using AI resources, doctors can better monitor patients, analyze results of different examinations, and take decisions with greater agility and precision. The positive side of telemedicine lies in making health accessible to the greatest number of people at any time and place, significantly reducing the travel time and costs for patients, in addition to providing contact with professionals from several other specialties. The health system reduces the demand for specialists and hospitals right at the beginning of care, as there is a decentralization of care, both in the prevention and in the treatment of diseases [34, 35].

In the same vein, the adoption of remote monitoring is also increasing, adding machine-learning algorithms that have been allowing health teams to monitor, manage, and interact with patients, considering that data are essential to providing relevant telemedicine diagnostics in the comfort of their own homes. For high-risk individuals, health professionals are relying on teleconsultation and remote monitoring, as doctors can use a large amount of potentially useful external information and compare or analyze patient data based on that, ensuring better results for patients, while significantly reducing costs. Naturally, this will require organization to ensure that the use of patient data remains a benefit and not a risk, which implies a strong ethical imperative [34, 35].

Telemedicine can help during the current pandemic by reducing the demand for other care, allowing hospitals to care for patients infected with COVID-19 and urgent and emergency cases, as well as avoiding potential unnecessary exposure to the coronavirus. With regard to other types of medical assistance, it can be clarified by remote assistance, without the need for a face-to-face consultation. In addition, the telemedicine tool can be used to monitor patients confirmed with COVID-19, who are in isolation at home [34, 35].

From a technical point of view, one of the main obstacles encountered during the COVID-19 crisis was to collecting samples, processing them, and sending them to the diagnostic suppliers (who were overloaded), then waiting for the results to come back and communicating them to the patients. In this context, a multitude of machine-learning-based applications in the Cloud have emerged that can be deployed on mobile devices (Mobile Health [mHealth]), many of which can capture and store patients' vital signs for instant access by health care teams and clinicians [36, 37].

Another highlight of machine-learning technology, given COVID-19, is the processing of data concerning spatial analysis, through factor analysis based on mathematical concepts. This analysis allows spatial evaluation of the object of study, and, using the concepts of dimension and vector base, it is possible to represent and spatially evaluate the chosen scheme, which can be used with data collected to visually map the hotspots of the epidemic. This allows integration of the dimensions that make up the object of study, allows documentation, coding, and analysis of data comprehensively in a quick and detailed way, forming a unitary structure; and evaluates the object of study from new variables, i.e., spatial variables and evaluating a hierarchical structure for a more complete evaluation of the object, obtaining statistically significant results by combining spatial algorithms [37, 38].

For transparency and reliability of the best evidence available currently, doctors often need recommendations and guidance regarding reliable treatments that do not yet exist in the peer-reviewed literature, for example. This was quite evident during the COVID-19 pandemic, as thousands of scientific publications and trials related to COVID-19 were carried out. It is practically impossible for anyone to assimilate this amount of information. In this sense, machine-learning-oriented tools enhance and accelerate the way in which doctors have access to information on this new disease, guiding them in the best decisions and closing the gaps between what doctors saw and what emerging research showed from smart document reading. This is the ability that new computer systems have: to recognize, analyze, and extract relevant information from documents automatically [38, 39].

Artificial intelligence has been an excellent ally in clinical surveillance systems known for providing timely and relevant patient updates and clinical alerts in real time, allowing identification of a wide range of acute and chronic health conditions more accurately. With this, doctors are able to identify patients at risk, bringing very positive impacts, both from the point of view of clinical results and the cost to institutions [39].

By integrating spatial information in the machine-learning and deep-learning processes, inference for object detection, classification, and image segmentation becomes possible. This also leads to a high processing computational demand. Using AI technologies as a support tool in the analytical process, it is possible to perform engineering and data transformation, and model statistical data, which require a lot of machine processing to support the analytical process by providing data to create real-time analysis with a large volume of data, and also making it possible to use image analysis efficiently [38, 39].

In the future, health areas are likely to establish pandemic and epidemic surveillance and response centers as part of their strategic scenario and policy-planning initiatives, as the challenge encountered at the international, national, and local levels was the lack of preparedness for the pandemic, which culminated in a different crisis situation region to region, with hospitals in the most affected areas completely overcrowded whereas others still had some capacity. This type of scenario would easily be overcome through the use of machine-learning tools, through self-service analytical machine-learning tools fed by data from government health agencies, making it possible not only to monitor outbreaks and diseases in different parts of the country but also to provide useful information through visual analysis panels that proactively monitor, analyze, and measure both the implications of demand and the supply of health care. In this context, data analysis fulfills the promise of improving the quality of care at a lower cost, enabling executives, business leaders, clinicians, and nurses to harness the power of machine-learning-oriented predictive and prescriptive analysis [40–44].

Thus, in order to make sense of an ever-growing “tsunami” of structured and unstructured data, and to automate repetitive operations that previously required manual processing, the vast potential of AI, machine learning, and natural language processing (NLP) should be used to apply advanced technologies, and even deep learning to transform clinical and commercial processes [42–44].

As the complexity of the data increases, it is imperative to adopt descriptive and predictive analyses, ranging from capturing patients’ vital signs, while learning machine learning and NLP to obtain the necessary information. However, there is a need to be able to ask the right questions, so that advances in technology do not come at the expense of ethics [42–44].

However, machine-learning models are specific to each context in which they are applied, as it is still very difficult to obtain machine-learning models that predict multi-class tasks with high performance, considering that almost everything in medicine is multiclass as it deals with diagnostic probabilities daily and does not deal with a "closed" diagnosis. In addition, there are still ethnic biases related to the amount of data referring to different populations, as there is also little explainability of some machine-learning models, something that is extremely necessary in health. Yet another challenge to be overcome is in dealing with the medical community's lack of knowledge about AI technology, causing a barrier to machine-learning-oriented applications, considering that both data science and AI will only really impact health when it reaches health professionals who really understand its potential and impact on the results of health diagnoses and prognoses [42–44].

1.4 Discussion

Machine learning is a sub-area of AI that allows predictions to be made about specific diseases and treatments, in a personalized way and in a short time. This technology is responsible for one of the greatest revolutions in human history, and has been successful in medicine, as it is possible to teach machines to make predictions and make decisions in an increasingly simple way and through increasingly accurate systems and tools.

From the care perspective, to assist the patient and provide technology so that the health professional can decide which path to follow regarding the treatment, it is possible using tools based on AI, such as machine learning, to extract knowledge of what has already been registered, by grinding these data so that they can "tell" how it is possible to improve the patient's journey, i.e., a symbiosis of technologies × human. People in their lives generate a large amount of health data including images, genomics, consultations, and wearables data. Such quantity and complexity make analysis by humans impractical. This also increases the need of advanced computational tools to support health professionals. Therefore, it is necessary to use machine-learning tools that transform these data into information, especially insights that allow more assertive decisions to be made.

From this, it is possible to reduce costs, improve management (improvement of administrative processes), and the service (possibility of getting to know the patient better) becomes more effective. This is due to the improvement of hardware with increased computational power and the increase in the amount of data collected causing a significant technological development in AI, clarifying that within AI is the sub-area of machine learning, and within that sub-area is found another sub-area related to deep learning. Deep learning has potential health implications, especially in image recognition, in which neural networks perform as seen for medical image classification.

Machine-learning-oriented algorithms are able to detect patterns in milliseconds, to segment tumors into thousands of images through the use of neural networks to perform tasks that include radiology; or even the majority of AI models currently proposing to perform tasks with respect to forecasting the spread during the COVID-19 pandemic; or in relation to the recognition (emergency with flu-like symptoms) of COVID-19 on radiographs or tomography.

Machine learning can be also used to identify mutational changes and support personalized medicine. This includes enhancing prevention mechanisms, enabling early diagnosis, developing better and more specific treatments, and reducing health costs. However, we emphasize that these improvements depend on proper communication of the clinical platforms and the analysis of clinical results.

The COVID-19 pandemic has been the biggest technological disruption factor in the global health industry, not only affecting lives, economies, and industries but triggering an unprecedented transformation. COVID19 has also accelerated the growing health dependency on data-driven AI/machine-learning technologies. As a result, health care providers prioritize aggregating more and more data sources for the purpose of creating accurate treatment plans, diagnoses, and therapeutic strategies. However, it is not yet possible to measure the extent of the change, but one thing is certain: digital health care will continue to evolve, given the emergence of machine-learning techniques that will require a paradigm shift, placing the use of data, whether old or in real time, in the foreground.

In the AI era, it is possible to solve these challenges of excess data through machine-learning techniques, neural networks, and NPL, considering that its potential of in health is huge. As previously mentioned, data on genetic mutations, and their cross-referencing with treatment strategies, can increase the chances of cure. However, the analysis of such data is complex and voluminous, requiring hundreds of hours if carried out manually or with inadequate computational tools.

It should also be considered that a very important part of machine-learning systems is the possibility of homogenizing the diagnosis and care for the patient, despite the heterogeneity of the training of professionals, as the technology, because of its characteristics (access to better scientific evidence for taking a decision), can contribute to better medicine on a daily basis, not interfering with the doctor–patient relationship, but promoting better care and the greatest benefit to the patient. In addition, having access to this volume of data makes it possible to "see" each person as unique and not just apply treatments according to what works for the majority, emphasizing that the technology is totally synergistic.

Comparatively, doctors carry out a great deal of traditional medicine by placing the "ear on the patient," through a stethoscope; however, machine-learning technologies allow "seeing" of the patient, increasing the capacity, and enhancing human performance in what it is not possible to program. Considering that the challenge in the area of modern health has become complex enough in that it is no longer possible for medical professionals to act alone, it is necessary to have multidisciplinary medical specialist teams, adding efforts with the AI-based technology available to achieve the objectives in faster, lower-cost, and higher-quality delivery. In other words, AI-oriented technology is the path to more sustainable, more personalized health, and, through the generation of data insights, even more humane.

1.5 Future Trends

A diagnostic chatbot equipped with AI is as good as a doctor; as technology has already changed the way in which patients and doctors communicate, this feature has revolutionized the experience of users and patients, transforming information that could be provided via forms into a pleasant conversation. If we consider that messaging applications are among those most frequently used, it is easy to understand the ease of adoption of medical chatbots, considering AI-oriented technologies for understanding natural language, text, or voice, and the use of intelligent algorithms. There are several possibilities for using chatbots in the health sector, from the most obvious, which is the scheduling of consultations, to the most complex ones, such as the analysis of test results, passing through responding to doubts, providing instructions for carrying out examinations, confirmation of presence in procedures, and even monitoring of patients with chronic diseases [45–47].

In essence, considering the premise of discovering a drug molecule that interacts with a particular cancer receptor, discovering new ways to detect and treat cancer is a computational problem. Machine-learning models are capable of analyzing millions of molecules to find a small set that are most likely to be used in a specific treatment condition. Machine-learning-oriented models examine how potential drug molecules would be absorbed into the body, metabolized, distributed, or even eliminated, and whether these potential molecules fit the particular cancer receptor for the right disease. This massive AI-oriented approach to computation plus machine learning speeds up the process of discovering drugs capable of advancing to clinical tests, which is applicable to the discovery of treatments to fight cancer or any other disease. Thus, more clinical trials mean more hope and options for patients looking for treatment for their particular type of cancer, and this increase in the speed with which candidate drugs can be discovered means that more drugs enter the clinical trial pipeline. All of this leads to precision medicine, with the ultimate goal being not simply offering patients treatment for a specific type of cancer but offering tailored therapy designed for individual cancers [48, 49].

An example of the use of computational power for precision medicine can be found in relation to individuals with breast cancer using machine learning, computing power, intelligent algorithms, and very intelligent models, such as neural networks, from sophisticated intensive computational analyses in real time, analysis of the patient's pathological report (digital examination), and personalization of its digital properties to provide a personalized diagnosis [49, 50].

From the current point of view, the practical application of AI is able to analyze lung radiographs and detect visual COVID-19 patterns, thus speeding up patient screening, considering that the solution automatically receives radiological images

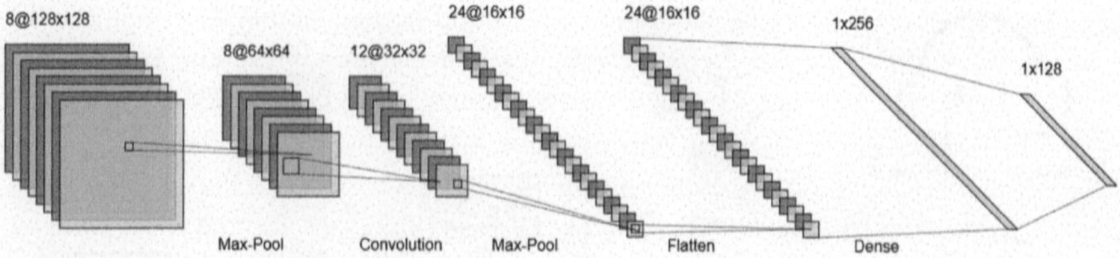

Fig. 1.4 Convolutional neural networks

on a PACS server in the Cloud sent by X-ray equipment. After that, the neural network determines which the chest radiographs are, performs an analysis of the images, and classifies them as positive or negative according to the presence of radiological alterations suggestive of COVID-19. From this pre-processing, a set of specific features is obtained, which serve as input into a series of deep neural networks, such as convolutional neural networks (Fig. 1.4), previously trained and organized. Each neural network generates a pre-diagnosis, determining the presence or absence of COVID-19, as well as the lesions that the disease may have caused in the patient. As the main impact of this project is the definition of a screening process for patients with symptoms of the disease in hospital emergencies, with a high probability of success, using only X-ray devices that already exist in the vast majority of hospitals, clinics, and service stations spread throughout Brazil and the world, there is less wear and tear on health professionals and their consequent use in other more strategic activities [51–53].

The Internet of Things (IoT) is known for being a collective term that describes any of the multiple networks of processors, actuators, sensors, and computers connected to the Internet, which makes it possible to generate connectivity, ease, and creation of devices integrated into everyday life. Today, some devices and operating systems allow daily monitoring of the status and other health data, as the service starts to look at and consider the individual in its entirety, so that the devices follow people and constantly measure the results, in a way that customization occurs that concerns the specific needs and issues of that patient. That is, through this connection between the device, user, and doctor, it is possible to monitor in real time the vital signs, number of steps, blood-glucose measurement, oximetry, calorie-burning, and limitless biometric information that can quickly assist in solving problems and diagnostics. At the same time, IoT tools help to improve and closely observe the deficiencies of everyday life, whether in sleep, weight loss, improving blood glucose, an athlete's performance, etc. In addition, when these data are captured and used more often, there is a lower margin of error and greater precision in resolving the case [54–56].

Artificial intelligence learning comes from the collection of large volumes of data that are analyzed and interpreted by the algorithms, resulting in automatic improvements; considering that only with the data generated by objects connected (Fig. 1.5) to the internet (IoT) can the AI-oriented algorithms cause the machines to learn and work. In this sense the IoT focuses on the medical needs. AI is

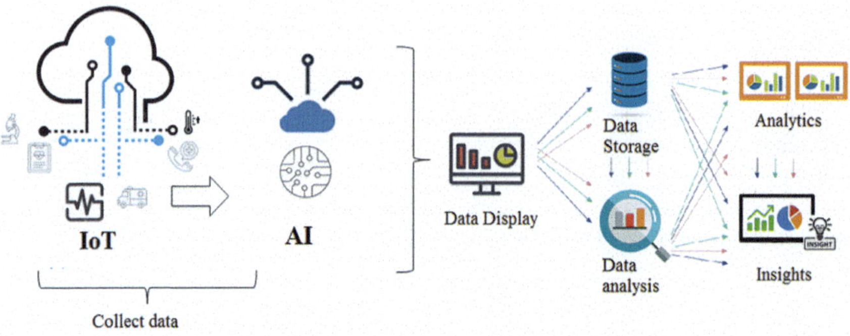

Fig. 1.5 Internet of Things (IoT) in health care. AI, artificial intelligence

able to analyze the collected data, and absorb the largest amount of data possible to offer something extremely personalized to that patient, without the need for a human performing this processing, to give immediate and automatic results. Still, considering that IoT devices are continually empowering human service, this increases personalization, creates indicators, and helps to increase patient engagement. When all of this is used assertively, it is possible to achieve a good relationship, with proximity and positive results [54–62].

1.6 Conclusions

The advancement of digital technologies has had several impacts on medicine, especially in times of pandemics; given the high rate of contamination by the coronavirus, telemedicine, for example, has become a safer alternative for medical care. However, the digitization of medicine is not restricted to online care. AI has been an important ally in urgent and emergency operations, allowing more efficient actions, as the technology optimizes the professional's routine, offering countless advantages to the health professional, with the use of electronic medical records, office management, and storage of the entire service history in the Cloud.

More and more data science and analytics tools, and even the use of predictive models and machine-learning algorithms, are of fundamental importance for health professionals and managers, as they have become indispensable in all areas of the health sector; thus, decision making is always carried out by managers and leaders with greater security, accuracy, and confidence, such as diagnoses, assistance in examinations, preventive programs, public-health problems, consultations, and surgeries, monitoring the expansion of diseases and combating outbreaks, and AI models for hospital management, clinics, and laboratories, with a focus on well-being and individual and collective health.

One of the main advantages of machine learning in medicine is in the area of diagnostics, which can verify whether the individual has a certain disease according to the symptoms they present. Offering greater precision in the analysis makes it possible to find patterns for each disease, and is faster both in the performance of examinations and in the availability of results. And all this generates several benefits in relation to the most effective screening process, disease control, preventing or delaying its progression, directly impacting the patient's quality of life, greater productivity of doctors and health services, the correct choice of effective treatments, reduction of operating costs and individual expenses, and even more quality, accessibility, agility, and effectiveness for patients, doctors, and organizations.

In this context, probability based models are able to extract patterns from the dataset and predict the occurrence of a specific clinical event. Machine learning facilitates the interpretation of medical examinations, pathology slides, and skin lesions, having the potential to positively impact preventive medicine and the discovery of new drugs, images of the retina, electrocardiograms, endoscopy, and vital signs, matching the drug and the dose to each patient, and even diagnose and treat mental illnesses, that is, customize medicine.

Additionally, predicting diseases, optimizing hospital operations, diagnosing cancer, and predicting success rates for new drugs, have effects that can be grouped into three levels taking into account (a) health systems, improving workflow and reducing potential medical errors; (b) doctors, predominantly through fast and accurate image interpretation; and even (c) patients, allowing personalized diagnosis and treatment. Through the support of activities guided by some machine learning related to (a) modeling and simulation of diseases based on the data, including with positive impacts on prevention; (b) improvement of the health system, public and private, through more accurate knowledge; as well as (c) the use of advanced AI technologies to aid diagnosis and medical decisions.

However, there are obstacles to be faced, one of which is the access to and quality of patient data used in the AI algorithm training process, or even developing an AI technology capable of anonymizing patient data; as well as identification of the patient in the examinations, allowing them to be shared while maintaining privacy. Considering the premise that machine-learning-oriented systems are used to support physicians to provide personalized treatments, the need of previous patient data can lead to a late diagnosis. Studies using technologies that work with preliminary data and insights are needed to confirm the potential of AI models to support a more personalized service.

References

1. França, R. P., Monteiro, A. C. B., Arthur, R., & Iano, Y. (2021). An overview of the machine learning applied in smart cities. In *Smart cities: A data analytics perspective* (pp. 91–111). Springer.
2. Holzinger, A. (2016). Machine learning for health informatics. In *Machine learning for health informatics* (pp. 1–24). Springer.
3. Monteiro, A. C. B., França, R. P., Carnielli, G. P., Iano, Y., & Arthur, R. (2020). General aspects of telemedicine: From emergence to use in the COVID pandemic 19. In *Engenharia Moderna: Soluções para Problemas da Sociedade e da Industria* (pp. 1–13). Atena.

4. Kushwaha, S., Bahl, S., Bagha, A. K., Parmar, K. S., Javaid, M., Haleem, A., & Singh, R. P. (2020). Significant applications of machine learning for COVID-19 pandemic. *Journal of Industrial Integration and Management, 5*(4), 453–479.
5. Punn, N. S., Sonbhadra, S. K., & Agarwal, S. (2020). COVID-19 epidemic analysis using machine learning and deep learning algorithms. *MedRxiv*. https://doi.org/10.1101/2020.04.08.20057679
6. Khuriwal, N., & Mishra, N. (2018, March). Breast cancer diagnosis using adaptive voting ensemble machine learning algorithm. In *2018 IEEMA engineer infinite conference (eTechNxT)* (pp. 1–5). IEEE.
7. Cho, S. B., & Won, H. H. (2003, January). Machine learning in DNA microarray analysis for cancer classification. In *Proceedings of the first Asia-Pacific bioinformatics conference on Bioinformatics 2003* (Vol. 19, pp. 189–198). Australian Computer Society, Inc.
8. Asri, H., Mousannif, H., Al Moatassime, H., & Noel, T. (2016). Using machine learning algorithms for breast cancer risk prediction and diagnosis. *Procedia Computer Science, 83*, 1064–1069.
9. Lu, J., Bu, P., Xia, X., Lu, N., Yao, L., & Jiang, H. (2021). Feasibility of machine learning methods for predicting hospital emergency room visits for respiratory diseases. *Environmental Science and Pollution Research, 28*, 29701–29709.
10. Rajkomar, A., Dean, J., & Kohane, I. (2019). Machine learning in medicine. *New England Journal of Medicine, 380*(14), 1347–1358.
11. Deo, R. C. (2015). Machine learning in medicine. *Circulation, 132*(20), 1920–1930.
12. Cleophas, T. J., Zwinderman, A. H., & Cleophas-Allers, H. I. (2013). *Machine learning in medicine* (Vol. 9). Springer.
13. Ahmad, M. A., Eckert, C., & Teredesai, A. (2018, August). Interpretable machine learning in healthcare. In *Proceedings of the 2018 ACM international conference on bioinformatics, computational biology, and health informatics* (pp. 559–560). ACM.
14. Callahan, A., & Shah, N. H. (2017). Machine learning in healthcare. In *Key advances in clinical informatics* (pp. 279–291). Academic Press.
15. Dua, S., Acharya, U. R., & Dua, P. (Eds.). (2014). *Machine learning in healthcare informatics* (Vol. 56). Springer.
16. Shailaja, K., Seetharamulu, B., & Jabbar, M. A. (2018, March). Machine learning in healthcare: A review. In *2018 Second international conference on electronics, communication and aerospace technology (ICECA)* (pp. 910–914). IEEE.
17. Ravì, D., Wong, C., Deligianni, F., Berthelot, M., Andreu-Perez, J., Lo, B., & Yang, G. Z. (2016). Deep learning for health informatics. *IEEE Journal of Biomedical and Health Informatics, 21*(1), 4–21.
18. Miotto, R., Wang, F., Wang, S., Jiang, X., & Dudley, J. T. (2018). Deep learning for healthcare: Review, opportunities and challenges. *Briefings in Bioinformatics, 19*(6), 1236–1246.
19. Dhillon, A., & Singh, A. (2019). Machine learning in healthcare data analysis: A survey. *Journal of Biology and Today's World, 8*(6), 1–10.
20. Dargan, S., Kumar, M., Ayyagari, M. R., & Kumar, G. (2019). A survey of deep learning and its applications: A new paradigm to machine learning. *Archives of Computational Methods in Engineering, 27*, 1071–1092.
21. Sughasiny, M., & Rajeshwari, J. (2018, August). Application of machine learning techniques, big data analytics in health care sector–A literature survey. In *2018 Second international conference on I-SMAC (IoT in social, mobile, analytics, and cloud)* (pp. 741–749). IEEE.
22. França, R. P., Monteiro, A. C. B., Arthur, R., & Iano, Y. (2020). An overview of deep learning in big data, image, and signal processing in the modern digital age. In *Trends in deep learning methodologies: Algorithms, applications, and systems* (pp. 63–87). Academic Press.
23. Yalçın, O. G. (2021). Introduction to machine learning. In *Applied neural networks with TensorFlow 2* (pp. 33–55). Apress.
24. Biswas, A., Saran, I., & Wilson, F. P. (2021). Introduction to supervised machine learning. *Kidney360, 2*, 878–880.

25. Parasa, N. A., Namgiri, J. V., Mohanty, S. N., & Dash, J. K. (2021). Introduction to unsupervised learning in bioinformatics. In *Data analytics in bioinformatics: A machine learning perspective* (pp. 35–49). Wiley.
26. Sutton, R. S., & Barto, A. G. (2018). *Reinforcement learning: An introduction*. MIT Press.
27. Sugiyama, M. (2015). *Introduction to statistical machine learning*. Morgan Kaufmann.
28. Krogh, A. (2008). What are artificial neural networks? *Nature Biotechnology, 26*(2), 195–197.
29. Walczak, S. (2019). Artificial neural networks. In *Advanced methodologies and technologies in artificial intelligence, computer simulation, and human-computer interaction* (pp. 40–53). IGI Global.
30. Monteiro, A. C. B., Iano, Y., França, R. P., & Arthur, R. (2020). Deep learning methodology proposal for the classification of erythrocytes and leukocytes. In *Trends in deep learning methodologies: Algorithms, applications, and systems* (pp. 129–156). Academic Press.
31. Minango, P., Iano, Y., Monteiro, A. C. B., França, R. P., & de Oliveira, G. G. (2019). Automatic skin lesions classification from dermoscopic images employing deep learning. *SET International Journal of Broadcast Engineering, 5*, 108–115.
32. Gao, C., Sun, H., Wang, T., Tang, M., Bohnen, N. I., Müller, M. L., et al. (2018). Model-based and model-free machine learning techniques for diagnostic prediction and classification of clinical outcomes in Parkinson's disease. *Scientific Reports, 8*(1), 1–21.
33. Kundu, T., & Saravanan, C. (2017, December). Advancements and recent trends in emotion recognition using facial image analysis and machine learning models. In *2017 International conference on electrical, electronics, communication, computer, and optimization techniques (ICEECCOT)* (pp. 1–6). IEEE.
34. Hollander, J. E., & Carr, B. G. (2020). Virtually perfect? Telemedicine for COVID-19. *New England Journal of Medicine, 382*(18), 1679–1681.
35. Bashshur, R., Doarn, C. R., Frenk, J. M., Kvedar, J. C., & Woolliscroft, J. O. (2020). Telemedicine and the COVID-19 pandemic, lessons for the future. *Telemedicine Journal and e-Health, 26*(5), 571–573.
36. Dai, X., Spasić, I., Meyer, B., Chapman, S., & Andres, F. (2019, June). Machine learning on mobile: An on-device inference app for skin cancer detection. In *2019 Fourth international conference on fog and mobile edge computing (FMEC)* (pp. 301–305). IEEE.
37. Istepanian, R. S., & Al-Anzi, T. (2018). m-Health 2.0: New perspectives on mobile health, machine learning and big data analytics. *Methods, 151*, 34–40.
38. Sim, I. (2019). Mobile devices and health. *New England Journal of Medicine, 381*(10), 956–968.
39. Elaziz, M. A., Hosny, K. M., Salah, A., Darwish, M. M., Lu, S., & Sahlol, A. T. (2020). New machine learning method for image-based diagnosis of COVID-19. *PLoS One, 15*(6), e0235187.
40. Zoabi, Y., Deri-Rozov, S., & Shomron, N. (2021). Machine learning-based prediction of COVID-19 diagnosis based on symptoms. *npj Digital Medicine, 4*(1), 3.
41. Sujath, R., Chatterjee, J. M., & Hassanien, A. E. (2020). A machine learning forecasting model for COVID-19 pandemic in India. *Stochastic Environmental Research and Risk Assessment, 34*, 959–972.
42. Monteiro, A. C. B., França, R. P., Estrela, V. V., Iano, Y., Khelassi, A., & Razmjooy, N. (2018). Health 4.0 as an application of Industry 4.0 in healthcare services and management. *Medical Technologies Journal, 2*(4), 262–276.
43. França, R. P., Iano, Y., Monteiro, A. C. B., & Arthur, R. (2020). Potential proposal to improve data transmission in healthcare systems. In *Deep learning techniques for biomedical and health informatics* (pp. 267–283). Academic Press.
44. França, R. P., Iano, Y., Monteiro, A. C. B., Arthur, R., Estrela, V. V., Assumpção, S. L. D. L., & Razmjooy, N. (2019). Potential model for improvement of the data transmission in healthcare systems. In *IV International symposium on immunobiologicals & VII Seminário anual científico e tecnológico*.
45. França, R. P., Iano, Y., Monteiro, A. C. B., & Arthur, R. (2020). A methodology for improving efficiency in data transmission in healthcare. *Internet of Things for Healthcare Technologies, 73*, 49.

46. Negrete, P. D. M., Iano, Y., Monteiro, A. C. B., França, R. P., de Oliveira, G. G., & Pajuelo, D. (2021). Classification of dermoscopy skin images with the application of deep learning techniques. In *Proceedings of the 5th Brazilian technology symposium* (pp. 73–81). Springer.
47. Monteiro, A. C. B., Iano, Y., França, R. P., & Arthur, R. (2018, October). Methodology of high accuracy, sensitivity and specificity in the counts of erythrocytes and leukocytes in blood smear images. In *Brazilian technology symposium* (pp. 79–90). Springer.
48. Monteiro, A. C. B., Iano, Y., França, R. P., & Arthur, R. (2020). Development of a laboratory medical algorithm for simultaneous detection and counting of erythrocytes and leukocytes in digital images of a blood smear. In *Deep learning techniques for biomedical and health informatics* (pp. 165–186). Academic Press.
49. Sinkala, M., Mulder, N., & Martin, D. (2020). Machine learning and network analyses reveal disease subtypes of pancreatic cancer and their molecular characteristics. *Scientific Reports, 10*(1), 1–14.
50. Yokoyama, S., Hamada, T., Higashi, M., Matsuo, K., Maemura, K., Kurahara, H., et al. (2020). Predicted prognosis of patients with pancreatic cancer by machine learning. *Clinical Cancer Research, 26*(10), 2411–2421.
51. Binder, A., Bockmayr, M., Hägele, M., Wienert, S., Heim, D., Hellweg, K., et al. (2021). Morphological and molecular breast cancer profiling through explainable machine learning. *Nature Machine Intelligence, 3*, 355–366.
52. Khelassi, A., Estrela, V. V., Monteiro, A. C. B., França, R. P., Iano, Y., & Razmjooy, N. (2019). Health 4.0: Applications, management, technologies and review. *Medical Technologies Journal, 2*, 262.
53. Monteiro, A. C. B. (2019). *Proposta de uma metodologia de segmentação de imagens para detecção e contagem de hemácias e leucócitos através do algoritmo WT-MO.*
54. França, R. P., Iano, Y., Monteiro, A. C. B., & Arthur, R. (2020). Lower memory consumption for data transmission in smart cloud environments with CBEDE methodology. In *Smart systems design, applications, and challenges* (pp. 216–237). IGI Global.
55. França, R. P., Monteiro, A. C. B., Arthur, R., & Iano, Y. (2020). An overview of the integration between cloud computing and Internet of Things (IoT) technologies. In *Recent advances in security, privacy, and trust for Internet of Things (IoT) and cyber-physical systems (CPS)* (pp. 1–22). CRC Press.
56. França, R. P., Borges, A. C., Monteiro, R. A., & Iano, Y. (2021). The fundamentals and potential of IoT for bioinformatics and healthcare. In *Translational bioinformatics applications in healthcare* (pp. 87–108). CRC Press.
57. França, R. P., Monteiro, A. C. B., Arthur, R., & Iano, Y. (2019, October). An overview of Internet of Things security from a modern perspective. In *Brazilian technology symposium* (pp. 639–652). Springer.
58. Khamparia, A., Singh, P. K., Rani, P., Samanta, D., Khanna, A., & Bhushan, B. (2020). An internet of health things-driven deep learning framework for detection and classification of skin cancer using transfer learning. *Transactions on Emerging Telecommunications Technologies, 32*, e3963.
59. Goyal, S., Sharma, N., Bhushan, B., Shankar, A., & Sagayam, M. (2021). IoT enabled technology in secured healthcare: Applications, challenges and future directions. In *Cognitive internet of medical things for smart healthcare* (pp. 25–48). Springer.
60. Sharma, N., Kaushik, I., Bhushan, B., Gautam, S., & Khamparia, A. (2020). Applicability of WSN and biometric models in the field of healthcare. In *Deep learning strategies for security enhancement in wireless sensor networks* (pp. 304–329). IGI Global.
61. Jindal, M., Gupta, J., & Bhushan, B. (2019, October). Machine learning methods for IoT and their future applications. In *2019 International conference on computing, communication, and intelligent systems (ICCCIS)* (pp. 430–434). IEEE.
62. Kumar, S., Bhusan, B., Singh, D., & Choubey, D. K. (2020, July). Classification of diabetes using deep learning. In *2020 International Conference on Communication and Signal Processing (ICCSP)* (pp. 651–655). Chennai, India: IEEE. https://doi.org/10.1109/ICCSP48568.2020.9182293

Chapter 2
Exploring Quantum-Resistant Cryptography Solutions for Health Data Exchange

Andreas Andreou, Constandinos X. Mavromoustakis, Evangelos K. Markakis, George Mastorakis, Evangelos Pallis, and Athina Bourdena

2.1 Introduction

The emergence of quantum computing technology poses a progressively heightened risk to the conventional foundations of classical cryptography. This nascent risk permeates vital sectors, notably HC, eliciting apprehensions regarding safeguarding confidential health-related data within complex HC infrastructures. With the ongoing advancements in quantum computing, its prodigious computational capabilities might jeopardize the efficacy of cryptographic techniques traditionally trusted for data security.

A. Andreou (✉) · C. X. Mavromoustakis
Department of Computer Science, University of Nicosia and University of Nicosia Research Foundation, Nicosia, Cyprus
e-mail: andreou.andreas@unic.ac.cy; mavromoustakis.c@unic.ac.cy

E. K. Markakis
Department of Electrical and Computer Engineering, Hellenic Mediterranean University, Heraklion, Crete, Greece
e-mail: markakis@pasiphae.eu

G. Mastorakis
Department of Management Science and Technology, Hellenic Mediterranean University, Agios Nikolaos, Crete, Greece
e-mail: gmastorakis@hmu.gr

E. Pallis
Department of Industrial Design and Production Engineering, School of Engineering, University of West Attica, Athens, Greece
e-mail: epallis@uniwa.gr

A. Bourdena
Department of Business Administration & Tourism, Hellenic Mediterranean University Heraklion, Iraklion, Greece
e-mail: bourdena@hmu.gr

© The Author(s), under exclusive license to Springer Nature Switzerland AG 2024
A. Bourdena et al. (eds.), *Intelligent Technologies for Healthcare Business Applications*, Signals and Communication Technology,
https://doi.org/10.1007/978-3-031-58527-2_2

The preservation of patient confidentiality and the secure exchange of health-related data remain of utmost importance within the HC sector. The swift digitization of medical documentation and an increasing dependence on interconnected frameworks underscores the imperative for rigorous cryptographic protections to ensure patient privacy, uphold data integrity, and authenticate information [1]. However, the imminent advent of quantum computing poses a significant challenge by potentially exploiting frailties in contemporary cryptographic methodologies, jeopardizing patient data's sanctity, and undermining the foundational trust that sustains HC infrastructures.

This chapter underscores the urgent requirement for quantum-resilient cryptographic approaches to address these burgeoning concerns. Through a meticulous examination of the susceptibilities introduced by quantum computing to prevailing cryptographic techniques, this investigation casts light on the imminent perils. Specifically, Shor's algorithm stands on the cusp of deciphering prevalent encryption protocols rooted in integer factorization [2]. In contrast, Grover's algorithm jeopardizes the safety of symmetric cyphers by facilitating expedited brute-force intrusions [3]. These vulnerabilities manifestly highlight the insufficiency of traditional cryptographic instruments when confronted with the superior capabilities of quantum computing.

Considering these vulnerabilities, the necessity for QRC measures becomes manifestly clear. The complexities ushered in by quantum computing, including the prospective expeditious decryption of classical encryptions, demand anticipatory actions. Such actions encompass rigorous exploration and adoption of QRA, demonstrating fortitude against quantum adversarial endeavours. Notably, the potential of LBC and hash-based paradigms rises as a beacon of optimism, proffering plausible solutions adept at counteracting the formidable computational prowess of quantum machines [4, 5].

Nevertheless, the transition to quantum-resistant solutions encompasses inherent intricacies. Contending issues such as performance overhead and harmonizing with extant systems constitute notable challenges. However, the advantages of incorporating QRC methodologies within HC systems are considerable. The security framework for health data exchange could be fortified by employing these measures to anticipate and thwart quantum adversarial endeavours [6]. That would engender heightened patient trust, fostering a more expansive and secure milieu for data dissemination amongst HC practitioners. Furthermore, these forward-thinking initiatives are congruent with emerging privacy statutes, ensuring regulatory adherence whilst vigilantly protecting delicate patient data.

The advent of quantum computing emerges as a pivotal impediment to health data integrity within HC infrastructures. The necessity to delve into QRC methodologies is propelled by the mandate to bolster extant security measures against quantum adversarial manoeuvres. This chapter emphasizes the quintessential function that QRA, including LBC and hash-based paradigms, holds in assuring health information's confidentiality, veracity, and authenticity. By meticulously addressing the obstacles, evaluating the merits, and championing the integration of quantum-resistant strategies, this discourse substantively contributes to the paramount objec-

Table 2.1 Glossary of abbreviations

Definition	Abbreviation
Health Care	HC
Quantum-Resistant Cryptography	QRC
Quantum-Resistant Algorithms	QRA
Lattice-Based Cryptography	LBC
Discrete Logarithm Problem	DLP
Elliptic Curve Discrete Logarithm Problem	ECDLP
Transport Layer Security	TLS
Secure SHell	SSH
Internet Protocol Security	IPSec
Digital Signature Algorithm	DSA
Elliptic Curve Digital Signature Algorithm	ECDSA
RSA Probabilistic Signature Scheme	RSA-PSS
RSA Optimal Asymmetric Encryption Padding	RSA-OAEP
Health Insurance Portability and Accountability Act	HIPAA
Secure Sockets Layer/Transport Layer Security	SSL/TLS
Public Key Infrastructure	PKI
Health and Human Services	HHS
Learning With Errors	LWE
Hash-Based Cryptographic	HBC
National Institute of Standards and Technology	NIST
Shortest Vector Problem	SVP
General Data Protection Regulation	GDPR
California Consumer Privacy Act	CCPA
Post-Quantum Cryptographic	PQC

tive of preserving patient privacy and data security in the quantum computing epoch [7].

To enhance clarity and facilitate comprehension, Table 2.1 provides a glossary of all the abbreviations utilized throughout this chapter.

2.2 Quantum Computing and Cryptographic Vulnerabilities

Quantum computing epitomizes a profound departure from classical computational paradigms by leveraging the tenets of quantum mechanics to execute intricate calculations at velocities unattainable by traditional computing methodologies. Quantum bits, commonly referred to as qubits, can coexist in numerous states concurrently, thereby bestowing quantum computers the capacity to process substantial volumes of information in parallel.

Shor's and Grover's algorithms stand as seminal quantum algorithms that imperil the integrity of classical cryptographic techniques [8, 9]. The former, conceived by the esteemed mathematician Peter Shor, exploits the inherent capabilities of quantum computers to factorize substantial numerical values into their prime constituents with remarkable efficiency. Such an advancement gravely undermines the security of predominant public key cryptographic systems, notably the Rivest–Shamir–Adleman (RSA) algorithm [10]. The foundation of RSA encryption is predicated upon the computational challenge associated with the factorization of vast numbers. However, with the introduction of Shor's algorithm, the computational duration necessary for such factorization could be significantly curtailed, thereby jeopardizing the sanctity of RSA encryption and the assurance of secure communication.

Grover's algorithm, meticulously devised by Dr Lov Grover, pertains to the challenge of searching within an unorganized database. This algorithm holds significant implications for symmetric-key cryptographic systems wherein the encryption key originates from a confidential key. Notably, Grover's algorithm can traverse a database comprising N entities in $\sqrt{N}$ operations, in stark contrast to classical computers, which necessitate N operations. Consequently, this suggests that brute-force assaults on symmetric cyphers might experience an augmentation in their speed, thereby diminishing the requisite effective key length essential for ensuring robust security.

These algorithms elucidate inherent susceptibilities within the prevailing cryptographic architecture, wherein classical cryptographic techniques underpin the cornerstone of data safeguarding. The fortification of these systems is contingent upon the computational impracticability of specific endeavours, such as the factorization of extensive numerical values or the exhaustive search through cryptographic keys. Shor's and Grover's algorithms harness the distinctive proficiencies of quantum computing apparatuses to address these challenges, thereby calling into question the foundational premises upon which many encryption and hash functions have been constructed.

The capacity of quantum computing to compromise classical cryptographic techniques is derived predominantly from algorithms such as Shor's and Grover's. Shor's algorithm jeopardizes public key cryptography through its adeptness at factorizing substantial numerical entities, whilst Grover's algorithm expedites brute-force assaults on symmetric-key systems. Such algorithms illuminate inherent fragilities in the security bedrock of extant cryptographic frameworks, thereby emphasizing the imperative necessity for QRC strategies in a time characterized by the escalating sophistication of quantum computing devices.

2.2.1 Shor's Algorithm and Its Implications for Cryptography

Shor's algorithm, a groundbreaking quantum computational methodology conceived by the distinguished mathematician Peter Shor, presents a formidable challenge to prevalent cryptographic systems predicated on the computational intricacy of integer factorization. Fundamentally, this algorithm harnesses the inherent attributes of quantum computers, notably their capability to manage numerous states concurrently, to adeptly address the complex task of decomposing substantial numerical values into their prime constituents.

Integer factorization, which entails disintegrating a composite number into its constituent prime factors, is a pivotal element in numerous cryptographic protocols, with the RSA encryption framework being particularly salient. The underpinning of RSA encryption is predicated on the premise that the factorization of expansive numerical entities into their prime components presents a formidable challenge for conventional computational systems, thereby rendering it an exemplary mechanism for ensuring secure communication.

Nevertheless, Shor's algorithm represents a seminal quantum advancement. This algorithm can expedite the factorization procedure exponentially by capitalizing on quantum parallelism and entanglement. By employing a quantum computer's qubits, Shor's algorithm facilitates the exploration of manifold possibilities concurrently, culminating in a substantial exponential diminution in the temporal duration requisite to ascertain the prime factors of extensive numerical values.

The ramifications of Shor's algorithm resonate profoundly within the domain of cryptography. Conventional cryptographic methodologies, predicated upon the anticipated intricacy of integer factorization—exemplified by RSA encryption and analogous protocols—may find themselves susceptible to an adequately potent quantum computational apparatus. Shor's algorithm can adeptly factorize expansive numerical entities hitherto deemed impervious, thereby subjecting encrypted information to potential decryption.

Discrete Logarithm Problem (DLP) and Elliptic Curve Discrete Logarithm Problem (ECDLP) form the cornerstone of several cryptographic protocols and systems that ensure security in digital communication [11, 12]. The ability of Shor's algorithm to efficiently solve these problems, when implemented on a quantum computer, poses potential challenges to many existing cryptographic schemes and underscores the need for Post-Quantum Cryptographic (PQC) methods [13]. When implemented on a quantum computer, Shor's algorithm poses a significant threat to the foundational security protocols that underpin much of today's secure digital communication. Notably, it can compromise the security of the Transport Layer Security (TLS), Secure SHell (SSH), and Internet Protocol Security (IPSec) protocols [14–16]. A majority of these protocols are reliant on cryptographic techniques such as the Diffie–Hellman key exchange, which is dependent on the computational difficulty of the DLP or the ECDLP [17].

Furthermore, digital signature algorithms like the Digital Signature Algorithm (DSA), Elliptic Curve Digital Signature Algorithm (ECDSA), and RSA Probabilistic Signature Scheme (RSA-PSS) are similarly susceptible to compromise by Shor's algorithm [18–20]. Encryption schemes are also vulnerable, including the ElGamal encryption and RSA Optimal Asymmetric Encryption Padding (RSA-OAEP) [21, 22]. Given these vulnerabilities, Shor's algorithm underscores a potential risk to a vast array of public key cryptography mechanisms that form the backbone of secure communications on the Internet, prompting the need for innovative cryptographic solutions resistant to quantum-based threats.

The proficiency of Shor's algorithm in adeptly factorizing extensive numerical entities presents a formidable challenge to classical cryptographic architectures, especially those anchored in integer factorization for their security measures. The algorithm's harnessing of quantum parallelism and entanglement has the potential to undermine the very bedrock of encryption frameworks such as RSA, thereby imperilling confidential data. That accentuates the pressing imperative for developing and adopting QRC strategies.

Shor's algorithm addresses a deeper, more abstract computational problem known as the abelian hidden subgroup problem. The essence of this problem is to identify a hidden subgroup H of an abelian group G from a function $f : G \to X$ which is consistent $f(x) = f(y) \Leftrightarrow x - y \in H$. Shor's quantum algorithm achieves this by leveraging the quantum Fourier transform to detect periodicities in functions [23]. This periodicity detection is pivotal for solving problems such as integer factorization and the discrete logarithm problem, as their underlying mathematical structures can be translated into an instance of the abelian hidden subgroup problem. Once the periodicity is found, one can deduce factors of a large number or the logarithm in the case of the DLP.

Mathematical Explanation

The factorization of a number n into its prime factors can be accomplished by initially selecting a number $m < n$. Then by using Shor's algorithm the period ω of the function (2.1) is determined. Thus, the function (2.1) becomes (2.2), where $m^{\omega} - 1$ is a multiple of n. Hence, $m^{\omega} - 1$ can be factorized as presented in (2.3).

$$f(x) = m^{x} mod(n) \ , \tag{2.1}$$

$$f(x) = m^{x+\omega} mod(n) \ , \tag{2.2}$$

$$f(x) = m^{\omega} - 1 = (m^{\omega/2} - 1)(m^{\omega/2} + 1) \ . \tag{2.3}$$

Paradigm

Factorization of 91 into its prime factors can be done as follows:

Step 1: Select a number $m = 6$ between 1 and 91.

Step 2: Since the Greatest Common Divisor (GCD) is 1, proceed to the next step. Otherwise m would be a factor.

Step 3: Apply the following process to determine ω:

$1 \times 6 mod(91) = 6$

$6 \times 6 mod(91) = 36$

$36 \times 6 mod(91) = 34$

$34 \times 6 mod(91) = 22$

$22 \times 6 mod(91) = 41$

$41 \times 6 mod(91) = 64$

$64 \times 6 mod(91) = 20$

$20 \times 6 mod(91) = 29$

$29 \times 6 mod(91) = 83$

$83 \times 6 mod(91) = 43$
$43 \times 6 mod(91) = 76$
$76 \times 6 mod(91) = 1.$

Step 4: Since the number of transformations is even $\omega = 12$, continue to the next step. If it was odd, different m must be selected.

Step 5: Since the remainder $r = 64$ in $(\omega/2)$th $=$ 6th transformation gives $64+1 \neq 91$, proceed to the next step. Otherwise, select different m.

Step 6: Determine the factors of n by finding the GCD$(r-1, n)$ =GCD$(63, 91) = 7$ and GCD$(r+1, n)$ =GCD$(65, 91) = 13$. Hence, 7 and 13 are the prime factors of 91.

To this point, it is important to note that the actual "quantum" part of Shor's algorithm is in step 4, finding the period ω. Classical algorithms struggle with this, but quantum Fourier transform allows quantum computers to determine the period exponentially faster than the best known classical algorithms.

Before we proceed Hadamard gates should be explained. The Hadamard gate is a one-qubit quantum gate which performs a specific linear transformation on a qubit. Its matrix representation is given by (2.4).

$$H = \begin{bmatrix} \frac{1}{\sqrt{2}} & \frac{1}{\sqrt{2}} \\ \frac{1}{\sqrt{2}} & -\frac{1}{\sqrt{2}} \end{bmatrix}. \tag{2.4}$$

When a qubit in the state $|0\rangle$ and $|1\rangle$ is subjected to a Hadamard gate, it is transformed to a superposition as presented in (2.5) and (2.6).

$$H|0\rangle = \begin{bmatrix} \frac{1}{\sqrt{2}} & \frac{1}{\sqrt{2}} \\ \frac{1}{\sqrt{2}} & -\frac{1}{\sqrt{2}} \end{bmatrix} \begin{bmatrix} 1 \\ 0 \end{bmatrix} = \begin{bmatrix} \frac{1}{\sqrt{2}} \\ \frac{1}{\sqrt{2}} \end{bmatrix} = \frac{1}{\sqrt{2}}(|0\rangle + |1\rangle) \tag{2.5}$$

$$H|0\rangle = \begin{bmatrix} \frac{1}{\sqrt{2}} & \frac{1}{\sqrt{2}} \\ \frac{1}{\sqrt{2}} & -\frac{1}{\sqrt{2}} \end{bmatrix} \begin{bmatrix} 0 \\ 1 \end{bmatrix} = \begin{bmatrix} \frac{1}{\sqrt{2}} \\ -\frac{1}{\sqrt{2}} \end{bmatrix} = \frac{1}{\sqrt{2}}(|0\rangle - |1\rangle). \tag{2.6}$$

These resulting states are known as quantum superpositions and are fundamental to the power of quantum computing. The Hadamard gate is particularly useful in quantum algorithms because it creates these superpositions from classical $|0\rangle$ and $|1\rangle$ states. The outcome of a Hadamard gate operation is a superposition of both possible states.

A broad overview of the quantum steps in Shor's algorithm follows:

Step 1: Begin with two quantum registers. The first register has N qubits, where $2^N > 91$ initialized to $|0\rangle$, and the second has $log_2(91)$ qubits initialized to $|1\rangle$. Thus the state after the initialization is $|0\rangle|1\rangle$.

Step 2: Apply Hadamard gates to each qubit in the first register to prepare a superposition with state (2.7).

$$\frac{1}{\sqrt{2^N}} \sum_{x=0}^{2^N-1} |x\rangle|1\rangle. \tag{2.7}$$

Step 3: Using a quantum circuit for modular exponentiation, transform each component of the superposition $|x\rangle|1\rangle \to |x\rangle|6^x mod 91\rangle$ with state (2.8).

$$\frac{1}{\sqrt{2^N}} \sum_{x=0}^{2^N-1} |x\rangle|6^x mod 91\rangle. \tag{2.8}$$

After this step, the second register collapses to one of the possible values of $6^x mod 91$. Let it collapse to the value y which corresponds to some set of x-values that form an arithmetic progression. This means our first register is now in a superposition of those x-values.

Step 4: Apply the Quantum Fourier Transform (QFT) to the first register to obtain the periods corresponding to the x-values' arithmetic progression.

Step 5: Measure the first register. The outcome will be some value z which can be related to the period ω. Specifically, the measurement outcome is closely related to a fraction of the form $z/2^N$, and the denominator of this fraction's simplest form is expected to be ω or a factor of it.

Step 6: Use continued fractions to find the best rational approximation of $z/2^N$.

Step 7: Considering $\omega = 12$, compute GCD$(6^{\omega/2} - 1, n)$ =GCD$(46655, 91) = 7$ and GCD$(6^{\omega/2} + 1, n)$ =GCD$(46657, 91) = 13$

2.2.2 *Grover's Algorithm and Quantum Attacks on Symmetric Ciphers*

Grover's algorithm, an avant-garde quantum computational methodology devised by Dr Lov Grover, pertains to the challenge of efficiently searching within an unorganized database at a rate surpassing that of classical algorithms. This algorithm exemplifies the prowess of quantum computing mechanisms in augmenting search procedures, bearing consequential ramifications for the realm of cryptography, especially concerning symmetric cyphers.

In classical computational paradigms, the search dilemma entails locating a particular element within an unordered collection of N entities. Employing traditional methodologies, this mandates, on average, $N/2$ comparisons equivalent to a linear search procedure. In contrast, Grover's algorithm proffers a quantum enhancement, executing the search in approximately $\sqrt{N}$ iterations, thereby bestowing a quadratic acceleration relative to classical computational algorithms.

Within cryptography, Grover's algorithm presents an innovative and disturbing viewpoint concerning symmetric cyphers [24]. Symmetric cyphers employ an identical key for both the encryption and decryption processes. The fortification of these cyphers is contingent upon the computational challenge associated with brute-force efforts to ascertain the precise encryption key correlating plaintext to ciphertext. Traditional brute-force assaults necessitate evaluating all conceivable keys and verifying the ensuing outcomes, which demands an exhaustive traversal through an expansive essential domain [25].

The algorithm can be aptly utilized for this objective. Although it does not proffer an exponential acceleration akin to Shor's algorithm in the context of factorization, Grover's algorithm possesses the potential to bisect the duration mandated for a brute-force exploration. For instance, should a conventional brute-force onslaught necessitate the evaluation of 2^k keys, it diminishes this to approximately $2^{k/2}$ operations. This quadratic enhancement might appear moderate; however, in scenarios encompassing extensive key domains, it could lead to a considerable contraction in the exertion and temporal investment necessary to compromise symmetric cyphers.

The ramifications of Grover's algorithm within the cryptographic domain suggest that symmetric keys necessitate a twofold increase in length to preserve an equivalent security threshold in the epoch of quantum computing. Whereas a classical brute-force assault demands examining 2^k keys, a quantum brute-force endeavour employing Grover's algorithm would mandate approximately $2^{k/2}$ operations. Consequently, cryptographic frameworks contingent upon symmetric cyphers must augment their key dimensions by a factor of 2 to counteract the vulnerabilities introduced by quantum computational apparatuses.

Grover's algorithm exemplifies the prowess of quantum computers in augmenting search procedures within unorganized databases. Such capabilities bear significant ramifications for the field of cryptography, especially concerning symmetric cyphers. Within this context, Grover's algorithm possesses the potential to bisect the duration requisite for a brute-force assault. Consequently, there emerges a compelling impetus to adopt extended key lengths to maintain established security benchmarks in light of the advancements in quantum computing.

It can be used to attack symmetric cryptographic systems. Classic brute-force attacks on n-bit symmetric cryptographic systems would take $O(2^n)$ time. However, as aforementioned with Grover's algorithm, this time is reduced to $O(2^{n/2})$, a quadratic speedup. As a result of Grover's algorithm, symmetric cryptographic systems, like AES, would need to double their key lengths to maintain the same level of security against quantum attacks. An AES-256, which is considered secure against classical attacks, would have the security of AES-128 against a quantum attacker.

Paradigm

Grover's algorithm is a quantum search algorithm that finds, with high probability, the unique input to a black box function that produces a particular output value, using just $O(\sqrt{N})$ evaluations of the function. Consider the function (2.9), where we need to determine w.

$$f : \{0, 1\}^n \rightarrow \{0, 1\}, x \in \{0, 1\}^n \Rightarrow f(x) = 0, \forall x \neq w, f(w) = 1. \tag{2.9}$$

Step 1: Prepare an equal superposition of all possible states (2.10), using Hadamard gates (2.11)

$$|s\rangle = \frac{1}{\sqrt{N}} \sum_{x=0}^{N-1} |x\rangle \tag{2.10}$$

$$|0\rangle^{\otimes n} \xrightarrow{H^{\otimes n}} |s\rangle. \tag{2.11}$$

Step 2: An oracle (black box) U_f is used, which flips the sign of the state for which $f(x) = 1$ as shown in Eq. (2.12).

$$U_f|x\rangle = (-1)^{f(x)}|x\rangle. \tag{2.12}$$

Step 3: The transformation (2.13) amplifies the amplitude of the correct answer.

$$U_s = 2|s\rangle\langle s| - I \ , \tag{2.13}$$

where I is the identity matrix.

Step 4: Repeat Steps 2 and 3 $\sqrt{N}$ times to maximize the probability of measuring the correct answer $|w\rangle$.

2.3 Health Data Exchange and Security Concerns

The exchange of health data is instrumental in contemporary HC, expediting the fluid interchange of medical particulars amongst HC practitioners, institutions, and patients. Such data transmission fosters prompt, synchronized, and exhaustive patient care. The facility of health data exchange grants medical professionals the capability to procure essential patient details, encompassing medical antecedents, diagnostic outcomes, pharmaceutical records, and therapeutic blueprints, regardless of their geographical disposition. That serves to refine diagnostic precision, curtail medical discrepancies, and bolster patient prognoses.

Health-affiliated information is of pronounced sensitivity, given its profoundly personal character. Data about patients encompasses individual, medical, and potentially indelicate particulars, which individuals intrinsically anticipate to be retained in confidentiality. Elements such as a patient's medical ailments, therapeutic interventions, and historical medical data remain sacrosanct, underpinning the fiduciary rapport between physician and patient. Furthermore, patient-centric data is circumscribed by rigorous legal stipulations advocating its safeguarding. Within the United States, the Health Insurance Portability and Accountability Act

(HIPAA) imposes exacting directives to assure the privacy and fortification of patients' medical records [26]. Infringements concerning patient data may culminate in reputational detriment, judicial repercussions, and an erosion of faith in medical infrastructures.

Cryptographic methodologies are invoked to fortify the confidentiality, integrity, and honesty of health-related data during its interchange. Encryption emerges as a paramount modality within this sphere. Data encryption transmutes intelligible data into an encoded schema utilizing cryptographic keys, rendering it incomprehensible to unauthorized entities. Robust protocols, such as Secure Sockets Layer/Transport Layer Security (SSL/TLS), are instituted to encrypt data conveyances across networks, ascertaining that data sustains its confidentiality throughout its transmission [27].

The Public Key Infrastructure (PKI) represents an additional cryptographic methodology [28]. PKI encompasses the deployment of paired public and private cryptographic keys. Public keys are designated for encryption purposes, whereas private keys facilitate decryption, imbuing the exchange mechanism with an augmented stratum of security. Digital signatures, which proffer a means to authenticate the integrity and intactness of data, are realized through cryptographic hash functions in conjunction with private keys.

The exchange of health data is indispensable to contemporary HC, augmenting patient care by facilitating the prompt and synchronized acquisition of medical particulars. The acute sensitivity associated with health-oriented data accentuates the imperative of upholding patient privacy, preserving confidentiality, and ensuring adherence to pertinent legal ordinances. Cryptographic methodologies, encompassing encryption, PKI, and digital signatures, are invoked to fortify the security of health data exchange, guaranteeing the safeguarding of patient data throughout its traversal within HC infrastructures.

In an increasingly interconnected digital era, the imperative of safeguarding and facilitating the fluid exchange of medical data cannot be overstated. It is essential to ensure that healthcare practitioners are granted access to precise, up-to-date information, regardless of the geographical location where the patient previously sought medical services. As depicted in Fig. 2.1, a strategic vision is presented for exchanging health data across diverse sectors, including instances when individuals journey overseas. A forward-thinking paradigm for health data interchange accentuates the harmonious relationship between avant-garde technological advancements and the foundational trust vested by patients. This model is anchored in data security, unambiguous transparency, and collaborative endeavours. Adherence to such principles propels us closer to a horizon where every medical determination is rooted in clarity, accuracy, and a focus on the holistic well-being of the patient.

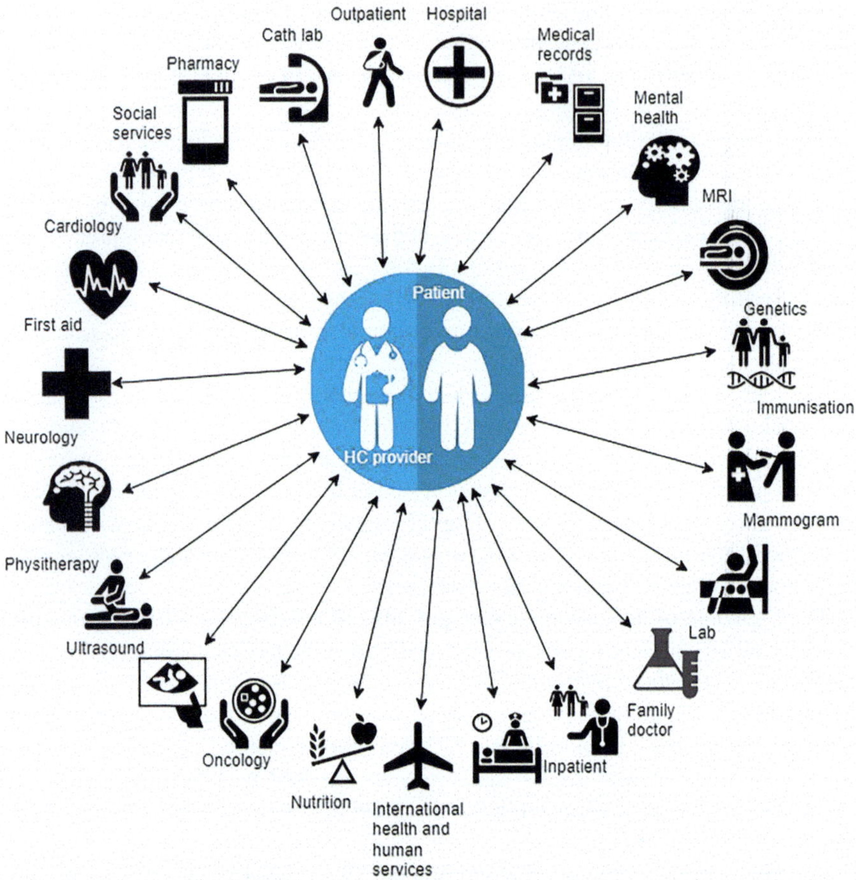

Fig. 2.1 Vision for data exchange

2.3.1 Importance of Health Data Exchange in Modern HC

Health data exchange is symbolic of a cornerstone within the modern HC milieu, assuming a cardinal role in guaranteeing adept and exhaustive patient care. The facility to fluidly disseminate medical particulars amongst HC practitioners and institutions equips medical professionals with the requisite tools to render informed decisions, proffer precise diagnoses, and administer prompt therapeutic interventions. This refined conduit for data interchange ameliorates extant knowledge lacunae, curtails superfluous repetitions, and amplifies the aggregate quality of patient care. Also, it permits diverse HC practitioners to procure a patient's exhaustive medical antecedents, diagnostic outcomes, and therapeutic blueprints. This holistic perspective engenders more expeditious and precise diagnostic processes, forestalling lags that might conceivably jeopardize patient prognoses.

As patients transition amongst disparate HC environments or specialist practitioners, disseminating medical data ascertains continuity in their care. Attending physicians have access to contemporary information, attenuating the potentiality of diagnostic inaccuracies or incongruous therapeutic interventions.

Procuring comprehensive and contemporaneous medical documentation diminishes the likelihood of medical oversights, including prescribing pharmaceuticals that exhibit adverse interactions or redundantly administering diagnostic assessments consequent to an informational deficit. Exhaustive health documentation empowers HC practitioners to render judicious determinations concerning therapeutic modalities, duly considering the patient's antecedent medical chronicle, hypersensitivities, and prospective hazards.

The dissemination of health data facilitates the intelligent identification of potential health perils, engendering efficacious preventative measures. HC practitioners can assiduously oversee chronic ailments and proffer bespoke therapeutic strategies. The facilitation of health data interchange curtails the necessity for redundant diagnostics and procedures. That not only refines the patient experience but also culminates in fiscal conservation for the patients and the overarching HC infrastructures.

The availability of disseminated medical data champions patient-centric medical provision. Patients are capacitated to engage proactively in their therapeutic blueprints, and HC practitioners can customize care, aligning with individual requisites and preferences.

Whilst the advantages of health data interchange remain incontrovertible, they demand an unwavering commitment to formidable data security. Given the delicate essence of medical intelligence, in tandem with the prospective ramifications of data transgressions, it becomes imperative to institute rigorous security protocols. Upholding patient privacy, ensuring confidentiality, and preserving data integrity are quintessential to sustaining confidence in HC infrastructures.

The amalgamation of these considerations accentuates the imperative for avant-garde data security protocols, which include encryption, fortified data transmission mechanisms, meticulous access controls, and stringent adherence to legal stipulations [29]. As HC infrastructures metamorphose into increasingly interconnected and data-centric establishments, the pivotal significance of protecting disseminated medical records is conspicuously manifest.

2.3.2 *Sensitivity of Health Data: Privacy, Confidentiality, and Legal Regulations*

The nature of health data is distinguished by its unparalleled sensitivity, stemming from the profoundly intimate and deeply personal particulars it encapsulates. Patient health records chronicle medical diagnoses and therapeutic regimens and delve into mental health antecedents, reproductive health specifics, and other personal peculiarities. Unauthorized divulgence of such data, bereft of consent, can profoundly influence an individual's dignity, esteem, and psychological equilibrium. Patients entrust their HC practitioners with this intelligence, operating under the presumption that it will remain inviolate and be deployed exclusively for therapeutic ends. The delicate character of health data mandates an augmented degree of vigilance and fortification to preserve patient confidentiality.

Given the paramount significance of preserving health data, legislative frameworks have been promulgated to fortify the security of patient information. The HIPAA exemplifies such legislative undertakings in the United States. HIPAA delineates rigorous standards for safeguarding patient health records, imposing exacting privacy and security protocols to which HC professionals, insurance corporations, and affiliated institutions are obliged to conform.

This regulation governs the utilization and dissemination of an individual's health information. It ascertains that patients retain autonomy over their data and are comprehensively informed regarding its intended use. The Security Rule mandates that covered entities institute protective measures to safeguard electronic health records. These provisions include data encryption, meticulous access controls, and periodic security evaluations.

Covered entities are responsible for formally notifying affected individuals, the Department of Health and Human Services (HHS), and, in certain circumstances, media outlets in case of a patient health information breach. Violations of HIPAA can lead to significant financial repercussions and penalties. Depending on the magnitude of the breach and the intent of the offending entity, repercussions can span from civil monetary penalties to criminal indictments.

These legal stipulations emphasize the paramount significance of preserving patient privacy and mandate establishing rigorous security protocols to deter unauthorized access, dissemination, or exploitation of health data. The HIPAA and other global regulatory frameworks are foundational pillars in engendering public trust. It achieves this by imposing accountability on entities to uphold the sanctity of patient confidentiality and ensure health data security.

The profound sensitivity associated with health data mandates rigorous privacy and security protocols to preserve patient confidentiality and sustain their trust. Legislative frameworks such as the HIPAA serve as a linchpin in asserting that HC establishments accord paramount importance to data protection. That underscores the ethical and legal obligation to shield patient health information assiduously.

2.4 The Need for QRC in HC

The imperative for QRC measures within HC emanates from the swift evolution of quantum computing and the resultant vulnerabilities it introduces to traditional cryptographic techniques. HC infrastructures intrinsically depend on the confidentiality, integrity, and accessibility of sensitive patient information. With the maturation of quantum computational capabilities, their inherent ability to undermine extant cryptographic paradigms may imperil the security mechanisms governing health data exchanges, endangering patient confidentiality, data integrity, and foundational trust in HC systems.

Quantum computational devices, characterized by their prodigious computational capacities, can subvert foundational security precepts intrinsic to classical cryptographic techniques. Algorithms, notably Shor's and Grover's, jeopardize salient components of cryptographic infrastructures, potentially empowering malicious actors to dismantle encryption mechanisms and expedite brute-force intrusions on symmetric encryption systems. If this burgeoning menace remains unchecked, it could culminate in the unsanctioned exposure of health-centric data, precipitating grave ramifications for patients and the broader HC community.

The ramifications of overlooking the emerging threats posed by quantum computing are profoundly significant. Health data about patients, which is unequivocally categorized as some of the most delicate information, stands at risk of being imperilled, precipitating unauthorized intrusions, identity misappropriations, and even the alarming spectre of medical identity deception. Furthermore, the fidelity of medical archives could be jeopardized, potentially catalyzing misdiagnoses, erroneous therapeutic strategies, and fragmentation in the orchestration of patient care. An erosion of patient confidence stemming from such security infractions might engender a hesitancy to divulge pivotal medical data, which could interfere with medical progress and adversely influence patient prognoses.

Anthem, a prominent health insurance entity, endured a data security infringement that divulged the personal particulars of approximately 78.8 million individuals in a particularly egregious breach within the HC sector. Whilst this specific incident was not attributed to quantum mechanisms, it starkly illustrates the inherent vulnerabilities in HC infrastructures and the consequential ramifications of deficient data security protocols.

A cybersecurity infringement targeting UCLA Health resulted in disclosing records of about 4.5 million patients [30]. This breach unveiled critical medical data, encompassing Social Security identifiers, birth dates, and comprehensive medical histories, accentuating the paramount significance of fortifying electronic health record systems.

The imperative to integrate QRC solutions becomes increasingly pronounced in light of the rapid and exponential advancements in quantum computing capacities. HC institutions need to anticipate a forthcoming era wherein traditional cryptographic techniques may fail to offer sufficient defence against emergent quantum adversities. By embracing QRA, HC infrastructures can guarantee patient data's confidentiality, integrity, and security, even when confronted with sophisticated quantum onslaughts. Such a forward-thinking strategy in security not only upholds patient privacy but also fortifies the structural integrity of HC frameworks, underscoring the indispensable role of QRC within the HC domain.

2.4.1 *Recognizing the Threat: Quantum Computers and Cryptanalysis*

The imminent advent of quantum computing poses profound challenges to the foundational cryptographic structures that anchor contemporary data security measures. Quantum computers can penetrate and dismantle the defensive bulwarks that have shielded sensitive data for generations. Cryptographic methodologies, hitherto deemed impregnable, stand vulnerable to quantum algorithms meticulously crafted to leverage their inherent weaknesses. This nexus of quantum computing and cryptography signifies the dawning of a transformative epoch, wherein the security milieu stands at the precipice of a fundamental metamorphosis.

Recognizing the impending peril quantum computing poses is paramount to enhancing and reinforcing data security in our contemporary landscape. Succumbing to complacency and opting to emphasize solely extant security measures without regard for future quantum threats constitute a precarious position. Overlooking the vulnerabilities that quantum algorithms could lay bare risks leaving critical data vulnerable to breaches. The consequences of such security infringements could be profound and extensive, whether pertaining to individual financial details, medical archives, or confidential governmental intelligence.

In light of this developing challenge, it is imperative to espouse a forward-looking stance. The opportune moment to respond is the present, before the materialization of quantum computers with adequate computational capabilities. Deferring action until the menace is imminent might render organizations susceptible to infringements that are arduous to counteract. Such anticipatory measures necessitate exploring, formulating, and deploying QRC strategies capable of resisting onslaughts from advanced quantum computational systems.

The imperative of allocating resources towards the research and development of QRA is of paramount significance. By maintaining a vanguard position and synchronizing with the evolving landscape of quantum computing, entities can safeguard their confidential data, thereby upholding the trust and confidence of stakeholders, collaborators, and the broader community.

The emergent peril presented by quantum computers necessitates a recalibration of prevailing perspectives. Recognizing this impending menace, instead of diminishing its significance, is imperative for preserving confidential data. Adopting anticipatory strategies by channelling investments into QRC mechanisms to fortify data confidentiality, integrity, and authenticity amidst an accelerating technological epoch is vital. Such a visionary stance guarantees the robustness of cryptographic infrastructures and epitomizes an unwavering dedication to maintaining the zenith of data security standards in the digital era.

One of the candidates for post-quantum cryptography standardization by NIST is the CRYSTALS-Kyber which is a lattice-based public key encryption scheme. ICSF currently supports Kyber-1024 Round 2. Kyber-1024 aims at security roughly equivalent to AES-256.

The following delineates an overview and highlights key concepts of the algorithm to augment the clarity and thoroughness of the procedure.

CRYSTALS-Kyber relies on module learning with rounding problems over polynomial rings. The main problem is to compute Eq. (2.14).

$$b = a \times s + emod(q), \forall a \in R_q, s \in S, e \in E, \tag{2.14}$$

where Rq denotes the polynomials modulo q, while S and E are sets that define certain properties of the secret key and error, respectively, such as bounded norm. To obtain the key, a sample secret key s is chosen uniformly at random from the set S. Then, a public polynomial a is selected from Rq. The public key is computed as $b = a \times s + emod(q)$. Hence, given a message denoted by m, the public key (a, b) and sample r from R_q the encryption are implemented by computing Eqs. (2.15) and (2.16). Thus, the ciphertext is (u, v).

$$u = a \times rmod(q) \tag{2.15}$$

$$u = b \times s + encode(m)mod(q). \tag{2.16}$$

Given the ciphertext (u, v), the message $m = decode(m')$ can be recovered by computing Eq. (2.17).

$$m' = v - u \times smod(q). \tag{2.17}$$

The security and efficiency of the scheme depend on the choice of R_q, S, E, and the encoding/decoding functions.

2.4.2 *Risk Assessment: Quantum Computing's Potential Impact on Health Data*

The emergence of quantum computing presents formidable challenges to health data security, warranting an exhaustive evaluation of potential susceptibilities. Quantum computational devices boast capabilities that have the potential to subvert traditional cryptographic techniques employed to fortify health data. The vulnerabilities susceptible to quantum exploitation may jeopardize the confidentiality, integrity, and accessibility of critical medical records.

Quantum computational devices, harnessing the power of Shor's algorithm, possess the potential to factorize substantial numerical values with efficiency, thereby undermining prevalent public key encryption algorithms, notably RSA. Such a development could leave encrypted health records susceptible to unsanctioned access and decryption, imperilling the confidentiality of patient data. Furthermore, quantum computational devices can potentially expedite the process of identifying collisions within hash functions, facilitating the generation of disparate inputs that yield identical hash values. Such a capability may precipitate unauthorized data modifications and compromise health records' integrity, undermining the very foundation of data veracity.

Using Grover's algorithm, quantum computers can expedite brute-force assaults on symmetric encryption keys, substantially diminishing the duration needed to ascertain the appropriate key. Such susceptibility has the potential to facilitate unauthorized decryption of health-related data, thereby jeopardizing its confidentiality and undermining its intrinsic integrity. In addition, they can undermine digital signature protocols, mechanisms that certify the provenance and integrity of electronic documents. Consequently, this might result in the fabrication of signatures on health-related documents, casting doubt on the authenticity of the data therein.

Blockchain technology, frequently employed for the secure preservation of health-related data, is predicated on cryptographic protocols. The advent of quantum computational capabilities threatens the integrity of these cryptographic mechanisms, potentially facilitating unauthorized data access, alterations to the stored information, or even the negation of transactions within the blockchain structure. HC records typically encompass susceptible personal data, and any compromise in the cryptographic infrastructures safeguarding such information could result in its inadvertent exposure. The unauthorized revelation of individual health diagnoses, therapeutic interventions, and medical chronicles could culminate in significant privacy infringements, engendering potential detrimental consequences.

Cryptographic shortcomings unveiled by the advent of quantum computing might jeopardize data, even if it remains encrypted over extended periods, spanning years or possibly decades. Data presumed secure in the present landscape might become vulnerable in forthcoming times, thus presenting a sustained peril to the sanctity of health data security.

The emergence of quantum computing possesses the potential to capitalize on extant weaknesses in secure communication protocols, thus facilitating unauthorized eavesdropping on transmissions of health data. Such unauthorized interceptions during the exchange of health-related information could grievously jeopardize the very principle of confidentiality.

The risks that quantum computing introduces to health data security are manifold and profound. Quantum computational devices can capitalize on extant frailties in encryption, hash functions, digital signatures, and other cryptographic methodologies. The consequential security breaches might imperil patient confidentiality, data integrity, and the overarching trust in HC infrastructures. It is imperative, therefore, to discern these susceptibilities, thereby facilitating the inception of quantum-resilient cryptographic methodologies capable of counteracting the emergent quantum menaces, ensuring the preservation of health data security amidst an ever-evolving technological milieu.

2.5 QRC Solutions

Given the escalating risk posed by quantum computers to conventional cryptographic techniques, the quest for quantum-resistant solutions assumes paramount importance. Algorithms are resistant to quantum capabilities, frequently denominated as PQC, and endeavour to furnish security notwithstanding potential quantum adversarial actions. Within the myriad of explored strategies, lattice-based cryptographic solutions and hash-based methodologies stand out as up-and-coming candidates.

LBC is predicated upon the intricate mathematical architecture of lattices, which are delineated as arrays of points within a multidimensional continuum. Such algorithms capitalize on the inherent challenges of resolving lattice problems, obstacles that persistently endure, even in the face of quantum computational prowess. The Learning With Errors (LWEs) and its counterpart, the Ring-LWE, are anchored in the complexity of deciphering noisy linear equation systems–schemes derived from LWE proffer encryption mechanisms, signature protocols, and key exchange methodologies [31, 32]. The NTRUEncrypt, a notable exemplar of lattice-based encryption algorithms, employs polynomial rings, thus facilitating expeditious critical formulation and encryption processes [33]. Conversely, Hash-Based Cryptographic (HBC) modalities are constructed upon the arduousness of identifying collisions within cryptographic hash functions [34]. Whilst conceptually lucid, these hash-based frameworks retain resilience against quantum incursions, bestowing capabilities for digital signatures and key exchange protocols.

The Merkle Tree is a cryptographic data structure wherein data collection is organized and hashed into a hierarchical tree format [35]. This arrangement facilitates the efficient validation of the authenticity of discrete data elements within the encompassing dataset. On the other hand, the Winternitz One-Time Signature Scheme employs the iterative application of a hash function to sign messages, presenting a quantum-resistant substitute to conventional digital signatures [36].

The pressing need to formulate and apply quantum-resistant methodologies has precipitated profound research and standardization endeavours. Institutions like the National Institute of Standards and Technology (NIST) have initiated contests to discern and codify PQC algorithms [37, 38]. NIST's PQC Standardization initiative aims to assess and choose QRA apt for diverse cryptographic usages, encompassing encryption, digital signatures, and key exchange procedures.

The current endeavours underscore the paramountcy of establishing a compendium of standardized, rigorously evaluated PQC algorithms. These algorithms are designed to exhibit resistance to quantum-based threats and an array of conventional attacks. The scholarly community is vigorously participating in the formulation, scrutiny, and refinement of these algorithms to guarantee their efficacy, proficiency, and robust security.

QRC methodologies, encompassing lattice-based cryptographic approaches and hash-based frameworks, exhibit the potential to counteract the vulnerabilities introduced by quantum computational capabilities. The prevailing research and standardization initiatives accentuate the collective pursuit to ready the computational sphere for the quantum epoch by furnishing secure replacements for conventional cryptographic techniques. The advent of such solutions guarantees that medical records and other categories of confidential data maintain their safeguarded status in a domain progressively susceptible to quantum-induced risks.

2.5.1 Overview of QRA

QRA refer to cryptographic protocols explicitly constructed to resist adversarial attempts using quantum computing. With the progression of quantum computing capabilities, conventional cryptographic methodologies demonstrate susceptibility, stemming from their foundational computational assumptions, which quantum computers possess the potential to compromise. Often termed PQC, these QRAs introduce a novel category of cryptographic primitives, ensuring security against adversarial actions from both traditional and quantum computing perspectives.

PQC recognizes the impending challenges quantum computers present to established cryptographic methodologies. This discipline encompasses the meticulous study, formulation, and deployment of innovative algorithms that ensure security in an environment dominated by advanced quantum computational capabilities. The terminology "post-quantum" emphasizes cryptographic techniques that remain efficacious after the inception of quantum computing, guaranteeing data protection in this evolving technological epoch.

The significance of PQC arises from the understanding that quantum computers can potentially render extant cryptographic paradigms ineffectual. Traditional encryption techniques, which hitherto depended upon the complexity of factoring sizable integers or addressing discrete logarithm problems, might be susceptible to efficient circumvention through quantum algorithms. Consequently, this exposes critical data to risks, jeopardizing its confidentiality, integrity, and authenticity.

PQC seeks to rectify this susceptibility by investigating alternate mathematical foundations impervious to quantum adversarial strategies. Such foundations may capitalize on mathematical challenges that inherently pose significant difficulty for classical and quantum computational frameworks, guaranteeing security irrespective of the prevailing computational prowess.

Within health data protection, PQC is indispensable in preserving the confidentiality of patient documentation, fortifying medical research, and bolstering trust in HC infrastructures. As HC institutions navigate towards digitized platforms and integrated network systems, the incorporation of quantum-resilient cryptographic mechanisms is imperative to shield patient confidentiality and data integrity from potential quantum-induced vulnerabilities.

The domain of QRA, frequently called PQC, emerges as a countermeasure to the prospective susceptibilities that quantum computers pose to conventional cryptographic techniques. It is centred on the conceptualization and implementation of cryptographic methodologies capable of resisting adversarial onslaughts from classical and quantum paradigms, affirming data security in an era influenced by quantum capabilities. This emphasis on anticipatory fortification of data protection assumes pronounced relevance in arenas like health data security, given the imperative to safeguard the inherently delicate nature of such information against nascent challenges.

2.5.2 LBC: Principles and Applications

LBC represents an avant-garde methodology in data protection, drawing extensively upon the sophisticated attributes of mathematical lattices. Lattices are constructs characterized by systematically arranged points within multidimensional spaces. The inherent complexity of particular lattice challenges, such as the Shortest Vector Problem (SVP) and LWE, underpins the security mechanisms within lattice-based cryptographic paradigms [39]. It is postulated that these problems remain computationally arduous for both traditional and quantum computational frameworks to address efficiently.

LBC can assume a cardinal role in defending health data against quantum-centric vulnerabilities. Moreover, it can be judiciously employed to secure electronic health records during the retention and transference phases. Medical histories, diagnostic outcomes, and patient therapeutic blueprints can be ciphered utilizing lattice-based protocols, guaranteeing that solely sanctioned entities retain the requisite decryption credentials.

Health data exchange infrastructures may judiciously adopt lattice-based encryption to facilitate the secure conveyance of data amongst HC practitioners, diagnostic laboratories, and insurance entities. This technological approach ascertains that patient-specific information retains its confidentiality and integrity during transmission, mitigating the likelihood of unsanctioned access or manipulation. The strategy can be harnessed to fortify patient identities, inhibiting unauthorized incursions into personal datasets. Such protective measures encompass safeguarding data, including Social Security numerals, residential coordinates, and additional identifying variables susceptible to malevolent exploitation for identity misappropriation. Furthermore, the signature protocols can be leveraged to validate health-centric documents and vouch for their undistorted state. Such a framework ensures that medical analyses, prescription directives, and therapeutic stratagems remain inviolate, reinforcing confidence in their integrity for patients and medical practitioners.

Amidst the ascendance of telehealth and remote patient surveillance, LBC can serve as an instrument to safeguard the real-time transmission of health metrics from wearable apparatuses to medical professionals. This mechanism upholds patients' physiological data discretion, concurrently facilitating distanced HC provisions. Together, as genetic diagnostics amplify in ubiquity, lattice-based encryption offers a robust solution to shield genomic datasets, which bear profound personal and sensitive connotations. This framework guarantees the seclusion of a patient's genetic profile whilst permitting scientific investigators to scrutinize consolidated datasets without unmasking individual identities.

The intrinsic robustness of LBC against quantum adversarial endeavours renders it a quintessential choice for fortifying health data in a timeframe wherein quantum computation menaces traditional cryptographic paradigms. By capitalizing on the mathematical intricacies inherent to lattices, health-related data can be insulated from unauthorized intrusion, manipulation, and security breaches, thereby perpetuating the sanctity of patient confidentiality and data integrity within HC infrastructures.

2.5.3 Hash-Based Schemes: Merkle Trees, Winternitz, and More

HBC paradigms present a distinguished alternative for quantum-resilient data safeguarding. Such paradigms are predicated on the computational challenge of identifying collisions–distinctive inputs that yield identical hash outcomes–in cryptographic hash functions. Intrinsically, hash-based methodologies exhibit resistance to quantum adversarial actions and can assume a paramount role in fortifying the exchange of health data and safeguarding other forms of sensitive information.

Merkle trees, an integral construct within HBC, ascertain data integrity and authenticity. Operating through the hashing of data segments, they engender a stratified architecture of hashed denominations. The apex hash, denominated as the Merkle root, epitomizes the entirety of the dataset. Any alterations to an individual data segment precipitate a domino effect in the associated hashes, a deviation readily discernible upon validation of the Merkle root. Such structures are adept at corroborating the authenticity of singular data entities within an expansive dataset, ensuring that medical documentation, diagnostic outcomes, and clinical reports sustain their original state during conveyance and retention.

The Winternitz One-Time Signature Scheme constitutes a hash-based, quantum-resilient signature paradigm. This mechanism necessitates the iterative application of hash functions to endorse a message, culminating in creating a concise signature that remains fortified against quantum adversarial endeavours. Winternitz signatures can be judiciously harnessed to validate the integrity of health-centric documents, thereby ascertaining their provenance and wholeness. This protocol can electronically endorse medical records, prescriptive directives, and clinical mandates, thereby inhibiting unsanctioned alterations.

Hash-based paradigms are indispensable in fortifying health data exchange, meticulously ensuring the confidentiality, integrity, and authenticity of sensitive medical records. Whether the corroboration of the virtue of patient dossiers via Merkle tree constructs or the electronic endorsement of health dossiers employing Winternitz signatures, hash-based methodologies proffer quantum-resilient alternatives adept at defending against the developing challenges of quantum computational devices. Within a milieu where traditional cryptographic techniques are confronted by vulnerabilities stemming from quantum advancements, hash-based schemes bestow a stalwart foundation for preserving health data. Their inherent robustness against quantum adversarial incursions renders them an eminently suitable selection for maintaining patient confidentiality and assuring the undistorted state of health-centric information throughout its transmission and archival.

2.6 Challenges and Considerations

QRC presents auspicious solutions; however, its integration into HC systems is accompanied by specific challenges. Several impediments must be surmounted to guarantee the successful incorporation of these algorithms. Notably, they tend to be more computationally demanding than classical equivalents. The deployment of these algorithms could consequently result in augmented processing durations and escalated resource utilization. Given that HC systems necessitate swift and efficient data interchange, any substantial performance diminution could obstruct the seamless operation of such systems.

The shift from classical to QRC represents a sophisticated endeavour. HC institutions are compelled to oversee the simultaneous operation of both cryptographic regimes throughout the transitional phase–Engender challenges associated with key administration, retrospective compatibility, and data security assurance during migration. HC architectures frequently encompass components, applications, and apparatuses necessitating flawless communication. Incorporating QRC into these frameworks whilst preserving compatibility with preexisting infrastructure poses considerable challenges. It is imperative to ensure that newly introduced cryptographic protocols can interface effectively with legacy systems to facilitate an unobstructed transition.

Research endeavours must concentrate on enhancing the efficacy of QRA. Implementations that efficaciously diminish computational overhead are quintessential to guarantee that the exchange of health-related data retains its promptness and reactivity. A phased migration tactic from classical to QRC is advisable to prevent undue disruption. This methodology entails commencing with nonessential systems and progressively broadening the application to include pivotal components.

Prudent management of cryptographic keys during the transition period is also imperative. A meticulously devised key management approach is pivotal in ensuring the sanctity of data encrypted via both classical and QRA. The standardization of QRA remains instrumental in ensuring seamless compatibility and interoperability within various HC systems. Endeavours made collaboratively to forge industry-wide standards will expedite and simplify the adoption process. HC professionals must receive adequate education concerning the ramifications of quantum computing and the subsequent transition to QRC. Such enlightenment programmes will cultivate a more profound understanding, facilitating informed decision-making and seamless incorporation. HC systems may consider integrating gateways or transition layers. These would adapt data encrypted with QRA into formats congruous with preexisting systems, ensuring data interchange whilst maintaining the heightened security attributes proffered by QRC.

Though promising for fortifying HC data security, it does not come without inherent challenges. It is paramount to strike a balance in performance considerations, orchestrate a seamless transition, assure interoperability, and refine key management to ensure the proficient incorporation of these sophisticated cryptographic methodologies into HC infrastructures. By methodically addressing these complexities, HC entities can adeptly integrate QRC whilst upholding the paramount principles of data integrity, confidentiality, and accessibility pertaining to patient information.

2.6.1 Performance and Computational Overhead of QRA

Whilst QRAs proffer heightened security face-to-face quantum threats, apprehensions emerge concerning their possible ramifications on system efficacy. Such algorithms frequently incorporate a degree of computational overhead, which might adversely influence the efficiency of data processing and transmission within HC infrastructures. Compared to their classical counterparts, these algorithms customarily entail intricate mathematical operations. These complicated procedures could engender extended processing durations, impeding the indispensable encryption, decryption, and authentication processes for exchanging HC data. Furthermore, there may be an augmented demand for computational resources, encompassing processing capacity and memory. Such difficulties could exert undue pressure on the HC systems' infrastructure, potentially culminating in diminished system responsiveness and an overall decline in efficiency.

Augmented computational requisites might result in heightened latency during data conveyance. Within the realm of HC, the prompt exchange of information is of paramount importance for efficacious patient care. Any latency engendered by the computational surplus of QRA could potentially impinge upon the calibre of HC provisions. HC infrastructures frequently grapple with extensive data volumes. If QRAs are not meticulously refined for scalability, they could amplify the predicaments of managing and processing voluminous datasets.

The delicate equilibrium between heightened security and system efficacy is a pivotal consideration. Although the primary objective remains to safeguard the confidentiality and integrity of HC data, it is equally imperative for HC systems to sustain an exemplary performance level to ensure punctual patient care delivery. Scholars and professionals are ardently endeavouring to optimize QRA to diminish their computational intricacy. Efficacious implementations possess the potential to assuage the consequential performance ramifications. Incorporating specialized hardware may be judiciously leveraged to expedite the operationalization of QRA. Such hardware-centric solutions can bolster system performance whilst steadfastly upholding security.

Hybrid methodologies, intertwining both classical and QRA, hold the potential to strike equilibrium between security and system efficacy. It is prudent to employ QRA for the critical constituents whilst allowing the less sensitive segments to hinge upon conventional cryptographic techniques. Continual scholarly investigations are indispensable to devise QRAs that proffer superior performance without any security derogation. Symbiotic endeavours within the cryptographic and HC fraternities are paramount to realizing this objective.

The performance implications tethered to QRA merit earnest contemplation, especially within domains of acute time sensitivity such as HC. Notwithstanding the presence of these concerns, they are by no means insuperable. Through sustained research, dedicated optimization initiatives, and specialized hardware deployment, one can judiciously achieve equilibrium between the augmented security proffered by QRC and the efficiency imperative for the unimpeded exchange of health data within HC infrastructures.

2.6.2 *Transition Strategies: Migrating to QRC*

The transition from conventional to QRC epitomizes a multifaceted undertaking that mandates meticulous strategizing and execution. HC infrastructures must astutely manoeuvre through this transition to ascertain the enduring security of patient-centric data. An incremental migration methodology, whereby QRAs are introduced progressively, is prudent. Commencing with noncritical systems and data of lesser sensitivity can serve as the initial phase, permitting HC entities to accrue expertise and assurance before the transposition of pivotal components.

Combining hybrid methodologies, which amalgamate classical and QRC techniques, might proffer a pragmatic middle ground. Components of heightened sensitivity can be safeguarded by employing QRA, whilst areas of lesser sensitivity might persevere with conventional methodologies. Operating classical and QRC infrastructures concomitantly during the transitional juncture can vouchsafe uninterrupted functionalities. This stratagem facilitates the phased transference of services devoid of abrupt discontinuities.

During the transition, the stewardship of cryptographic keys emerges as a formidable challenge. Diverse algorithms may present variegated key stipulations, and organizations must ascertain that these keys are kept secure and adeptly managed throughout the entire migration trajectory. Upholding compatibility with extant systems, which leverage traditional cryptographic methodologies, remains paramount. The transitional phase should not engender communication disruptions amongst strategies that have not yet embraced QRA.

QRA may infuse computational overhead, thereby influencing the performance of systems. It is indispensable for organizations to deliberate upon prospective latency in data processing and transmission and earnestly engage in the optimization of these algorithms. Both HC professionals and IT personnel must undergo comprehensive training concerning the novel cryptographic protocols and their consequent implementation. Augmenting awareness about the ramifications of quantum computing and the metamorphosis to QRC remains crucial. Frequently, HC systems are contingent upon third-party services and vendors. The transition mandates meticulously considering these services' compatibility with the emergent cryptographic algorithms.

The QRA chosen should exhibit robust resilience against prospective advancements in both quantum and classical computational realms. It is paramount to guarantee the enduring security and viability of the elected solutions. The metamorphosis of cryptographic methodologies may have implications for adherence to statutes, such as HIPAA. Consequently, HC institutions must ascertain that innovative cryptographic solutions harmoniously concur with legal mandates. Pertaining to systems that archive historical data encrypted via conventional techniques, a coherent strategy for migrating and transforming data to contemporary algorithms is essential to preserve the security integrity of antecedent records.

The shift from conventional to QRC mechanisms within HC infrastructures necessitates meticulous strategizing and contemplation of diverse facets. Employing tactics such as incremental migration, combined solutions, and concomitant implementations can significantly facilitate an untroubled transition. It is imperative to confront and resolve challenges encompassing key stewardship, retrospective compatibility, performance ramifications, educational outreach, and adherence to regulatory mandates to unequivocally safeguard the integrity, confidentiality, and accessibility of patient data throughout this transformative endeavour.

2.7 Conclusion and Discussion

The present chapter accentuates the imperative requirement for HC infrastructures to confront the looming menace of quantum computing vis-à-vis conventional cryptographic paradigms. With the progression of quantum computational technology, safeguarding delicate health-related data disseminated within HC frameworks faces unparalleled perils. The necessity of this predicament is of paramount significance, particularly when one contemplates the potential ramifications of jeopardized patient confidentiality and the sanctity of data.

Quantum computing's capacity to decipher traditional cryptographic methodologies, including but not limited to integer factorization and symmetric cyphers, jeopardizes the integrity of health data circulated amongst HC practitioners. The advent of algorithms, notably Shor's and Grover's, poses formidable challenges, given their proficiency in expeditiously decrypting encryption and hash functions. It is thus imperative that extant mechanisms designed for the protection of health data undergo evolution to retain their efficacy in this nascent quantum epoch.

In contemporary HC, exchanging health data is a cornerstone, facilitating the meticulous coordination of patient care and fostering medical research endeavours. Given the inherent sensitivity of health-centric information, it is paramount to employ stringent security protocols to preserve patient confidentiality, privacy, and adherence to regulatory mandates, such as HIPAA, within the United States. The imperativeness of assimilating QRC methodologies is accentuated, and its significance cannot be sufficiently emphasized. Empirical case studies, drawn from historical cryptographic infringements within the HC domain, elucidate the potentially grave ramifications of any laxity in addressing quantum challenges with enthusiasm. Synergistic undertakings remain indispensable in actualizing quantum-resistant strategies designed to counteract quantum aggressions and guarantee uninterrupted data exchange and impeccable patient care.

The efficacious introduction of quantum-resistant methodologies necessitates concerted collaboration amongst HC practitioners, information technology specialists, regulatory entities, and technological vendors. In the face of the dynamic evolution of quantum threats, an anticipatory stance is crucial in shielding health-centric data. HC institutions must channel investments towards enlightenment, capacitation, and infrastructural enhancements, ensuring that QRC mechanisms are seamlessly integrated into their overarching data defence matrix.

Amid the rapid advancements in quantum computational technology, the imperativeness of fortifying patient health data remains unequivocal. Synergistic endeavours towards assimilating QRC modalities are paramount in sustaining patient confidence, adhering to privacy mandates, and guaranteeing the unimpaired dissemination of health-related information. The present moment offers a prime juncture to confront the challenges of quantum computational threats. Consequently, it is of utmost importance that HC frameworks convene to instate stalwart quantum-resistant strategies, thereby bolstering data security measures and safeguarding patients' holistic well-being in this emergent quantum epoch.

Acknowledgments The research work was supported by the project entitled "Smart and Health Ageing through People Engaging in supporting Systems" with acronym SHAPES, which has received funding from the European Union's Horizon 2020 research and innovation programme under grant agreement No. 857159.

References

1. Andreou, A., Mavromoustakis, C. X., Mastorakis G., Do, D. T., Batalla, J. M., Pallis, E., & Markakis, E. K. (2021). In *Towards an optimized security approach to IoT devices with confidential HC data exchange*. Multimedia Tools and Applications (Vol. 80, pp. 31435–31449). Springer.
2. Bhatia, V., & Ramkumar, K. R. (2020). An efficient quantum computing technique for cracking RSA using Shor's algorithm. In *2020 IEEE 5th international conference on computing communication and automation (ICCCA)* (pp. 89–94). IEEE.
3. Preston, R. H. (2022). Applying Grover's algorithm to hash functions: A software perspective. In *IEEE transactions on quantum engineering* (Vol. 3, pp. 1–10). IEEE.
4. Khalid, A., McCarthy, S., O'Neill, M., & Liu, W. (2019). Lattice-based cryptography for IoT in a quantum world: Are we ready?. In *2019 IEEE 8th international workshop on advances in sensors and interfaces (IWASI)* (pp. 194–199). IEEE.
5. Haraty, R. A., Boukhari, B., & Kaddoura, S. (2021). An effective hash-based assessment and recovery algorithm for HC systems. In *Arabian journal for science and engineering* (pp. 1–14). Springer.

6. Andreou, A., Mavromoustakis, C. X., Mastorakis, G., Batalla, J. M., Sahalos, J. N., Pallis, E., & Markakis, E. (2021). Robust encryption to enhance IoT confidentiality for HC ecosystems. In *2021 IEEE 26th international workshop on computer aided modeling and design of communication links and networks (CAMAD)* (pp. 1–6). IEEE.
7. Muthukrishnan, H., Suresh, P., Logeswaran, K., & Sentamilselvan, K. (2022). Exploration of quantum blockchain techniques towards sustainable future cybersecurity. In *Quantum blockchain: An emerging cryptographic paradigm* (pp. 317–340). Wiley.
8. LaPierre, R., & LaPierre, R. (2021). Shor algorithm. In *Introduction to quantum computing* (pp. 177–192). Springer.
9. Park, G., Zhang, K., Yu, K., & Korepin, V. (2023). Quantum multi-programming for Grover's search. *Quantum Information Processing, 22*(1), 54. Springer.
10. Sihotang, H. T., Efendi, S., Zamzami, E. M., & Mawengkang, H. (2020). Design and implementation of Rivest Shamir Adleman's (RSA) cryptography algorithm in text file data security. *Journal of Physics: Conference Series, 1641*(1), 012042. IOP Publishing.
11. Boudot, F., Gaudry, P., Guillevic, A., Heninger, N., Thomé, E., & Zimmermann, P. (2020). Comparing the difficulty of factorization and discrete logarithm: A 240-digit experiment. In *Proceedings of the Advances in Cryptology–CRYPTO 2020: 40th Annual International Cryptology Conference, CRYPTO 2020, Santa Barbara, CA, USA, August 17–21, 2020, Part II 40* (pp. 62–91). Springer International Publishing.
12. Larasati, H. T., & Kim, H. (2021). Quantum cryptanalysis landscape of Shor's algorithm for elliptic curve discrete logarithm problem. In *Information security applications: 22nd international conference, WISA 2021, Jeju Island, South Korea, August 11–13, 2021, Revised Selected Papers 22* (pp. 91–104). Springer International Publishing.
13. Paquin, C., Stebila, D., & Tamvada, G. (2020). Benchmarking post-quantum cryptography in TLS. In *Proceedings of the Post-Quantum Cryptography: 11th International Conference, PQCrypto 2020, Paris, France* (pp. 72–91). Springer International Publishing.
14. Li, P., Su, J., & Wang, X. (2020). iTLS: Lightweight transport-layer security protocol for IoT with minimal latency and perfect forward secrecy. *IEEE Internet of Things Journal, 7*(8), 6828–6841.
15. Ylonen, T. (2019). SSH key management challenges and requirements. In *2019 10th IFIP international conference on new technologies, mobility and security (NTMS)* (pp. 1–5). IEEE.
16. Uddin, M. R., Evan, N. A., Alam, M. R., & Arefin, M. T. (2021). Analysis of Generic Routing Encapsulation (GRE) over IP Security (IPSec) VPN Tunneling in IPv6 Network. In *Proceedings of the ubiquitous communications and network computing: 4th EAI international conference, UBICNET 2021* (pp. 3–15). Springer International Publishing.
17. Mitra, S., Das, S., & Kule, M. (2021). Prevention of the man-in-the-middle attack on Diffie–Hellman key exchange algorithm: A review. In *Proceedings of international conference on frontiers in computing and systems: COMSYS 2020* (pp. 625–635). Springer Singapore.
18. Chou, T., Niederhagen, R., Persichetti, E., Randrianarisoa, T. H., Reijnders, K., Samardjiska, S., & Trimoska, M. (2023). Take your meds: Digital signatures from matrix code equivalence. In *International conference on cryptology in Africa* (pp. 28–52). Springer Nature Switzerland.
19. Yuvaraj, N., Praghash, K., & Karthikeyan, T. (2022). Data privacy preservation and trade-off balance between privacy and utility using deep adaptive clustering and elliptic curve digital signature algorithm. *Wireless Personal Communications, 124*(1), 655–670.
20. Farooq, S. M., Hussain, S. S., & Ustun, T. S. (2019). Performance evaluation and analysis of IEC 62351-6 probabilistic signature scheme for securing GOOSE messages. *IEEE Access, 7*, 32343–32351.
21. Reegan, A. S., & Kabila, V. (2021). Highly secured cluster based WSN using novel FCM and enhanced ECC-ElGamal encryption in IoT. *Wireless Personal Communications, 118*, 1313–1329.
22. Zhong, Y. (2022). An Overview of RSA and OAEP Padding. In *Highlights in Science, Engineering and Technology* (Vol. 1, pp. 82–86).
23. Waidyasooriya, H. M., Oshiyama, H., Kurebayashi, Y., Hariyama, M., & Ohzeki, M. (2022). A scalable emulator for quantum Fourier transform using multiple-FPGAs with high-bandwidth-memory. *IEEE Access, 10*, 65103–65117.

24. Anand, R., Maitra, A., Maitra, S., Mukherjee, C. S., & Mukhopadhyay, S. (2021). Quantum resource estimation for FSR based symmetric ciphers and related Grover's attacks. In *Proceedings of the progress in cryptology–INDOCRYPT 2021: 22nd international conference on cryptology in India, Jaipur, India, December 12–15, 2021* (pp. 179–198). Springer International Publishing.
25. Somsuk, K., & Sanemueang, C. (2019). The new modified methodology to solve ECDLP based on brute force attack. In *Recent advances in information and communication technology 2018: Proceedings of the 14th international conference on computing and information technology (IC2IT 2018)* (pp. 255–264). Springer International Publishing.
26. Mean, W. D. T., Rule, H. P. (2022). Health Insurance Portability and Accountability Act of 1996 (HIPAA).
27. Paris, I. L. B. M., Habaebi, M. H., & Zyoud, A. M. (2023). Implementation of SSL/TLS security with MQTT protocol in IoT environment. In *Wireless Personal Communications* (pp. 1–20).
28. Viriyasitavat, W., Xu, L. D., Sapsomboon, A., Dhiman, G., & Hoonsopon, D. (2022). Building trust of Blockchain-based Internet-of-Thing services using public key infrastructure. *Enterprise Information Systems, 16*(12), 2037162.
29. Khan, S., Zafar, S., Iftekhar, N., Biswas, S., & Tripathi, G. (2021). Inculcating Dynamic Trust Management across Internet through avant-garde Approach. In *Proceedings of the 2nd International Conference on ICT for Digital, Smart, and Sustainable Development, ICIDSSD 2020, 27–28 February 2020, Jamia Hamdard, New Delhi, India.*
30. Choi, S. J., & Johnson, M. E. (2021). The relationship between cybersecurity ratings and the risk of hospital data breaches. *Journal of the American Medical Informatics Association, 28*(10), 2085–2092.
31. Espitau, T., Joux, A., & Kharchenko, N. (2020). On a dual/hybrid approach to small secret LWE: A dual/enumeration technique for learning with errors and application to security estimates of FHE schemes. In *Progress in Cryptology–INDOCRYPT 2020: 21st international conference on cryptology in India, Bangalore, India, December 13–16, 2020, proceedings 21* (pp. 440–462). Springer International Publishing.
32. Chen, H., Dai, W., Kim, M., & Song, Y. (2021). Efficient homomorphic conversion between (ring) LWE ciphertexts. In *International conference on applied cryptography and network security* (pp. 460-479). Cham: Springer International Publishing.
33. Yu, H., Zhang, C., & Jiang, H. (2021). A FPGA-Based heterogeneous implementation of NTRUEncrypt. In *Advances in parallel and distributed processing, and applications: Proceedings from PDPTA'20, CSC'20, MSV'20, and GCC'20* (pp. 461–475). Springer International Publishing.
34. Suhail, S., Hussain, R., Khan, A., & Hong, C. S. (2020). On the role of hash-based signatures in quantum-safe internet of things: Current solutions and future directions. *IEEE Internet of Things Journal, 8*(1), 1–17.
35. Zhu, H., Guo, Y., & Zhang, L. (2021). An improved convolution Merkle tree-based blockchain electronic medical record secure storage scheme. *Journal of Information Security and Applications, 61*, 102952.
36. Majenz, C., Manfouo, C. M., & Ozols, M. (2021). Quantum-access security of the Winternitz one-time signature scheme. arXiv preprint arXiv: 2103.12448.
37. Turan, M. S., McKay, K., Chang, D., Calik, C., Bassham, L., Kang, J., & Kelsey, J. (2021). Status report on the second round of the NIST lightweight cryptography standardization process. In *National Institute of Standards and Technology Internal Report.*
38. Fregly, A., Harvey, J., Kaliski Jr, B. S., & Sheth, S. (2023). Merkle tree ladder mode: Reducing the size impact of NIST PQC signature algorithms in practice. In *Cryptographers' Track at the RSA Conference* (pp. 415–441). Springer International Publishing.
39. Dable-Heath, E., Casa, L., Porter, C., Mintert, F., & Ling, C. (2023). Quantum algorithmic solutions to the shortest vector problem on simulated coherent Ising machines. arXiv preprint arXiv:2304.04075.

Chapter 3
Artificial Intelligence-Enabled 6G Mobile Systems

Ahrar Bin Aslam, Faiza Iqbal, Unzela Talpur, Zafi Sherhan Syed, and Faisal Karim Shaikh

3.1 Introduction

In recent times, the rapid growth of mobile communication networks has changed the way we interact with the world. From the initial development of 1G networks to the 4G and 5G [1], the mobile industry has consistently pushed the boundaries of innovation by deploying voice communication to allow high-speed data transfer [2], connectivity, and advancement of smart devices [3]. The evolution of mobile communication systems is paving a path to enhanced performance, efficiency, and user experience [4, 5, 6]. Innovative technologies including the Internet of Everything (IoE), holographic communication, extended reality, and others have emerged; however, their growing network requirements place limitations on 5G's capacity to fulfill these demands [7]. This served as inspiration for the creation of 6G networks, as it will be more efficient, intelligent, reliable, meet the network demands of emerging applications, and will overcome the limitations faced by 5G. In comparison to its predecessor, 5G, 6G wireless networks are expected to have higher data rates of up to 1 Tbps, ultra-low end-to-end latency of less than 0.1 ms, and increased reliability of more than 99.99% [8]. Due to its significance for the future of wireless communication networks, numerous studies have been conducted on its potential application, use cases, architecture, vision, and enabling technologies [9, 10–13].

A. B. Aslam · F. Iqbal · U. Talpur · Z. S. Syed (✉) · F. K. Shaikh
Department of Telecommunication Engineering, Mehran University of Engineering and Technology, Jamshoro, Pakistan
e-mail: 18tl04@students.muet.edu.pk; 23msds004@students.muet.edu.pk; 23msds005@students.muet.edu.pk; zafisherhan.shah@faculty.muet.edu.pk; faisal.shaikh@faculty.muet.edu.pk

© The Author(s), under exclusive license to Springer Nature Switzerland AG 2024

A. Bourdena et al. (eds.), *Intelligent Technologies for Healthcare Business Applications*, Signals and Communication Technology,
https://doi.org/10.1007/978-3-031-58527-2_3

6G will incorporate AL, ML, and edge computing to make it more intelligent, enhanced, and adaptable. The integration of these technologies will enable 6G to cater wide range of applications such as energy-efficient smart cities [14], metaverse [15], intelligent transportation system [16], industry 5.0 [17], smart healthcare [18], and many more. AI in 6G is poised to play a vital role in shaping the future of wireless communications [19, 20] by making it more intelligent and enabling intelligent resource management, enhancing security, better network optimization, etc. It would enable technologies that benefit society, such as in the healthcare sector where it would be a key component of augmented reality (AR) and virtual reality (VR) for conducting remote surgeries, and will also help in smart patient monitoring using AI-powered robots [21].

In this chapter, we discuss the significance of AI in 6G wireless communication technology and how it would be beneficial in revolutionizing our world. By examining recent studies, we understand how AI can make devices intelligent and enhance their security. We discuss the various AI techniques, their role in 6G's IoT for a smarter world, and how it address the security issues associated with 6G networks. In addition, we also provide a brief review of the applications of AI in 6G for the healthcare sector.

The remainder of the chapter is structured as follows. Section 3.2 discusses the comparative analysis of earlier mobile generations to 6G networks. Section 3.3 provides a detailed survey of AI techniques used for the development and enhancement of 6G networks. Section 3.4 explores the convergence of AI and Internet of Things titled Artificial Internet of Things (AIoT). Section 3.5 investigates various risks associated with 6G networks and the use of AI in mitigating them. Section 3.6 consists of different ways in which AI-enabled 6G networks can be used in the healthcare sector. To conclude the chapter, in Sect. 3.7 we provide a brief conclusion of our study.

3.2 Comparative Analysis of 4G, 5G, and 6G Networks

In this section, we shall provide a comparative analysis of the modern wireless communication technologies, exploring key features, and investigate the growing demands of modern communication technologies, which have prompted the need to move from older technologies to emerging ones.

3.2.1 Fourth Generation of Wireless Communication Technology (4G)

The fourth generation of wireless communication technology (4G) also known as long-term evolution (LTE) is a successor of the third generation of wireless communication technology (3G), providing higher speeds and lower latency [22]. The International Telecommunication Union-Radio Communication Sector (ITU-R)

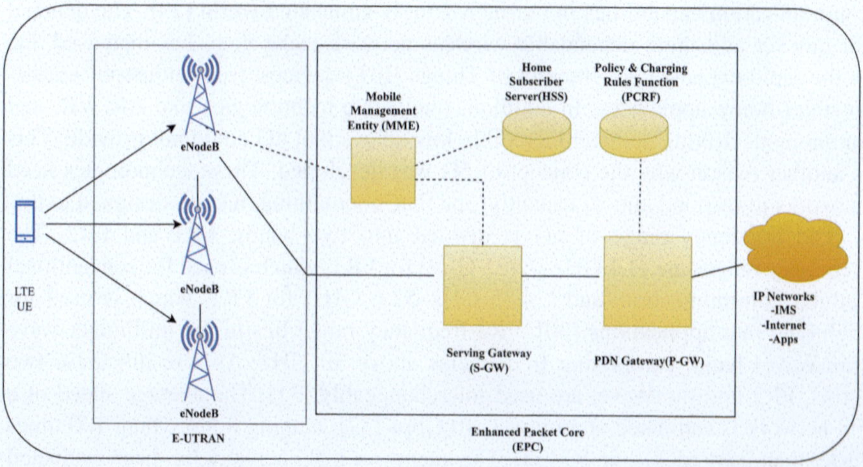

Fig. 3.1 4G System architecture according to 3GPP Release 8 [27]

created a set of standards known as International Mobile Telecommunications Advanced (IMT-Advanced) that networks must meet to be considered as 4G. According to IMT- Advanced, a 4G network enables a mobile device to exchange data at 100 Mbps for high mobility and at 1 Gbps for low mobility communication [23].

Due to its enhanced speed to its predecessor, users can enjoy high-definition mobile TV, video streaming, faster Internet browsing, video conferencing, gaming, etc. The 4G wireless communication technology utilizes the sub-6 GHz frequency range and the frequency ranges from 700 MHz to 3 GHz [24]. The sub-6 GHz frequency range refers to the frequencies below 6 GHz. The average latency of a 4G network is estimated at around 50 ms, and its capacity is quite low as compared to its successors 5G and 6G, as it can support around 2000 devices per 0.38 square mile or roughly 1 square kilometer [25].

Orthogonal frequency division multiplexing (OFDM) and multiple input multiple output (MIMO) are used by LTE to provide higher data rates [26]. LTE-Advanced (LTE-A) is a further enhancement in the 4G LTE technology, providing even higher data rates and reduced latency.

The system architecture of 4G wireless communication technology is illustrated in Fig. 3.1.

3.2.2 *Fifth Generation of Wireless Communication Technology (5G)*

The fifth generation of wireless communication technology (5G) is a successor of 4G, providing even higher speeds and reduced latency [28]. The need for 5G arises from the growing demand for faster, more reliable, and more efficient wireless communication capabilities in our increasingly connected world [29]. The demand for quicker and more dependable wireless network technology has increased due to the rapid expansion of Internet of Things (IoT) devices, from industrial sensors to smart home appliances. In addition, innovative technologies like AR, VR, and autonomous driving demand incredibly low delays that 4G could not provide. This is another reason why the concept of 5G was developed. These technologies need networks to respond almost instantly, and that's something 5G was designed to do.

The frequency range of 5G is divided into two bands, FR1 and FR2. The frequency ranges are (4.1 GHz–7.125 GHz) for FR1, which is used for conventional cellular communication, and (24.25 GHz–52.6 GHz) for FR2, which is used for high data rate applications [30]. FR2 frequency range lies in the millimeter-wave (mmWave) band, comprising frequencies above 30 GHz. As a result, these two terms, FR2 and mmWave, are used interchangeably [31]. The average speed of a 5G network is estimated at around 1–10 Gbps [32], making it more than 100 times faster than its predecessor 4G [33]. The latency of a 5G network has been evaluated to be less than 10 ms [34]. 5G can provide services to 100,000 to 1,000,000 devices per square kilometer, making its capacity significantly greater than 4G [35].

The three primary use cases of the 5G technology are enhanced mobile broadband (eMBB), ultra-reliable low latency communication (URLLC), and massive machine-type communications (mMTC) [36]. eMBB transforms wireless data transmission by providing super-fast Internet, enabling seamless streaming and high-quality video conferencing. It is useful for applications that require high data rates. URLLC ensures devices communicate with minimal delays, crucial for applications like autonomous vehicles and real-time surgery. It paves the way for real-time interactions that were previously unattainable. mMTC has a connection density of 10^6 devices per square kilometer in an urban environment [37], facilitating smart cities and homes, and driving efficiency and innovation. It is fundamental to building a highly connected world where devices can effortlessly communicate and share data. Overall, these use cases redefine mobile communication's speed, reliability, and connectivity for a more advanced and connected world.

A variety of applications are made possible by 5G such as smart cities [35], enhanced mobile Internet [38], IoT [39], streaming quality 4K and 8K video content [40], advancements in industry 4.0 and automation [35], autonomous vehicles [41], and the immerse experiences of AR and VR [42].

Figure 3.2 shows the system architecture of 5G wireless communication technology, which is customized to fulfill the needs of complex and demanding 5G applications.

3.2.3 Sixth Generation of Wireless Communication Technology (6G)

The sixth generation of wireless communication technology (6G) is the successor of 5G and is expected to be available for users in around 2030 [44]. Even

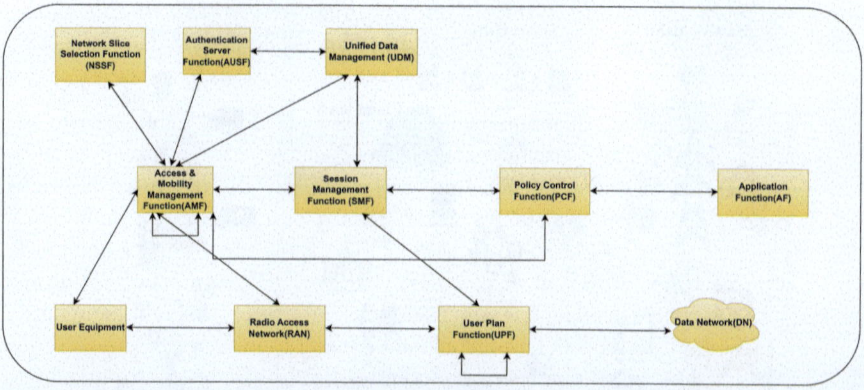

Fig. 3.2 5G System architecture according to 3GPP Release 15 [43]

though 5G wireless networks are still in the early stage of development and have improved data rates, reduced latency, and increased capacity [33], network demands are increasing every passing day due to increased interconnectivity and introduction of emerging technologies. To satisfy the rising network demands, there is a requirement for even higher data rates, lower latency, and increased capacity. Therefore, researchers and companies are already looking toward enhancing their capabilities with 6G, for data-intensive applications such as autonomous vehicles [45]. The 6G wireless communication technology will integrate techniques like AI, ML, and edge computing [46] to create an entirely new kind of Internet.

The W-band, which spans above 75 GHz to 110 GHz, the D-band, which ranges from 110 GHz to 175 GHz, as well as bands between 275 GHz and 300 GHz are among the frequency ranges being considered for 6G. In addition, the 6G technology would utilize the tera-hertz (THz) frequencies ranging from 0.3 to 10 THz [47]. With estimated speeds of 1 to 10 Tbps, 6G is expected to be significantly faster than its preceding generations [48]. 6G would make considerable improvements over the 5G with the latency reduced to 10–100 μs from 10 ms and 50 ms of 5G and 5G, respectively. 6G would also enable 10,000,000 devices to be connected per square kilometer, whereas the area traffic capacity would increase to 1 Gb/s/m^2 [48]. The system architecture of 6G wireless communication technology provides a visual representation of the potential infrastructure of the next generation of wireless communication and is illustrated in Fig. 3.3.

The device at the outer layer of the architecture is used to gather data in the communication network to provide connectivity. The devices including cellular users, IoT nodes, smart cells, massive MIMO devices, device-to-device (D2D), and vehicle-to-everything (V2X) devices by default have a certain level of intelligence to intelligently manage interference, smart sensing, and smart selection of channels. The links represent the wireless connectivity among devices.

The second layer consists of an AI-enabled cloud, edge devices, and a cloud-based radio access network (RAN) designed to carry out intelligent tasks, including

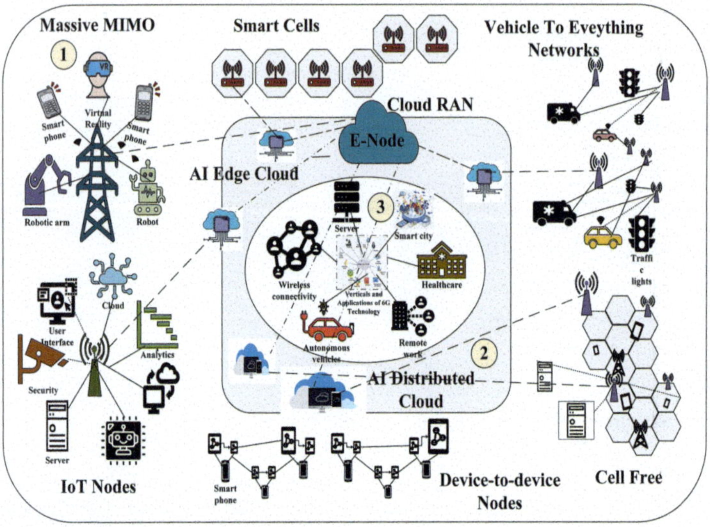

Fig. 3.3 6G System architecture according to [49]

Table 3.1 Parameters comparison of 4G, 5G, and 6G communication systems according to [50]

Parameters	4G	5G	6G
Peak data rate	1 Gbps	10 Gbps	1 Tbps
Max frequency	6 GHz	90 GHz	10 THz
End-to-end latency	100 ms	10 ms	1 ms
Mobility	350 km/h	500 km/h	1000 km/h
Maximum spectral efficiency	15 bps/Hz	30 bps/Hz	100 bps/Hz
THz communication	No	Very limited	Extensively
Artificial intelligence	No	Limited	Fully
Autonomous vehicle support	No	Limited	Fully
XR	No	Limited	Fully
Satellite integration	No	Limited	Fully

user management, the allocation of resources, and the overall optimization of the network's performance. These components collectively work to ensure that the network operates efficiently and effectively, meeting the demands of modern communication scenarios.

The third layer in this diagram represents the applications and verticals of 6G network architecture to receive and provide services from the other two layers. This interaction allows for providing a variety of services, shaping end-users' experiences, and ensuring smooth communication across the entire system.

Table 3.1 presents the overall comparison of different parameters for the three technologies: 4G, 5G, and 6G. It offers a comprehensive overview of the different characteristics of these wireless communication generations.

3.3 Artificial Intelligence Techniques in 6G Communication Systems

In this section, we shall discuss several AI techniques that may be used in 6G networks. AI is an emerging field and plays a significant role in the evolution of 6G technology. It can be employed in 6G networks to personalize 6G services and has the potential to empower machines to automate tasks, elevate decision-making processes, and enable them to take valuable insights from complex problems [51]. Our analysis is based on the proposal of AI in 6G wireless communication networks.

Sheth et al. [52] presented a complete survey on 6G architecture and deployment of AI in 6G technology for various applications such as object localization, security, and privacy. In addition, they also discussed a use case of UAV-enabled intelligent transportation system (ITS) which can achieve safe lane changing, optimal traffic signal control, emergency warning notification, and smart parking. In spite of the advantages of the current ITS, it faces several challenges, such as bandwidth limitations, managing data from numerous vehicles in close proximity, privacy and security concerns, existing scheduling and channel allocation algorithms are inefficient, and the decentralization characteristic lacks a fixed central system for reliable communication. They proposed an AI-enabled 6G architecture and utilizing its visible light communication (VLC) can eliminate bandwidth constraints. Optimization of channel allocation can be made possible with CNNs. In the data link layer of their architecture, they placed AI techniques like principal component analysis (PCA) and ISOMAP to streamline data flow by extracting relevant information. Decentralization security can be enhanced through AI integration in 6G. They also proposed that RL algorithms can efficiently allocate resources among vehicles and the central system, boosting overall efficiency.

The integration of wireless devices has been increasing rapidly, and the main aim of the AI-enabled 6G network is to automate the tasks done by machines working with human intelligence and high precision. By integrating AI techniques in 6G networks, various challenges have been solved, which were previously faced by traditional existing networks including achieving seamless connectivity, meeting assured quality of service (QoS) requirements and handling vast amounts of data generated by IoT devices.

Several studies have been conducted by scientists and researchers in which they have incorporated AI techniques in 6G technology to enhance the connectivity and efficiency of wireless networks. A few of those studies have been discussed below.

3.3.1 Machine Learning

Machine learning (ML) is a branch of AI that allows computers to learn from data, recognize patterns, resolve issues, and anticipate outcomes without being programmed in advance. The process involves training the machine on a data set, and it makes predictions based on the new data given to it.

There are three types of ML, namely, supervised, unsupervised, and reinforcement learning [53]. As the next phase of wireless communications generation, 6G presents a wide range of possibilities as well as challenges, and ML techniques may be essential in maximizing the capabilities of 6G networks.

Several studies have been carried out by researchers, utilizing ML for the improvement and enhancement of 6G technology. In [54], P. Rekkas et al. provided an extensive summary of the usage of ML algorithms, including supervised, unsupervised, and reinforcement learning (RL) to enhance the performance of deep learning (DL) algorithms such as convolutional neural network (CNN) and long short-term memory (LSTM) [55] for various 6G applications like optimization problems where they introduced a model based on deep reinforcement learning (DRL) actor-critic approach. This model aims to optimize tasks like resource allocation, beam selection, channel estimation, anomaly detection, and tackling joint network control challenges. To improve accuracy up to 96.7%, they also suggested a deep Q-learning approach in the detection of faults or anomalies within 6G networks.

Tang et al. [56] advocated the use of advanced ML techniques in vehicular communications and networking. They proposed that ML could be applied to enhance the effectiveness of detection of breaches and data encryption in automotive networks. The use of ML for intelligent beamforming methods in mmWave communication and for enhancing the effectiveness of proactive detection in automotive network security are both addressed in the study. They also investigated the ML-based approaches including DL-based channel estimation for multiradio access, CNN for vehicular traffic prediction, recurrent neural network (RNN) for network resource allocation, support vector machine (SVM) for intrusion detection in vehicular networks, and decision trees (DT) for vehicular network security.

3.3.1.1 Supervised Learning

Supervised learning is an ML approach where algorithms are trained on a labeled data set [57]. For supervised learning to be applied in any application, there should be a substantial amount of data [58]. It is mostly employed in tasks involving classification and regression. Some of the algorithms within this approach include k-nearest neighbor (KNN), Naive Bayes, SVM, backpropagation, and DT [59].

In [60], Ahmed et al. emphasized the importance of supervised ML models for effective quality of experience (QoE) monitoring and provided a detailed overview of implementing QoE measurement and predictive solutions for video streaming using supervised ML. They also provide a comparative analysis of different supervised ML algorithms based on five performance metrics, including root mean squared error (RMSE), mean absolute error (MAE), R-squared (R2), Pearson linear correlation coefficient (PLCC), and Spearman rank correlation coefficient (SRCC). Their analysis revealed that complex supervised ML algorithms such as Random Forest and Gradient Boosting outperform simpler ML models like DT and KNN because QoE prediction is a challenging non-linear problem.

In the study [61], Mahmood et al. presented a detailed review of the supervised learning techniques, including regression, SVM, and KNN, for 6G applications. Regression algorithms can be applied in the localization of devices, outrage analysis, target detection, and the design of energy-efficient systems. Additionally, the study proposed that some of the use cases for applying SVM would be spectrum sensing, target tracking, resource management, pattern recognition, and fault detection in the sensor network. On the other hand, KNN is applied in resource allocation, indoor localization, and device clustering.

In [62], Daba and Abdul-Latif proposed the application of SVM in 6G communication networks to detect signals in the presence of noise in the channel. The study examined the bit error rate metric performance of SVM compared to that of a conventional M-ary signal model detector employing m-ary phase shift keying (MPSK) modulation. It was discovered that SVM performs better than traditional detectors, which need about 7 bits of coding to produce results that are comparable to SVM.

3.3.1.2 Unsupervised Learning

Unsupervised learning algorithms are trained on unlabeled data set [57], which means the input data predicts results with no information on output labels. One of the common techniques of unsupervised ML is clustering [63]. The most widely used unsupervised algorithms include principal component analysis (PCA) and k-means. Rekkas et al. [64] presented a thorough review of the significance of unsupervised ML techniques for various 6G applications, such as optimization problems, user mobility estimation, channel estimation, security, UAV networks, MIMO, and fault detection.

To identify abnormalities in 6G networks, the authors in [65] evaluated five distinct unsupervised learning techniques: local outlier factor (LOF), k-means clustering, local outlier probabilities (LoOP), fuzzy c-means clustering, and Kohonen's self- organizing maps (SOM). The results demonstrate that fuzzy c-means and k-means are not as effective as SOM-based techniques in identifying faults in 6G networks. To address fault detection, another paper [66] proposed the k-aware k-means clustering technique, a modification of the conventional k-means clustering. In this modified version of k-means, the model uses an unsupervised learning phase to understand the smallest cluster in the data and then updates this understanding by identifying outliers. This process helps the model automatically determine the optimal number of clusters ($K \leq$ value), resulting in a high prediction accuracy of 99.7%.

3.3.1.3 Reinforcement Learning

Reinforcement learning is a method of ML where agents learn to make choices by engaging with their surroundings. The agent receives rewards for favorable actions and penalties for unfavorable ones. As there is no data set associated with the desired output and indirect supervision is required to understand the system's optimal performance, RL is regarded as a hybrid of supervised and unsupervised learning [67]. RL algorithms can be classified into two main categories, value-based algorithms, such as Q-learning and state-action-reward-state-action (SARSA), and policy-based algorithms, which include policy gradient (PG), proximal policy optimization (PPO), and actor-critic (A2C) [68].

For fault detection in 6G networks, a deep Q-learning method has been proposed, which can achieve an accuracy of up to 96.7% while making use of a limited number of features [69]. Regarding the enhancement of data rate optimization, two novel transmission systems utilizing RL techniques have been introduced: reinforcement learning channel-aware transmission (RL-CAT) and reinforcement learning pCAT (RL-pCAT) [70]. They can achieve data rate improvements of up to 181% in the uplink and 270% in the downlink compared to conventional probabilistic models.

A study conducted by Su et al. [71] proposed a deep Q-learning approach for cooperative communications in the 6G wireless network. The goal of the model is to efficiently select the best relay from various nodes without needing a network model. This approach's results revealed that it outperforms existing approaches in performance probability, energy consumption, and convergence time.

3.3.2 *Natural Language Processing*

Natural language processing (NLP) is a sub-field of AI with the help of which it has become easy to do interaction between computers and human languages. It enables computers to understand human language. Due to the increased focus on human-machine interaction and smart devices, NLP would be important in the development of 6G technology in applications such as voice assistants, language translation, smart customer support, etc.

In our earlier research [72], we proposed that NLP applied to COVID-19-related YouTube vlogs can be utilized to aid public health practitioners in public health screening of COVID-19 and other viral diseases. Our methodology encompassed the utilization of word clouds, lexical analysis, and Latent Dirichlet Allocation (LDA) Topic Modeling to extract insights into people's personal experiences with the virus. Notably, we identified key terms, such as symptoms, generic terms, medical equipment, etc. These findings are important in assisting public health officials in their efforts to detect and mitigate the transmission of such diseases.

In another of our prior studies [73], NLP was utilized to differentiate between praise and insult in Reddit comments. We evaluated the classification performance using Term-Frequency Inverse Document Frequency (TF-IDF) features and then employed two distinct deep learning methods: Keras Embedding and Global vectors for word representation (GloVe). In summary, our approach achieved accuracy rates of 83% for TF-IDF, 89% for GloVe, and an impressive 93% for Keras Embeddings. Despite being slightly below the 97.8% baseline accuracy, our solution's compact size of 28 MB, compared to the 340 MB of the baseline XLNet model, makes it highly suitable for real-time applications.

In [74], Sana and Strinati focused on the implementation of semantic communication within 6G networks that enable the receiver to receive the intended message. Semantic communication helps to transmit only relevant information sufficient for the receiver to understand meaningful information ensuring better bandwidth utilization.

In [75], the research uses text mining and natural language processing to analyze patents related to 6G satellite communication. They employ techniques like LDA, ontology matching, k-means clustering, technology function matrix (TFM), and the s-curve to understand the technology landscape. The study identifies major technology leaders and sub-technologies, aiming to discover trends and potentials in satellite communication. The paper presents a strategic research plan for technology-savvy countries, with a focus on Taiwan. It emphasizes the role of AI technologies in 6G satellite communication and its impact on various applications.

3.3.3 Deep Learning

Deep learning (DL) is a sub-field of ML that uses artificial neural networks to model data and solve complex problems. These neural networks are inspired by the structure of the human brain designed with neural nodes connected as a network [76], therefore allowing them to process enormous amounts of data and make precise predictions of complex and intricate problems. Over the past few years, DL has arrived as an efficient AI technique in wireless communication networks [77].

The study by Chen et al. [78] focuses on the DL approach for image recognition in detecting driver's behavior within 6G and IoT networks. Their research contributes to comparing several CNN techniques to detect and specify improper driving behavior.

In [79], Ozpoyraz et al. unveiled the latest advancements in DL-based physical layer methods for potential application in 6G wireless networks. It explored four key concepts, massive MIMO systems, sophisticated multi-carrier waveform designs, reconfigurable intelligent surface-empowered communications, and physical layer security. They presented recent breakthroughs in DL and their comparison with existing approaches. Overall, the article aimed to showcase the importance of DL-based physical layer methods for 6G applications.

In [80], Jagganath et al. offered the need to design signal processing algorithms for 6G wireless networks by leveraging DL techniques to fulfill its physical layer requirements. Their research introduced a method called deep unfolded signal processing to achieve this objective.

In the research of Zhang et al. [81], new methods were suggested to push forward the development of 6G communication. These approaches involve combining block-structured and end-to-end DL, integrating model-driven and data-driven DL, using both online and offline training, employing ubiquitous learning, and utilizing explainable DL techniques.

3.3.4 Computer Vision

Computer vision is a sub-field of AI and computer science that enables computers to understand and comprehend meaningful information from images. Some of the key applications (image processing, object recognition, and facial recognition) of computer vision in various industries include AR and VR, healthcare, and autonomous systems.

In [82], a DL method integrated into 6G wireless systems known as optimizing computer vision with AI-enabled technology (OCV-AI) is proposed along with a framework for the 6G network employed with DL techniques for pattern recognition and smart management systems. In addition, the study also highlighted the importance of DL-based computer vision for advanced analytics and intelligent systems.

The current beam management technique 5G new radio (NR) has a beam sweeping period of 20ms [83]. This results in latency, increased power consumption, and wastage of resources, making it unsuitable for 6G. To address these challenges, the article [84] introduced a novel method of beam management using computer vision. In this approach, a camera attached to the base station captures the image and it is processed using a DL object detector. This allows the system to identify the mobiles located in a particular area in 3D space. This technique achieves higher beamforming gain and lower latency, as this technique allows the base station to directly adjust the beam direction without quantization codebook and feedback delay, making it vital for 6G. As compared to 5G NR, the proposed method achieves 40% more beamforming gain and a 40% decrease in beam training overhead.

The research by Rubio et al. [85] introduced the use of large intelligent surfaces (LIS) for radio sensing for 6G networks. The researchers made use of communication signals in the environment and processed them using LIS to create a radio map that indicated the physical locations of the passive devices such as the scatterers and humans. To extract meaningful insights from the radio maps, computer vision and ML techniques such as template matching, component labeling, and k-means clustering were utilized. To assess the accuracy of this method, the researchers used it for active and passive user detection in an indoor environment. The results indicated that it could detect 98% of the passive and 100% of the active users and could also work in low signal-to-noise ratio (SNR) conditions.

Beamforming is essential for THz communication as the wavelengths are exceedingly small making them susceptible to signal impairments such as attenuation and scattering. The current beam management methods consist of beam training overheads and increasing latency, which is not helpful for advanced wireless networks like 6G. To enhance beam management, Jiang et al. [86] proposed an ML framework based on an encoder-decoder architecture beam tracking method which could predict the future of beams based on previously collected visual data collected from cameras on base stations. The method was tested on a large DeepSense 6G data set [87]. The results of the evaluation revealed an accuracy of 64.47% and a normalized power of 97.66%. Additionally, it required less than 1% of the beam training overhead as compared to the previous methods. The results indicated that the proposed vision-aided beam tracking solution performs exceptionally well in real-world scenarios.

The high reliability and low latency of millimeter wave and sub-terahertz depends upon the sensitivity of these signals to blockages, as these signals rely on line of sight communication (LOS) between the base stations and the user equipment and any blockage in the LOS would affect the latency and reliability of these signals. To cater to this issue, the article [88] presents a DL neural network architecture that utilizes RGB images and beamforming vectors to learn and predict the signal link blockages in the future. This method is evaluated on a publicly available data set [89] achieving an impressive accuracy of 86% in predicting future link blockages.

3.4 Artificial Intelligence-Enabled IoT in 6G Communication Systems

In this section, we shall delve into the comprehensive details of how AI-enabled IoT can be implemented in 6G wireless communication networks. We will discuss its advantages and the wide range of applications that would be essential for enhancing 6G technology.

The integration of AI technologies with the IoT ecosystem is known as AIoT (Artificial Intelligence of Things). It involves using AI algorithms and techniques to improve the capabilities and intelligence of IoT devices, systems, and applications. AIoT enables IoT devices to process, analyze, and act on data in a more intelligent and autonomous manner, resulting in increased efficiency, better decision-making, and improved user experiences. Some of the key aspects of AIoT are data analysis and insights, predictive analysis, real-time decision-making, context awareness, energy efficiency, edge computing, security, and anomaly detection.

Overall, AI in IoT contributes significantly to the IoT ecosystem's improvements and capabilities. It gives IoT devices intelligence [90], autonomy [91], and adaptive behavior, increasing their value, efficiency, and ability to alter numerous businesses and domains. The two combined will pave the way to a new era of solutions and experiences that transform businesses across numerous industries, creating new opportunities altogether.

AIoT in 6G is the combination of AI with the Internet of Things in the framework of a sixth-generation wireless network. The goal of AIoT in 6G is to use the combined power of AI and IoT to create a more intelligent, efficient, and responsive network environment. Incorporating AI into sixth-generation wireless networks provides interesting solutions for addressing increasingly complicated network optimization problems [92]. Researchers are also looking into other technologies, like quantum communications in 6g for strong security against various cyber-attacks [93], and the THz band will play an important role in improving the capabilities of future 6G networks [94]. It is expected that 6G will revolutionize itself from "connected things" to "connected intelligence," which can evolve the serving network autonomously and intelligently [95].

The development of communication systems for future IoT within the context of 6G wireless networks obtains significant momentum by leveraging the capabilities of AI/ML. Through the integration of AI/ML, IoT can achieve massive connectivity with lower latency than 1 ms [96]. This relationship between AI/ML and IoT lays the groundwork for intelligent IoT in 6G wireless networks [97]. Next, we discuss comprehensively the integration and implementation of AIoT in 6G wireless communication networks.

Li et al. [98] used collective reinforcement learning (CRL), which allows IoT devices to collaborate and collectively improve their AI models and learning capabilities. In CRL, intelligent nodes learn from their own experiences in local states and share their training models with one another. This collective learning approach allows each node to freely share knowledge, increasing the training efficiency and accuracy of AI algorithms. Some of the AI-enhanced techniques for 6G IoT networks mentioned in the article were computation resource allocation via DRL to optimize the allocation of computation resources in distributed software-defined industrial IoT systems. DRL helps improve system energy efficiency by making intelligent decisions about resource allocation based on the current environment and workload. Additionally, the research explored, resource management optimization via dueling deep q-network (DQN) to optimize resource management, specifically for caching and computing tasks in delay-tolerant IoT scenarios. It helps to enhance data processing efficiency and reduce network overhead by intelligently managing resources. RL and DRL algorithms focus on training an individual agent to make decisions by interacting with its environment. The agent learns from the feedback it receives based on its actions, with the goal of maximizing a reward signal. RL and DRL are commonly used in IoT applications but rely heavily on massive pre-defined data sets based on the local environment. Federated learning (FL) is a decentralized approach to AI training, where multiple IoT devices collaborate to collectively learn a global model without sharing raw data centrally. Each device trains its local model based on its own data and then communicates updates to a central server, which aggregates and disseminates the global model back to all devices. FL addresses privacy and security concerns, but it may still rely on predefined environments.

The study of Ferrag et al. [99] proposed a technique for cyber threat-hunting (CTH) in 6G-enabled IoT networks involving the use of Generative AI. The specific AI technique suggested is the application of a novel generative adversarial network (GAN) and transformer-based model for CTH in 6G-enabled IoT systems. The GAN is a type of generative AI model that consists of two neural networks, a generator, and a discriminator, which work together to generate new data that closely resembles the real data. The transformer-based model, on the other hand, is a form of neural network architecture that was developed originally for NLP applications, but it has been adapted for other tasks, including cybersecurity. Their analysis of a novel cyber security data set indicated that the transformer-based security model for CTH achieved a remarkable accuracy of 95% in detecting IoT attacks.

To address the security challenges related to the 6G IoT networks, Mao et al. [100] introduced an AI-based security method that focuses on IoT devices. Their approach predicts future harvesting power using the extended Kalman filtering (EKF) method, allowing the system to anticipate the available energy for IoT devices. A mathematical model is employed during each energy-aware cycle to compute the required energy for various security methods. Based on this analysis, the system chooses the most advanced level of security protection that matches the given service needs while minimizing energy consumption.

The research of Zhang et al. [10] provides a detailed overview of IoT implementation in 6G using AI and introduces the concept of super IoT as a significant component of the future of wireless communication. Leveraging symbiotic radio and satellite-assisted communications, super IoT aims to achieve seamless, efficient connectivity between many IoT devices. Additionally, the study highlights the importance of ML techniques as promising candidates for AI in the context of 6G IoT. Among the potential AI techniques for deploying IoT in 6G are NLP which is the development of automated intelligent assistants and chatbots is a specific application in the IoT [99], FL which is a Federated Deep Learning Intrusion Detection System that employs the GAN architecture to detect cyber attacks in smart IoT systems [101], and DRL which can be used to optimize the allocation of computing resources in a mobile edge computing (MEC) environment, such as edge computing resources [102, 103].

In [104], an AI-based algorithm named the QoS-based joint energy, and entropy optimization (QJEEO) algorithm is presented to produce energy-efficient communication. To improve the efficiency of multimedia transmission on 6G networks, this algorithm optimizes both energy usage and entropy (information content). The study demonstrates how energy-efficient communication and customer satisfaction may be increased during multimedia transmission in 6G-based networks by utilizing IoT devices and AI approaches such as the QJEEO algorithm and correlation model. The goal is to improve the quality and efficiency of multimedia content distribution, which will lead to higher customer satisfaction and overall network performance. Satellite networks are used to provide flawless coverage and downlink multicast transmissions for IoT devices in remote places. However, the 6G era has stringent service standards for throughput and latency, which causes issues due to transmission latency, route loss, and IoT terminal energy constraints.

The study [105] explored the use of UAVs and satellites to provide edge and cloud computing capabilities to wireless-powered IoT devices. Utilizing THz frequency bands enables swift communication between UAVs and IoT devices. The key consideration of computation offloading is tackled through DL techniques because AI can address dynamics efficiently while avoiding the time-consuming iterations of traditional mathematical methods and has been identified as one of the key technologies for 6G [20, 106, 107]. The LSTM model is employed to predict future harvesting power based on historical data, leveraging its efficiency in sequential variable forecasting [108].

The study by Mahmood et al. [61] highlighted various AI methods and algorithms focused on improving and securing IoT networks and services. At the physical layer in IoT devices, algorithms such as CNN, RNN, deep neural network (DNN), and expectation maximization are utilized for tasks such as modulation recognition, channel estimation, and signal detection. These AI-driven technologies contribute to increased efficiency in terms of their energy, level of security, and overall effectiveness and dependability of IoT-enabled THz communication networks. ML techniques such as DNN, k-means clustering, Q-learning, and DRL are applied at the MAC layer in IoT-based communication for tasks such as channel allocation, power management, and beamforming design. In the 6G future, AI-powered beamforming and power management systems can increase the performance in terms of energy and reliability of IoT devices and networks. For the network layer, ML techniques such as k-means clustering, DNN, DRL, and Q-learning can be utilized to develop strategies for smart mobility management, traffic clustering, user association, and routing in IoT networks. These AI techniques help in the efficiency of IoT network operations and the enhancement of user experience in the 6G IoT ecosystem. In the transport layer, techniques such as DNN, KNN, Bayesian network, DRL, k-means clustering, and Q-learning for tasks such as traffic caching, prediction, and computational offloading can be applied in 6G IoT networks. AI algorithms such as CNN, SVM, LSTM, and DL can be utilized in IoT devices to discover attack trends and design preventive schemes. Their study concluded that AI/ML algorithms can be applied in different layers of THz communication networks to optimize various tasks and operations, ensuring high QoE and QoS for future wireless network applications in 6G IoT.

In the research of Janbi et al. [109], AI-enhanced IoT in 6G is achieved through the concept of distributed artificial intelligence-as-a-service (DAIaaS). It involves the integration of AI capabilities into the Internet of Everything (IoE) environment, which encompasses all interconnected devices and systems. The main idea is to leverage the power of 6G networks, which promise to support ubiquitous AI services and to enable smarter and more efficient decision-making across various applications and scenarios.

Liang et al. [110] explored the potential of integrating blockchain technology in modern supply chain management to enhance communication, particularly in the context of 6G. In addition, they develop a multi-head attention (MHA)-based gate recurrent unit (GRU) for inbound logistics task prediction which demonstrates higher efficiency and accuracy for the series, since it has improved fitting and prediction accuracy compared to other ML methods, aligning with the demands of future wireless applications in 6G-enabled networks.

In [111], Siddiqui et al. introduced a novel 6G intelligent IoT model to process massive data efficiently and optimize communication channels. It also introduced an AI-based 6G air interface architecture to enhance communication processes within the paradigm.

Figure 3.4 illustrates the AIoT applications that can be integrated into 6G technology enabling a highly efficient and intelligent network capable of providing services to billions of devices.

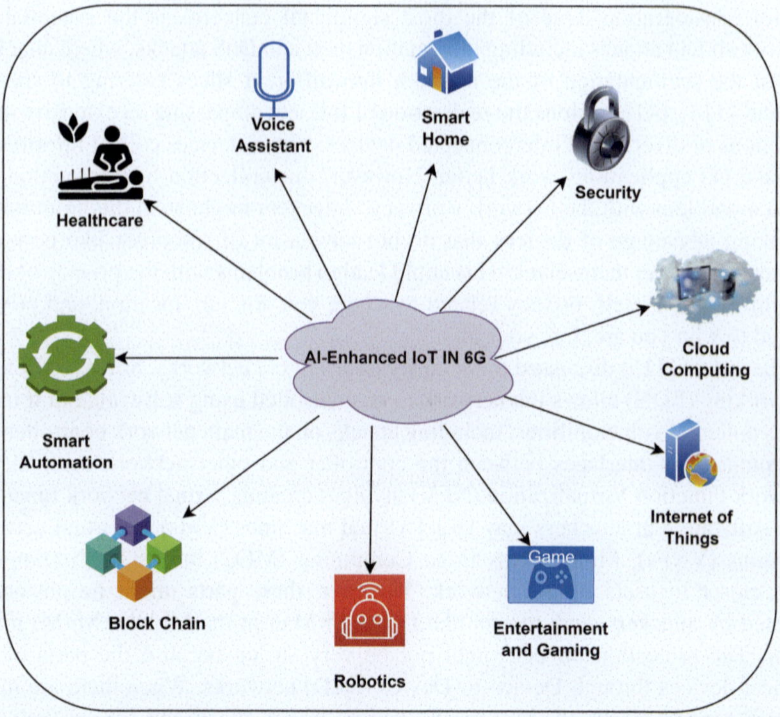

Fig. 3.4 AIoT applications in 6G technology

3.5 Artificial Intelligence-Enabled Security in 6G Communication Systems

Artificial intelligence security, also referred to as AI Security, is an essential and rapidly evolving topic in technology. There are enormous advantages to be achieved by integrating ML approaches into AI-driven security systems in terms of protecting digital information and protecting against multiple risks [112]. In our previous work [113], we proposed a novel machine learning-based intrusion detection solution for Vehicular Ad Hoc Networks (VANETs). We investigated a Random Forest classifier-based framework for detecting application layer Denial of Service (DoS) and Distributed Denial of Service (DDoS) attacks, which are harmful to VANETs. Furthermore, it incorporated the Local Interpretable Model-Agnostic Explanations (LIME) technique for enhanced prediction and model interpretability. The results were impressive, with a 99.84% accuracy rate achieved in intrusion detection, demonstrating the promising potential of this approach to bolster VANET security and prevent intrusion-based threats effectively.

While 6G communication networks offer promising advancements in communication technology, they also present a range of security challenges that require careful consideration. One of the most significant concerns is the potential for network slicing attacks including information theft and DoS attacks, where attackers exploit the segmentation of the network into different slices catering to specific services [114]. 6G envisions the realization of IoE, encompassing an extensive array of billions of diverse and interconnected devices. These devices collect information to make 6G applications work better. However, this collection of information can cause a problem with the network's privacy. Attackers might steal this information by taking advantage of devices that do not have a lot of resources like power or memory to protect themselves. This could lead to problems with the privacy of data, i.e., information itself, privacy related to where you are, i.e., location, and privacy related to who you are, i.e., your identity.

The article [115] discussed the security issues in 6G networks. Software Defined Networking (SDN) allows the network to be controlled using software, but it introduces potential vulnerabilities, including attacks on the main network controller and communication interfaces between the controller and other network components. Network Function Virtualization (NFV) involves creating virtual network functions with software, but attackers may target virtual machines (VMs) or virtual network functions (VNFs). Multi-access Edge Computing (MEC) brings small computer parts closer to users of the network. However, these parts might be physically targeted by attackers, and attacks like DDoS or Man-in-the-Middle (MitM) might occur. The protection on 6G might not be very strong because the parts of 6G connect devices through Device-to-Device (D2D) networks. When there are many devices connected closely in a mesh, devices might attack and spread their bad actions more easily. This makes the whole network more at risk. The big area of the Internet cannot protect each small network inside it very well because there are so many devices in those small networks. This makes it challenging to keep the network safe [116]. Another challenge in 6G networks occurs when attackers target molecular communication security by dropping the transmitted data or altering the information between sender and receiver such as Bio Denial-of-Service (Bio-DoS attacks) [117].

Security and privacy are interconnected concepts. Security pertains to safeguarding the integrity of data, whereas privacy focuses on concealing the identities related to that information. In the realm of 6G networks, the landscape of security and privacy is evolving rapidly. With the emergence of SDN and NVF safeguarding, these advanced networks demand innovative strategies. One promising solution is the integration of AI, specifically ML techniques to bolster defense mechanisms. The concept of multilayered intrusion detection and prevention, powered by DRL and DNN, effectively encounters a range of attacks including IP spoofing, DDoS, and host location hijacking. By leveraging the capabilities of AI in 6G, these techniques play a vital role in combating intricate threats to the network [118]. ML also finds its role in addressing the challenge of DDoS attacks. Approaches like Decision Trees and Random Forest enable rapid detection and precise identification of DDoS attacks [119].

6G requires a huge amount of user data from lots of devices, but there is a problem with privacy. People do not know how their data is being handled outside the systems. For example, smart systems that use unique features like faces or fingerprints might need to know private things about you. Also, small devices like sensors that share personal data with the AI cloud can be targeted by attackers. To fix these issues, there are several AI techniques used to resolve these challenges in 6G networks including edge-based federated learning that preserves data privacy by imposing physical control to maintain data closer to the user [120]. Another way to perform mathematical operations without unlocking your data is homomorphic encryption (HE) [121], and differential privacy can help protect private information when using super-fast 6G networks that keep the network safe from being stolen and misused.

AI has been recognized as a game-changing method for the development of 6G systems, due to its capacity to accommodate increasingly complex and diversified demands while simultaneously strengthening security measures [122]. It can provide a powerful response for solving security concerns by continuously analyzing network traffic patterns and user behavior in real-time enabling advanced threat detection and prevention. It can detect anomalies and potential cyber threats using ML algorithms, enabling network operators with quick and proactive solutions to limit risks.

Some significant security challenges associated with 6G networks revolve around the human-centric nature of 6G applications emphasizing the significance of security and privacy; therefore, they should be given top priority [50]. Hence, AI will be a vital part of ensuring that user data is authenticated and secured. Additionally, the wireless interface is more prone to security threats such as eavesdropping, and the success of integrating AI in future wireless networks like 6G will be highly reliant upon the security provided [123]. Furthermore, to address these challenges, 6G networks would require more advanced security methods, intelligent threat detection technologies, and AI would be essential in developing such techniques which would automatically detect security anomalies, potential threats, and be more advanced than cryptographic techniques [115].

In tandem with AI, the intelligent 6G network will enable virtual personalized mobile communication. Henceforth, the network will transform from the centralized type to the 3-centralized making it user, data, and fully-content centralized. Due to 6G's de-cellular and user-centric ultra-dense network (UUDN) architecture, interference becomes a main cause of concern, and AI will play a key role in addressing this problem [124].

Along with AI and quantum computing, blockchain and FL will also play an important part in securing the 6G networks. As AI evolves and integrates with 6G networks, it will reinforce the foundation for a future communication environment that is extremely safe, trustworthy, and robust. In the subsequent discussion, we provide a thorough overview of the implementation of AI-based security in 6G networks.

To make communication secure and maintain its privacy and confidentiality, Hakeem et al. [114] proposed a 6G security architecture. As the previous legacy networks such as 2G, 3G, 4G, and 5G have several security advancements over time, the technology is evolving rapidly and the evolving 6G technology may have new security issues and challenges that need to be addressed. The article offers security requirements of various 6G applications including autonomous vehicles, massive IoT, AR, VR, and video streaming. They highlight several security issues including data processing, traffic analysis, threat detection, and data encryption due to massive traffic processing in 6G. To address these challenges, they suggested decentralized security systems that enable localized, dynamic traffic management, which lessens the burden on centralized security infrastructure and enhances reaction to security threats. Furthermore, the study also explores the AI/ML layers and examines the proposed security solution for each layer.

In [125], the privacy, anonymity, data protection, and safeguarding of 6G networks by integrating AI techniques are discussed. In addition to outlining their vision for 6G security and security key performance indicators (KPIs) such as AI robustness, protection level, cost to deploy security functions coverage of security functions, and autonomicity level, the authors also describe a hypothetical attack scenario with reference to the predicted 6g network architecture. They also discuss the privacy and security concerns raised by the 6G specifications and potential 6G uses. They explained the security considerations of 6G technologies including distributed AI and ML, distributed ledger technology (DLT), visible light communication, THz, and quantum computing.

In [126], Kazmi et al. described the upcoming 6G cellular communication paradigm and its security implications. They described traditional and new innovative security concepts of 6G networks by integrating AI algorithms, quantum computing, and federated learning. FL is a method of ML that allows training models across decentralized devices and nodes to maintain the security and localization of data. Numerous studies believed that creating an AI framework through an ML data-driven approach would make it difficult for data processing of centralized systems.

In [127], Liu et al. proposed that FL would be an efficient solution to this problem due to its distributed and privacy-preserving nature, enabling popular AI adoption in 6G networks. 6G networks aim to push the boundaries of performance in diverse aspects in reference to the capabilities of the previous generation of wireless communication. AI-enabled 6G networks will make tremendous improvements in cellular technology.

In this regard, Gui et al. [128] discussed the innovations provided by 6G networks as compared to traditional cellular networks based on analysis of related studies in this domain. With the aim of improvements in 6G networks, they provided a detailed discussion on the core services of 6G technologies to enhance the performance of wireless networks, and these services are mobile broad bandwidth and low latency (MBBLL), massive broad bandwidth machine type (mBBMT), massive low latency machine type (mLLMT), and 6G-Lite. To support secure 6G services in this review, the KPI includes spectrum efficiency, capacity, intelligence, security, connectivity, latency, and data rate. Orchestration is an essential component of network and service provisioning in the context of present-day complex systems such as cloud computing, virtualized infrastructure, and SDN.

The research conducted by Siriwardhana et al. [115] focused on the role of AI in the orchestration and management of wireless networks in the context of 6G. They explained the role of AI in securing 6G network infrastructure. The paper presented a survey on challenges faced for data privacy protection and implementation of automated machine ethics in AI-enabled 6G network architecture. Blockchain is a decentralized distributed ledger technology that works on the principle of distributed data storage. It enables point-to-point transmission, encryption algorithms, and several other communication technologies. It plays a significant role in enhancing various aspects of 6G networks in terms of security, privacy, confidentiality, integrity, and network management. Integration of blockchain in 6G network can bring numerous benefits and novel applications to the security paradigm.

AI application on blockchain-based data security scheme for 6G network has been proposed by Li et al. [106]. This survey introduced 6G network architecture with integration of air, space, ground, and underwater network connectivity. They also discussed AI applications within the 6G network including indoor positioning and autonomous vehicles. With the integration of blockchain technology in 6G network, they demonstrate that data privacy and safety can be enhanced in the context of intelligent services such as indoor navigation which evaluate and optimize the quality of wireless network services. In addition to this, the author addresses several unresolved issues related to data security in forthcoming 6G networks in the article's conclusion. These concerns center on locating potential weaknesses, reducing security threats, and investigating innovative techniques to improve data protection and privacy.

3.6 Artificial Intelligence-Enabled 6G in Healthcare

The outbreak of the COVID-19 pandemic highlighted the global healthcare system's vulnerabilities. The hospitals did not have enough supplies for a large number of patients during the pandemic, and many individuals around the world were unable to receive the necessary medical care because they did not have access to critical medical care once the pandemic was declared. The pandemic raised awareness about the benefits of telemedicine, which includes receiving medical care via technology rather than visiting a hospital. This also reduces the chance of viral spread because people do not have to go to the hospital to see a doctor or receive specialist treatment. Our study believes that AI-enabled 6G technology can significantly contribute to the healthcare industry. Incorporating AI systems with 6G technology in the healthcare sector can undoubtedly bring enormous benefits when it comes to remote patient monitoring, virtual consultations, and AI-driven diagnosis. Especially in situations where real-time diagnosis and treatment are crucial, even a little mistake or delay can cause profound consequences for patients. 6G networks provide high accuracy and reliability and will enable convenient remote surgical procedures [129].

3.6.1 Advancements in Telemedicine and Digital Healthcare

In [130], Srinivasu et al. introduced a reference layered communication framework that will leverage the current communication network trends. 6G networks deployed with AI in virtual healthcare systems can help manage remote surgeries with ultra-low latency. The 6G-based intelligent networks assist and monitor patients with treatments at a time. The technology used in the healthcare sector must assist individuals with intelligent diagnosis, patient-centric treatment, and a range of other healthcare services both in the hospital and remotely, and AI-enabled 6G networks rely heavily on Intelligence IoT to store and process data more efficiently by offering ultra- low latency, high bandwidth, improvised QoS [131]. Their framework comprises of several layers that provide services like ultra-massive machine-type communications (umMTC) [132], extremely reliable and low latency communication (ERLLC) [133], and long-distance and high mobility communications (LDHMC) [134] with 6G features including high data rate, extremely high reliability, large scale antenna, AI, energy efficient, ultra-low latency, and massive connectivity.

In the new era of smart healthcare, sensors are either outwardly or inwardly connected to our bodies. This method employs smart gadgets like smartphones, wireless glucometers, and smartwatches as well as networks like body area networks. These devices collect health data from a variety of sources, including sensors, body implants, and medical systems [135]. Smart healthcare provides correct information and answers to doctors, nurses, family members, and patients. This decreases medical errors and lowers healthcare costs. With multiple healthcare devices connected and collecting various data, this vast amount of health information can improve well-being, aid in future illness management, and allow for early diagnosis of health problems. To properly handle these devices, hospitals require advanced communication networks capable of handling enormous amounts of data with minor delays. 6G-powered IoT networks will provide advanced capabilities for smart healthcare soon, including low latency, high data rates, high reliability, density, and energy efficiency.

A case study of remote robotic surgery on how 6G would enable wireless features in the healthcare sector in the future has been carried out in [130]. Doctors from different hospitals would be able to perform remote robotic surgeries. The cellular tower would directly interact with satellites and satellites will communicate; in this way, hospitals will be connected to this cellular tower to exchange data over a 6G framework.

The article [136] presented the approach toward 6G-enabled smart healthcare systems. They focused on three domains 6G, security, and smart health. They described various use cases for intelligent healthcare services enabled by 6G which could provide accurate and fast disease diagnoses. AR, holographic, and haptic methods can help evaluate a patient's internal organs in high resolution without intrusive painful procedures. Another discussed use case is interaction with disabled persons; to improve the quality of life of disabled individuals, the technology of AI and 6G helps in converting emotions, perceptions, and thoughts to physical orders by digitizing all five senses, haptic communication, and brain-computer interface (BCI), which expand prospects to communicate with impaired individuals. Real-time health pro-visioning has revolutionized the healthcare industry by enabling faster and more accurate diagnosis, treatment and monitoring, using exceptionally reliable networks on-body sensors, nanodevices, and implants, which may gather and transmit psychological and textual information in real-time by interacting with intra-body actuators like insulin pumps and cardioverters.

Some of the key applications used in healthcare are AR, VR, and Holographic communications. In [21], Khattak et al. presented a survey on 6G and AI applications in the healthcare sector, where 6G is offering 3D services with the help of holographic communication which will change the landscape of smart healthcare systems. Smart healthcare systems use transmission enabled with high-resolution multimedia, i.e., audio and video. They present a comprehensive survey on how AR and VR facilitate a view of a patient's internal anatomy helping doctors to precisely adjust specific areas of a patient's body and expand and enhance visibility with valuable insights during medical procedures that involve a critical degree of risk.

Another paper [137] presented a review on Holograms; the 3D image processing technology provides realistic images of objects allowing surgeons to interact with patients in a virtual environment. Similarly, AR and VR contribute to healthcare by increasing speed and reliability with secure wireless communication.

3.6.2 Challenges of AI-Enabled 6G Networks for Healthcare

The use of AI-enabled 6G technology in healthcare has great potential, but it also comes with numerous challenges that require careful consideration. As the number of connected healthcare devices and applications proliferates, generating vast and diverse data streams, the establishment of a robust communication network infrastructure becomes imperative. Overcoming challenges encompasses reliable and scalable connectivity for varied data sizes, timely health data exchange, and support for advanced applications like remote surgeries. Privacy concerns arise with the application of blockchain in healthcare, while the expanding attack surface in 6G networks raises security risks. The integration of AI and machine learning techniques offers immense potential, yet implementation complexities persist. Amid these challenges, evaluating user satisfaction and managing QoE remain pivotal aspects in the AI-enabled 6G healthcare landscape. The 6G network has some limitations like privacy and security factors, the cost of maintaining the network, and the health impact of 6G technology on humans. It has some network bandwidth issues as it requires a wider bandwidth to offer diverse services. With the advancement of technology in the context of 6G network systems, complexity and security issues have arisen, such as securing billions of smart health devices [114]. Security via cryptography techniques plays a critical role in ensuring the confidentiality, integrity, and privacy of sensitive health-related data in various digital healthcare systems and applications. The number of connected healthcare devices and applications is expected to generate huge amounts of data in varying sizes and formats. Consequently, the substantial volume of health-related data has the potential to significantly enhance human well-being and facilitate early-stage diagnostics. To effectively cater to the diverse range of healthcare devices and sensor-driven applications, the establishment of a robust and scalable communication network infrastructure becomes an absolute necessity. The challenges in supporting an increased number of interconnected healthcare devices and managing their data include ensuring reliable and scalable connectivity for the variable data generated by these devices. It also involves facilitating timely and accurate exchange of health-related data. Furthermore, enabling advanced healthcare applications such as remote surgeries and real-time diagnostics, which demand ultra-low latency and high reliability, remains crucial. Initially, 5G networks provided latency of 1–5 milliseconds, a figure further reduced to less than 1 millisecond with the emergence of 6G networks [138]. 6G technology is expected to address these challenges by offering attributes such as high throughput greater than 100 Gbps, ultra-low latency of less than 1 ms, exceptional reliability of 9 s, and spectral efficiency of 100 bps/Hz which are vital for enabling seamless and efficient communication in healthcare industry [139].

E-Health, facilitated by digital and communication technologies [140], has simplified healthcare services, providing direct patient access, remote medical advice, easy access to medical records, appointment booking, and automated reminders. While blockchain offers a distributed ledger system, it may not be suitable for storing sensitive healthcare data due to transparency [141]. 6G communication technology, especially with edge technology, can enhance privacy and security [142]. However, portable cryptographic systems increase security risks. Leveraging AI and machine learning in 6G networks can improve service quality but present implementation challenges [21]. In addition, managing QoE in 6G-powered healthcare involves addressing user satisfaction, energy efficiency, interference, and AI/ML deployment.

3.7 Conclusion

The chapter highlighted that the potential AI can bring to the upcoming 6G wireless networks. Through a comprehensive comparison of 4G and 5G with 6G, we have emphasized the role of AI in elevating 6G networks to unprecedented levels of efficiency, reliability, and intelligence. The techniques of AI that can be integrated into the 6G network architecture to make it work intelligently, connect the world, facilitate connectivity, and fulfill the growing network demands of society are also discussed in this overview. Furthermore, in this chapter, we discussed AI-enhanced IoT in 6G and the security techniques used in AI-enabled 6G networks. Finally, we examined different ways in which AI-powered 6G networks can be used in healthcare.

References

1. Sharma, P. (2013). Evolution of mobile wireless communication networks-1G to 5G as well as future prospective of next generation communication network. *International Journal of Computer Science and Mobile Computing, 2*(8), 47–53.
2. Bhandari, N., Devra, S., & Singh, K. (2017). Evolution of cellular network: From 1G to 5G. *International Journal of Engineering and Techniques, 3*(5), 98–105.
3. Baldomero Coll-Perales, B., Gozalvez, J., & Maestre, J. L. (2019). 5G and beyond: Smart devices as part of the network fabric. *IEEE Network, 33*(4), 170–177.
4. Jokela, T., Koivumaa, J., Pirkola, J., Salminen, P., & Kantola, N. (2006). Methods for quantitative usability requirements: A case study on the development of the user interface of a mobile phone. *Personal and Ubiquitous Computing, 10*, 345–355.
5. Mshvidobadze, T. (2012). Evolution mobile wireless communication and lte networks. In *2012 6th International Conference on Application of Information and Communication Technologies (AICT)* (pp. 1–7). IEEE.
6. Viswanathan, H., & Weldon, M. (2014). The past, present, and future of mobile communications. *Bell Labs Technical Journal, 19*, 8–21.
7. De Alwis, C., Kalla, A., Pham, Q. V., Kumar, P., Dev, K., Hwang, W. J., & Liyanage, M. (2021). Survey on 6G frontiers: Trends, applications, requirements, technologies and future research. *IEEE Open Journal of the Communications Society, 2*, 836–886.
8. Chavhan, S., et al. (2022). Shift to 6G: Exploration on trends, vision, requirements, technologies, research, and standardization efforts. *Sustainable Energy Technologies and Assessments, 54*, 102666.
9. David, K., & Berndt, H. (2018). 6G vision and requirements: Is there any need for beyond 5G? *IEEE Vehicular Technology Magazine, 13*(3), 72–80.
10. Zhang, L., Liang, Y. C., & Niyato, D. (2019). 6G visions: Mobile ultra-broadband, super internet-of- things, and artificial intelligence. *China Communications, 16*(8), 1–14.
11. Saad, W., Bennis, M., & Chen, M. (2019). A vision of 6G wireless systems: Applications, trends, technologies, and open research problems. *IEEE Network, 34*(3), 134–142.
12. Mahmoud, H. H. H., Amer, A. A., & Ismail, T. (2021). 6G: A comprehensive survey on technologies, applications, challenges, and research problems. *Transactions on Emerging Telecommunications Technologies, 32*(4), e4233.
13. Hakeem, S. A. A., Hussein, H. H., & Kim, H. (2022). Vision and research directions of 6G technologies and applications. *Journal of King Saud University-Computer and Information Sciences, 34*(6), 2419–2442.
14. Kamruzzaman, M. (2022). Key technologies, applications and trends of Internet of Things for energy- efficient 6G wireless communication in smart cities. *Energies, 15*(15), 5608.
15. Tang, F., Chen, X., Zhao, M., & Kato, N. (2022). The roadmap of communication and networking in 6G for the metaverse. *IEEE Wireless Communications*, 1–10.
16. Song, W., Rajak, S., Dang, S., Liu, R., Li, J., Chinnadurai, S.: Deep learning enabled irs for 6G intelligent transportation systems: A comprehensive study. IEEE Transactions on Intelligent Transportation Systems (2022), 24(11), 12973–12990.
17. Maddikunta, P. K. R., Pham, Q. V., Prabadevi, B., Deepa, N., Dev, K., Gadekallu, T. R., Ruby, R., & Liyanage, M. (2022). Industry 5.0: A survey on enabling technologies and potential applications. *Journal of Industrial Information Integration, 26*, 100257.
18. Kharche, S., & Kharche, J. (2023). 6G intelligent healthcare framework: A review on role of technologies, challenges and future directions. *Journal of Mobile Multimedia, 19*(3), 603–644.
19. Ahammed, T. B., Patgiri, R., & Nayak, S. (2023). A vision on the artificial intelligence for 6G communication. *ICT Express, 9*(2), 197–210.
20. Letaief, K. B., Chen, W., Shi, Y., Zhang, J., & Zhang, Y. J. A. (2019). The roadmap to 6G: AI empowered wireless networks. *IEEE Communications Magazine, 57*(8), 84–90.

21. Khattak, S. B. A., Nasralla, M. M., & Rehman, I. U. (2022). The role of 6G networks in enabling future smart health services and applications. In *2022 IEEE International Smart Cities Conference (ISC2)* (pp. 1–7). IEEE.
22. Abioye, A., Joseph, M., & Ferreira, H. C. (2015). Comparative study of 3G and 4GLTE network. *Journal of Advances in Computer Networks, 3*(3), 247–250.
23. Series, M. (2003). *Framework and overall objectives of the future development of imt-2000 and systems beyond imt-2000*. Rec. ITU-R, M. 1645.
24. Barb, G., & Otesteanu, M. (2020). 4G/5G: A comparative study and overview on what to expect from 5G. In *2020 43rd International Conference on Telecommunications and Signal Processing (TSP)* (pp. 37–40). IEEE.
25. Mishra, L., Vikash, V., & S. (2021). Seamless health monitoring using 5G NR for internet of medical things. *Wireless Personal Communications, 120*(3), 2259–2289.
26. Gopal, B., & Kuppusamy, P. (2015). A comparative study on 4G and 5G technology for wireless applications. *IOSR Journal of Electronics and Communication Engineering, 10*(6), 2278–2834.
27. 3rd Generation Partnership Project (3GPP). (2010). *Technical Specification 32.450 v9.1.0, KPIs for E-UTRAN (Release 9)*. Technical Specification 32.450, 3GPP.
28. Hossain, S. (2013). 5G wireless communication systems. *American Journal of Engineering Research (AJER), 02*, 344–353.
29. Attaran, M. (2023). The impact of 5G on the evolution of intelligent automation and industry digitization. *Journal of Ambient Intelligence and Humanized Computing, 14*, 5977–5993. https://doi.org/10.1007/s12652-020-02521-x
30. Dilli, R. (2020). Analysis of 5G wireless systems in fr1 and fr2 frequency bands. In *2020 2nd International Conference on Innovative Mechanisms for Industry Applications (ICIMIA)* (pp. 767–772). IEEE.
31. Lopez, A. V., Chervyakov, A., Chance, G., Verma, S., & Tang, Y. (2019). Opportunities and challenges of mmWave NR. *IEEE Wireless Communications, 26*(2), 4–6.
32. Attaran, M. (2021). The impact of 5G on the evolution of intelligent automation and industry digitization. *Journal of Ambient Intelligence and Humanized Computing*, 1–17.
33. Al-Falahy, N., & Alani, O. Y. (2017). Technologies for 5G networks: Challenges and opportunities. *IT Professional, 19*(1), 12–20.
34. Minopoulos, G., Kokkonis, G., Psannis, K. E., & Ishibashi, Y. (2019). A survey on haptic data over 5G networks. *IJFGCN, 12*(2), 37–54.
35. Rao, S. K., & Prasad, R. (2018). Impact of 5G technologies on industry 4.0. Wireless Personal Communications, *100*, 145–159.
36. Chen, K. C., Zhang, T., Gitlin, R. D., & Fettweis, G. (2018). Ultra-low latency mobile networking. *IEEE Network, 33*(2), 181–187.
37. Pokhrel, S. R., Ding, J., Park, J., Park, O. S., & Choi, J. (2020). Towards enabling critical mMTC: A review of URLLC within mMTC. *IEEE Access, 8*, 131796–131813.
38. Abdullah, D. M., & Ameen, S. Y. (2021). Enhanced mobile broadband (eMBB): A review. *Journal of Information Technology and Informatics, 1*(1), 13–19.
39. Li, S., Da Xu, L., & Zhao, S. (2018). 5G Internet of Things: A survey. *Journal of Industrial Information Integration, 10*, 1–9.
40. Ramadan, E., Narayanan, A., Dayalan, U. K., Fezeu, R. A., Qian, F., & Zhang, Z. L. (2021). Case for 5G-aware video streaming applications. In *Proceedings of the 1st Workshop on 5G Measurements, Modeling, and Use Cases* (pp. 27–34).
41. Hakak, S., Gadekallu, T. R., Maddikunta, P. K. R., Ramu, S. P., Parimala, M., De Alwis, C., & Liyanage, M. (2022). Autonomous vehicles in 5G and beyond: A survey. *Vehicular Communications, 39*, 100551.
42. Sukhmani, S., Sadeghi, M., Erol-Kantarci, M., & El Saddik, A. (2018). Edge caching and computing in 5G for mobile AR/VR and tactile internet. *IEEE Multimedia, 26*(1), 21–30.
43. 3rd Generation Partnership Project (3GPP). (2018). *System architecture for the 5G system*. Technical Specification TS 23.501, 3GPP.

44. Liu, G., Huang, Y., Li, N., Dong, J., Jin, J., Wang, Q., & Li, N. (2020). Vision, requirements and network architecture of 6G mobile network beyond 2030. *China Communications, 17*(9), 92–104.
45. Andreou, A., Mavromoustakis, C. X., Batalla, J. M., Markakis, E. K., & Mastorakis, G. (2023). UAV-assisted RSUs for V2x connectivity using Voronoi diagrams in 6G+ infrastructures. *IEEE Transactions on Intelligent Transportation Systems, 24*, 15855–15865.
46. Lovén, L., Leppänen, T., Peltonen, E., Partala, J., Harjula, E., Porambage, P., Ylianttila, M., & Riekki, J.: (2019). Edgeai: A vision for distributed, edge-native artificial intelligence in future 6G networks. In *6G Wireless Summit, March 24-–26, 2019 Levi, Finland*
47. Sarkar, P., & Saha, A. (2023). Evolution of 6G and terahertz communication. In *Optical to Terahertz Engineering* (pp. 45–58). Springer.
48. Khiadani, N. (2020). Vision, requirements and challenges of sixth generation (6G) networks. In *2020 6th Iranian Conference on Signal Processing and Intelligent Systems (ICSPIS)* (pp. 1–4). IEEE.
49. Bhat, J. R., & Alqahtani, S. A. (2021). 6G ecosystem: Current status and future perspective. *IEEE Access, 9*, 43134–43167. https://doi.org/10.1109/ACCESS.2021.3054833
50. Chowdhury, M. Z., Shahjalal, M., Ahmed, S., & Jang, Y. M. (2020). 6G wireless communication systems: Applications, requirements, technologies, challenges, and research directions. *IEEE Open Journal of the Communications Society, 1*, 957–975.
51. Yang, H., Alphones, A., Xiong, Z., Niyato, D., Zhao, J., & Wu, K. (2020). Artificial-intelligence-enabled intelligent 6G networks. *IEEE Network, 34*(6), 272–280.
52. Sheth, K., Patel, K., Shah, H., Tanwar, S., Gupta, R., & Kumar, N. (2020). A taxonomy of AI techniques for 6G communication networks. *Computer Communications, 161*, 279–303.
53. Kaur, J., Khan, M. A., Iftikhar, M., Imran, M., & Haq, Q. E. U. (2021). Machine learning techniques for 5G and beyond. *IEEE Access, 9*, 23472–23488.
54. Rekkas, V. P., Sotiroudis, S., Sarigiannidis, P., Wan, S., Karagiannidis, G. K., & Goudos, S. K. (2021). Machine learning in beyond 5G/6G networks – State-of-the-art and future trends. *Electronics, 10*(22), 2786.
55. Hochreiter, S., & Schmidhuber, J. (1997). Long short-term memory. *Neural Computation, 9*(8), 1735–1780.
56. Tang, F., Kawamoto, Y., Kato, N., & Liu, J. (2019). Future intelligent and secure vehicular network toward 6G: Machine-learning approaches. *Proceedings of the IEEE, 108*(2), 292–307.
57. Alpaydin, E. (2020). *Introduction to machine learning*. MIT Press.
58. Chen, M., Challita, U., Saad, W., Yin, C., & Debbah, M. (2019). Artificial neural networks-based machine learning for wireless networks: A tutorial. *IEEE Communications Surveys & Tutorials, 21*(4), 3039–3071.
59. Bhavsar, H., & Ganatra, A. (2012). A comparative study of training algorithms for supervised machine learning. *International Journal of Soft Computing and Engineering (IJSCE), 2*(4), 2231–2307.
60. Ahmad, A., Mansoor, A. B., Barakabitze, A. A., Hines, A., Atzori, L., & Walshe, R. (2021). Supervised-learning-based QoE prediction of video streaming in future networks: A tutorial with comparative study. *IEEE Communications Magazine, 59*(11), 88–94.
61. Mahmood, M. R., Matin, M. A., Sarigiannidis, P., & Goudos, S. K. (2022). A comprehensive review on artificial intelligence/machine learning algorithms for empowering the future IoT toward 6G era. *IEEE Access, 10*, 87535–87562.
62. Daba, J., & Abdul-Latif, O. M. (2020). Supervised machine learning classifiers for diversity combined signals in 6G massive mimo receivers. *Universal Journal of Electrical and Electronic Engineering, 7*(6), 320–327.
63. Morocho-Cayamcela, M. E., Lee, H., & Lim, W. (2019). Machine learning for 5G/B5G mobile and wireless communications: Potential, limitations, and future directions. *IEEE Access, 7*, 137184–137206.
64. Rekkas, V. P., Sotiroudis, S., Sarigiannidis, P., Karagiannidis, G. K., & Goudos, S. K. (2021). Unsupervised machine learning in 6G networks-state-of-the-art and future trends. In *2021*

10th International Conference on Modern Circuits and Systems Technologies (MOCAST) (pp. 1–4). IEEE.

65. Hashmi, U. S., Darbandi, A., & Imran, A. (2017). Enabling proactive self-healing by data mining network failure logs. In *2017 International Conference on Computing, Networking and Communications (ICNC)* (pp. 511–517). IEEE.
66. Mohamed, A., Ruan, H., Abdelwahab, M. H. H., Dorneanu, B., Xiao, P., Arellano-Garcia, H., Gao, Y., & Tafazolli, R. (2020). An inter-disciplinary modelling approach in industrial 5G/6G and machine learning era. In *2020 IEEE International Conference on Communications Workshops (ICC Workshops)* (pp. 1–6). IEEE.
67. Nawaz, S. J., Sharma, S. K., Wyne, S., Patwary, M. N., & Asaduzzaman, M. (2019). Quantum machine learning for 6G communication networks: State-of-the-art and vision for the future. *IEEE Access, 7*, 46317–46350.
68. Mollel, M. S., Abubakar, A. I., Ozturk, M., Kaijage, S. F., Kisangiri, M., Hussain, S., Imran, M. A., & Abbasi, Q. H. (2021). A survey of machine learning applications to handover management in 5G and beyond. *IEEE Access, 9*, 45770–45802.
69. Zhang, P., Wu, M., & Zhu, X. (2021). Research on network fault detection and diagnosis based on deep Q learning. In *Wireless and Satellite Systems: 11th EAI International Conference, WiSATS 2020, Nanjing, China, September 17–18, 2020, Proceedings, Part II* (pp. 533–545). Springer.
70. Sliwa, B., & Wietfeld, C. (2020). A reinforcement learning approach for efficient opportunistic vehicle- to-cloud data transfer. In *2020 IEEE Wireless Communications and Networking Conference (WCNC)* (pp. 1–8). IEEE.
71. Su, Y., Lu, X., Zhao, Y., Huang, L., & Du, X. (2019). Cooperative communications with relay selection based on deep reinforcement learning in wireless sensor networks. *IEEE Sensors Journal, 19*(20), 9561–9569.
72. Aslam, A. B., Syed, Z. S., Khan, M. F., Baloch, A., & Syed, M. S. S. (2023). Leveraging natural language processing for public health screening on youtube: A covid-19 case study. arXiv preprint arXiv:2306.01164.
73. Tariq, N., Syed, Z. S., & Saba, E. (2023). Praise or insult? Identifying cyberbullying using natural language processing. In *2023 7th International Multi-Topic ICT Conference (IMTIC)* (pp. 1–7). IEEE.
74. Sana, M., & Strinati, E. C. (2022). Learning semantics: An opportunity for effective 6G communications. In *2022 IEEE 19th Annual Consumer Communications & Networking Conference (CCNC)* (pp. 631–636). IEEE.
75. Trappey, A. J. C., et al. (2022). Transdisciplinary technology mining of advanced 6G satellite communication innovations. In *Transdisciplinarity and the Future of Engineering* (pp. 566–575). IOS Press.
76. Abdellah, A., & Koucheryavy, A. (2020). Survey on artificial intelligence techniques in 5G networks. *The Journal of Telecommunications and Information Technology SPbSUT Russ, 8*, 1–10.
77. Dai, L., Jiao, R., Adachi, F., Poor, H. V., & Hanzo, L. (2020). Deep learning for wireless communications: An emerging interdisciplinary paradigm. *IEEE Wireless Communications, 27*(4), 133–139.
78. Chen, M. Y., Fan, M. H., & Huang, L. X. (2021). AI-based vehicular network toward 6G and IoT: Deep learning approaches. *ACM Transactions on Management Information System (TMIS), 13*(1), 1–12.
79. Ozpoyraz, B., Dogukan, A. T., Gevez, Y., Altun, U., & Basar, E. (2022). Deep learning-aided 6G wireless networks: A comprehensive survey of revolutionary PHY architectures. *IEEE Open Journal of the Communications Society.*
80. Jagannath, A., Jagannath, J., & Melodia, T. (2021). Redefining wireless communication for 6G: Signal processing meets deep learning with deep unfolding. *IEEE Transactions on Artificial Intelligence, 2*(6), 528–536.
81. Zhang, S., Liu, J., Rodrigues, T. K., & Kato, N. (2021). Deep learning techniques for advancing 6G communications in the physical layer. *IEEE Wireless Communications, 28*(5), 141–147.

82. Kamruzzaman, M., & Alruwaili, O. (2022). AI-based computer vision using deep learning in 6G wireless networks. *Computers and Electrical Engineering, 102*, 108233.
83. 3GPP. (2017). *Study on new radio access technology: Physical layer aspects*. Tech. Rep. TR 38.802.
84. Ahn, Y., Kim, J., Kim, S., Shim, K., Kim, J., Kim, S., & Shim, B. (2022). Towards intelligent millimeter and terahertz communication for 6G: Computer vision-aided beamforming. *IEEE Wireless Communications*.
85. Vaca-Rubio, C. J., Ramirez-Espinosa, P., Kansanen, K., Tan, Z. H., & de Carvalho, E. (2023). Radio sensing with large intelligent surface for 6G. In *ICASSP 2023–2023 IEEE International Conference on Acoustics, Speech and Signal Processing (ICASSP)* (pp. 1–5). IEEE.
86. Jiang, S., & Alkhateeb, A. (2022). Computer vision aided beam tracking in a real-world millimeter wave deployment. In *2022 IEEE Globecom Workshops (GC Workshops)* (pp. 142–147). IEEE.
87. Alkhateeb, A., Charan, G., Osman, T., Hredzak, A., Morais, J., Demirhan, U., & Srinivas, N. (2023). Deepsense 6G: A large-scale real-world multi-modal sensing and communication dataset. *IEEE Communications Magazine*.
88. Charan, G., Alrabeiah, M., & Alkhateeb, A. (2021). Vision-aided dynamic blockage prediction for 6G wireless communication networks. In *2021 IEEE International Conference on Communications Workshops (ICC Workshops)* (pp. 1–6). IEEE.
89. Alrabeiah, M., Hredzak, A., Liu, Z., & Alkhateeb, A. (2020). Viwi: A deep learning dataset framework for vision-aided wireless communications. In *2020 IEEE 91st Vehicular Technology Conference (VTC2020-Spring)* (pp. 1–5). IEEE.
90. McCarthy, J. (2007). What is Artificial Intelligence. Available from http://jmc.stanford.edu/artificial-intelligence/what-is-ai/index.html
91. Li, B., Feng, Y., Xiong, Z., Yang, W., & Liu, G. (2021). Research on AI security enhanced encryption algorithm of autonomous IoT systems. *Information Sciences, 575*, 379–398.
92. Mastorakis, G., Mavromoustakis, C. X., Batalla, J. M., & Pallis, E. (2020). *Convergence of artificial intelligence and the Internet of Things*. Springer.
93. Dang, S., Amin, O., Shihada, B., & Alouini, M. S. (2020). What should 6G be? *Nature Electronics, 3*(1), 20–29.
94. Akyildiz, I. F., Jornet, J. M., & Han, C. (2014). Terahertz band: Next frontier for wireless communications. *Physical Communication, 12*, 16–32.
95. Zhou, Y., Liu, L., Wang, L., Hui, N., Cui, X., Wu, J., Peng, Y., Qi, Y., & Xing, C. (2020). Service-aware 6G: An intelligent and open network based on the convergence of communication, computing and caching. *Digital Communications and Networks, 6*(3), 253–260.
96. Hassan, B., Baig, S., & Asif, M. (2021). Key technologies for ultra-reliable and low-latency communication in 6G. *IEEE Communications Standards Magazine, 5*(2), 106–113.
97. Jameel, F., Sharma, N., Khan, M. A., Khan, I., Alam, M. M., Mastorakis, G., & Mavromoustakis, C. X. (2020). *Machine learning techniques for wireless-powered ambient backscatter communications: Enabling intelligent IoT networks in 6G era* (pp. 187–211). Convergence of artificial intelligence and the Internet of Things.
98. Li, M., Yu, F. R., Si, P., Zhang, Y., & Qian, Y. (2022). Intelligent resource optimization for blockchain-enabled IoT in 6G via collective reinforcement learning. *IEEE Network, 36*(6), 175–182.
99. Ferrag, M. A., Debbah, M., & Al-Hawawreh, M. (2023). Generative ai for cyber threat-hunting in 6G-enabled IoT networks. arXiv preprint arXiv:2303.11751.
100. Mao, B., Kawamoto, Y., & Kato, N. (2020). AI-based joint optimization of QoS and security for 6G energy harvesting Internet of Things. *IEEE Internet of Things Journal, 7*(8), 7032–7042.
101. Tabassum, A., Erbad, A., Lebda, W., Mohamed, A., & Guizani, M. (2022). FEDGAN-IDS: Privacy-reserving ids using GAN and federated learning. *Computer Communications, 192*, 299–310.
102. Sami, H., Otrok, H., Bentahar, J., & Mourad, A. (2021). AI-based resource provisioning of IoE services in 6G: A deep reinforcement learning approach. *IEEE Transactions on Network and Service Management, 18*(3), 3527–3540.

103. Manogaran, G., Mumtaz, S., Mavromoustakis, C. X., Pallis, E., & Mastorakis, G. (2021). Artificial intelligence and blockchain-assisted offloading approach for data availability maximization in edge nodes. *IEEE Transactions on Vehicular Technology, 70*(3), 2404–2412.
104. Sodhro, A. H., Pirbhulal, S., Luo, Z., Muhammad, K., & Zahid, N. Z. (2020). Toward 6G architecture for energy-efficient communication in IoT-enabled smart automation systems. *IEEE Internet of Things Journal, 8*(7), 5141–5148.
105. Mao, B., Tang, F., Kawamoto, Y., & Kato, N. (2021). Optimizing computation offloading in satellite-UAV-served 6G IoT: A deep learning approach. *IEEE Network, 35*(4), 102–108.
106. Li, W., Su, Z., Li, R., Zhang, K., & Wang, Y. (2020). Blockchain-based data security for artificial intelligence applications in 6G networks. *IEEE Network, 34*(6), 31–37.
107. Ali, S., Saad, W., Rajatheva, N., Chang, K., Steinbach, D., Sliwa, B., Wietfeld, C., Mei, K., Shiri, H., Zepernick, H.J., et al. (2020). 6G white paper on machine learning in wireless communication networks. arXiv preprint arXiv:2004.13875.
108. Zhou, Y., Fadlullah, Z. M., Mao, B., & Kato, N. (2018). A deep-learning-based radio resource assignment technique for 5G ultra dense networks. *IEEE Network, 32*(6), 28–34.
109. Janbi, N., Katib, I., Albeshri, A., & Mehmood, R. (2020). Distributed Artificial Intelligence-as-a-Service (DAIaaS) for smarter IoE and 6G environments. *Sensors, 20*(20), 5796.
110. Liang, W., Zhang, L., & Kadoch, M. (2022). 6G IoT tracking-and machine learning-enhanced blockchained supply chain management. *Electronics, 12*(1), 40.
111. Siddiqui, M., Khurshid, K., Rashid, I., & Khan, A. A. (2020). Artificial intelligence based 6G intelligent IoT: Unfolding an analytical concept for future hybrid communication systems. In *Proceedings of 2020 the 10th International Workshop on Computer Science and Engineering (WCSE 2020)* (pp. 122–129).
112. Sandeep, S., Ahamad, S., Saxena, D., Srivastava, K., Jaiswal, S., & Bora, A. (2022). To understand the relationship between machine learning and artificial intelligence in large and diversified business organisations. *Materials Today: Proceedings, 56*, 2082–2086.
113. Hassan, F., Yu, J., Syed, Z. S., Ahmed, N., Al Reshan, M. S., & Shaikh, A. (2023). Achieving model explainability for intrusion detection in vanets with lime. *PeerJ Computer Science, 9*, e1440.
114. Abdel Hakeem, S. A., Hussein, H. H., & Kim, H. (2022). Security requirements and challenges of 6G technologies and applications. *Sensors, 22*(5), 1969.
115. Siriwardhana, Y., Porambage, P., Liyanage, M., & Ylianttila, M. (2021). AI and 6G security: Opportunities and challenges. In *2021 Joint European Conference on Networks and Communications & 6G Summit (EuCNC/6G Summit)* (pp. 616–621). IEEE.
116. Suraci, C., Pizzi, S., Molinaro, A., & Araniti, G. (2021). MEC and D2D as enabling technologies for a secure and lightweight 6G eHealth system. *IEEE Internet of Things Journal, 9*(13), 11524–11532.
117. Shen, Q., Wu, J., Li, J., Zhang, X., & Wang, K. (2021). Communication modeling for targeted delivery under bio-dos attack in 6G molecular networks. In *ICC 2021-IEEE International Conference on Communications* (pp. 1–6). IEEE.
118. Abdulqadder, I. H., Zhou, S., Zou, D., Aziz, I. T., & Akber, S. M. A. (2020). Multi-layered intrusion detection and prevention in the SDN/NFV enabled cloud of 5G networks using AI-based defense mechanisms. *Computer Networks, 179*, 107364.
119. Santos, R., Souza, D., Santo, W., Ribeiro, A., & Moreno, E. (2020). Machine learning algorithms to detect DDoS attacks in SDN. *Concurrency and Computation: Practice and Experience, 32*(16), e5402.
120. Nguyen, D. C., Ding, M., Pham, Q. V., Pathirana, P. N., Le, L. B., Seneviratne, A., Li, J., Niyato, D., & Poor, H. V. (2021). Federated learning meets blockchain in edge computing: Opportunities and challenges. *IEEE Internet of Things Journal, 8*(16), 12806–12825.
121. Bandi, A., & Yalamarthi, S. (2022). Towards artificial intelligence empowered security and privacy issues in 6G communications. In *2022 International Conference on Sustainable Computing and Data Communication Systems (ICSCDS)* (pp. 372–378). IEEE.
122. Kato, N., Mao, B., Tang, F., Kawamoto, Y., & Liu, J. (2020). Ten challenges in advancing machine learning technologies toward 6G. *IEEE Wireless Communications, 27*(3), 96–103.

123. Challita, U., Ryden, H., & Tullberg, H. (2020). When machine learning meets wireless cellular networks: Deployment, challenges, and applications. *IEEE Communications Magazine, 58*(6), 12–18.
124. Chen, S., Liang, Y. C., Sun, S., Kang, S., Cheng, W., & Peng, M. (2020). Vision, requirements, and technology trend of 6G: How to tackle the challenges of system coverage, capacity, user data-rate and movement speed. *IEEE Wireless Communications, 27*(2), 218–228.
125. Porambage, P., Gür, G., Osorio, D. P. M., Liyanage, M., Gurtov, A., & Ylianttila, M. (2021). The roadmap to 6G security and privacy. *IEEE Open Journal of the Communications Society, 2*, 1094–1122.
126. Kazmi, S. H. A., Hassan, R., Qamar, F., Nisar, K., & Ibrahim, A. A. A. (2023). Security concepts in emerging 6G communication: Threats, countermeasures, authentication techniques and research directions. *Symmetry, 15*(6), 1147.
127. Liu, Y., Yuan, X., Xiong, Z., Kang, J., Wang, X., & Niyato, D. (2020). Federated learning for 6G communications: Challenges, methods, and future directions. *China Communications, 17*(9), 105–118.
128. Gui, G., Liu, M., Tang, F., Kato, N., & Adachi, F. (2020). 6G: Opening new horizons for integration of comfort, security, and intelligence. *IEEE Wireless Communications, 27*(5), 126–132.
129. Nova, S. N., Rahman, M. S., & Chakraborty, C. (2021). Patients' health surveillance model using IoT and 6G technology. In *Green Technological Innovation for Sustainable Smart Societies: Post Pandemic Era* (pp. 191–209). Springer.
130. Srinivasu, P. N., Ijaz, M. F., Shafi, J., Woźniak, M., & Sujatha, R. (2022). 6G driven fast computational networking framework for healthcare applications. *IEEE Access, 10*, 94235–94248.
131. Jameel, F., Javaid, U., Sikdar, B., Khan, I., Mastorakis, G., & Mavromoustakis, C. X. (2020). *Optimizing blockchain networks with artificial intelligence: Towards efficient and reliable IoT applications* (pp. 299–321). Convergence of artificial intelligence and the Internet of Things.
132. Kharel, B., López, O. L. A., Alves, H., & Latva-Aho, M. (2021). Ultra-reliable communication for critical machine type communication via cran-enabled multi-connectivity diversity schemes. *Sensors, 21*(23), 8064.
133. Mumtaz, S., Menon, V. G., & Ashraf, M. I. (2021). Guest editorial: Ultra-low-latency and reliable communications for 6G networks. *IEEE Communications Standards Magazine, 5*(2), 10–11.
134. Long, W., Chen, R., Moretti, M., Zhang, W., & Li, J. (2021). A promising technology for 6G wireless networks: Intelligent reflecting surface. *Journal of Communications and Information Networks, 6*(1), 1–16.
135. Chaudhary, V., Kaushik, A., Furukawa, H., & Khosla, A. (2022). Towards 5th generation AI and IoT driven sustainable intelligent sensors based on 2d MXenes and borophene. *ECS Sensors Plus, 1*(1), 013601.
136. Batista, E., Lopez-Aguilar, P., & Solanas, A. (2023). Smart health in the 6G era: Bringing security to future smart health services. *IEEE Communications Magazine*.
137. Al-Ansi, A. M., Al-Ansi, A., et al. (2023). An overview of artificial intelligence (AI) in 6G: Types, advantages, challenges and recent applications. *Buletin Ilmiah Sarjana Teknik Elektro, 5*(1), 67–75.
138. Ahad, A., & Tahir, M. (2023). Perspective – 6G and IoT for intelligent healthcare: Challenges and future research directions. *ECS Sensors Plus, 2*(1), 011601.
139. Ziegler, V., & Yrjola, S. (2020). 6G indicators of value and performance. In *2020 2nd 6G wireless summit (6G SUMMIT)* (pp. 1–5). IEEE.
140. Eysenbach, G., et al. (2001). What is e-health? *Journal of Medical Internet Research, 3*(2), e833.
141. Biswas, S., Sharif, K., Li, F., & Mohanty, S. (2020). Blockchain for e-Health-care systems: Easier said than done. *Computer, 53*(7), 57–67.
142. Srivastava, V., Mahara, T., & Yadav, P. (2021). An analysis of the ethical challenges of blockchain-enabled e-healthcare applications in 6G networks. *International Journal of Cognitive Computing in Engineering, 2*, 171–179.

Chapter 4
S-UAV Multiple Redundant Routing Scheme for Crisis Scenario

Grace Khayat, Constandinos X. Mavromoustakis, George Mastorakis, Evangelos Pallis, Evangelos K. Markakis, and Athina Bourdena

4.1 S-UAV Introduction

Unmanned aerial vehicles (UAVs), often named drones, have invaded almost every aspect of our lives including security, rescue missions, crisis prevention, etc. [1]. UAVs are highly used in heterogeneous transportation systems because of their high data rate and ultralow routing delay [2]. Every drone has dedicated data collection with computing capabilities to perform tasks instantly [3, 4]. UAVs that are typically

G. Khayat (✉) · C. X. Mavromoustakis
Department of Computer Science, University of Nicosia and University of Nicosia Research Foundation, Nicosia, Cyprus
e-mail: khayat.g@live.unic.ac.cy; mavromoustakis.c@unic.ac.cy

G. Mastorakis
Department of Management Science and Technology, Hellenic Mediterranean University, Agios Nikolaos, Crete, Greece
e-mail: gmastorakis@hmu.gr

E. Pallis
Department of Industrial Design and Production Engineering, School of Engineering, University of West Attica, Athens, Greece
e-mail: epallis@uniwa.gr

E. K. Markakis
Department of Electrical and Computer Engineering, Hellenic Mediterranean University, Heraklion, Crete, Greece
e-mail: markakis@pasiphae.eu

A. Bourdena
Department of Business Administration & Tourism, Hellenic Mediterranean University Heraklion, Iraklion, Greece
e-mail: bourdena@hmu.gr

© The Author(s), under exclusive license to Springer Nature Switzerland AG 2024

A. Bourdena et al. (eds.), *Intelligent Technologies for Healthcare Business Applications*, Signals and Communication Technology,
https://doi.org/10.1007/978-3-031-58527-2_4

equipped with a variety of sensors are in high demand in time-sensitive situations like hurricanes, tsunamis, or wildfires thanks to 6G infrastructure [5, 6].

A group of UAVs that are flying together to accomplish a single objective form a swarm of unmanned aerial vehicles (S-UAVs) [7, 8]. The UAVs are controlled either manually or autonomously and categorized as completely or partially autonomous. S-UAVs can also be classified as single-layered, in which case each drone serves as its leader, or it may be multilayered, in which case a designated leader present at each tier reports to the leader at the upper layer [9].

4.2 S-UAV Communication

The communication in S-UAVs can be decentralized or centralized. A centralized communication relies on a base station that communicates with all UAVs. By depending on nearby nodes, decentralized communication, sometimes referred to as ad hoc communication, removes communication range limits [10]. Two types of communication exist in S-UAVs and are represented in Fig. 4.1. UAVs communicate with each other as UAV-to-UAV communication, abbreviated as U-T-U communication. UAV-to-Infrastructure communication, abbreviated as U-T-I, is one-to-one communication between the UAV and the base station [11].

Since S-UAV networks are extremely susceptible to disconnections, ad hoc communication is the most preferred method of packet transmission [12]. In Fig. 4.2, three ad hoc S-UAV communication types are depicted. A network that does not depend on infrastructure is a single-group swarm ad hoc network. The gateway UAV, one of the swarm's UAVs, is in charge of communicating with the base station. The other UAVs are merely data-relay nodes [13]. Multigroup swarm ad hoc network is formed of UAV groups, each with a distinct goal. Finally, a multilayer swarm ad hoc network is a swarm of nearby UAVs which functions as an ad hoc network and communicates with the infrastructure through the nearest gateway UAV [14].

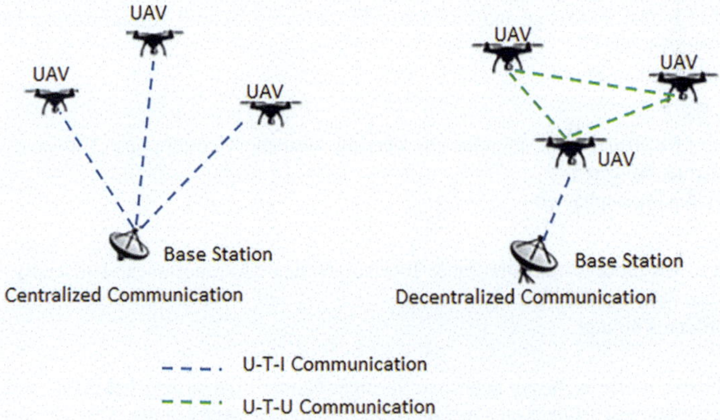

Fig. 4.1 S-UAV communication

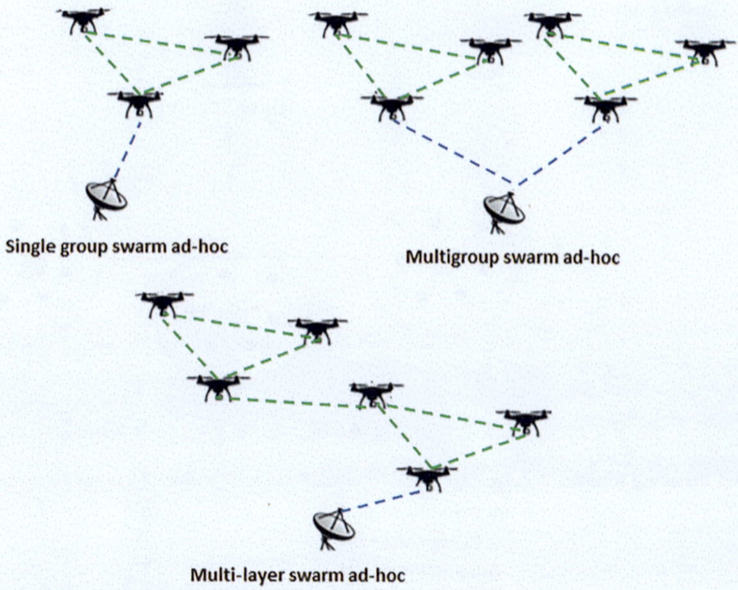

Fig. 4.2 S-UAV architectures

4.3 S-UAV Cluster Routing Schemes

Cluster routing schemes increase network scalability, decrease overhead, maximize throughput, and increase battery life [15, 16]. Nodes are grouped according to specific factors such as residual energy, distance, speed, and direction [17]. The network is classified into cliques known as clusters, as shown in Fig. 4.3. A cluster head (CH) and cluster members (CMs) make up each cluster. All intercluster communication, whether it is between CHs or between the CH and the infrastructure, is the responsibility of the CH. When the CH receives packets from the CMs, it packs them for base station upload [18, 19]. The packets received by the base station, which is supposed to be connected to the Internet, are uploaded and analyzed by the control station. The control station interprets the sensed data, and depending on the network's application, an action might be triggered if needed; otherwise, the data might just be informational [20]. A key player in cluster routing schemes is the CH due to its major role in packet routing. Since the selection of the CH highly impacts the performance of the cluster routing scheme, it has been a continuous field of research. Every cluster routing scheme has its process for selecting the CH that will optimize the routing scheme [21].

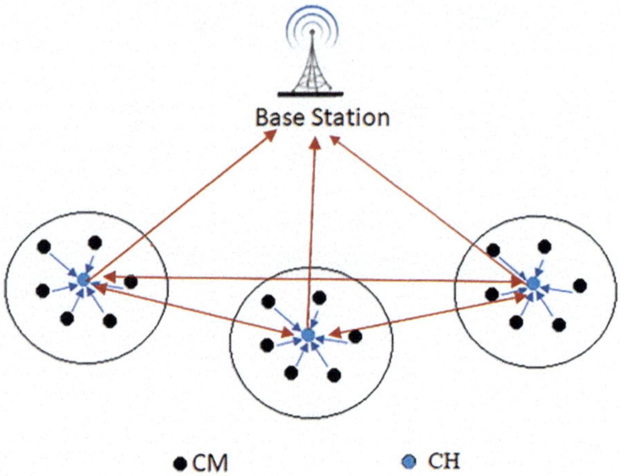

Fig. 4.3 Cluster routing scheme

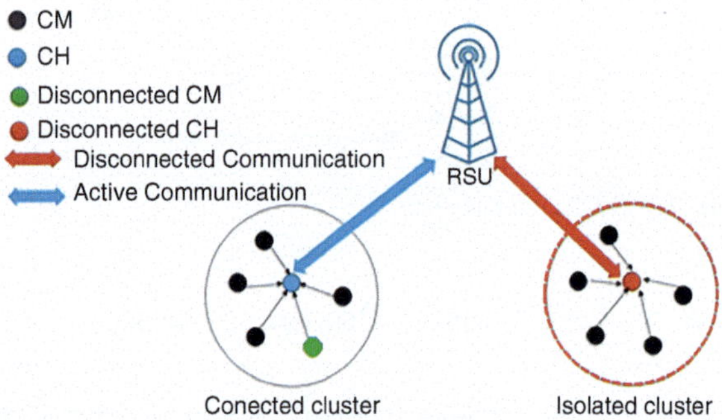

Fig. 4.4 Clustering scheme in S-UAV

4.4 S-UAV in Crisis Scenario

In crisis scenarios, UAVs are frequently utilized for monitoring and rescue operations. Since the CH is the primary point of contact in a clustering scheme if the nonoperational UAV serves as the CH, then the result will be an isolated cluster as shown in Fig. 4.4 [19, 22].

4.5 S-UAV Cluster Routing Schemes

If the primary CH is nonfunctional, a redundant CH will immediately take over the primary CH's roles to make sure that all intercluster routing continues to be legitimate [23]. The choice of the primary and secondary CHs should be made carefully because of the significant role they have [24]. This chapter represents a redundant cluster routing scheme developed by a weighted indicator with the following four metrics:

- The separation
- The rewarding indicator
- The energy
- The velocity

$$I_{(n,m)} = -\alpha D_{(n,m)} - \beta R_{(n,m)} - \phi E_{(n,m)}) - \mu V_{(n,m)} \tag{4.1}$$

where:

- $I_{(n,m)}$ is the clustering indicator of UAV m in regard to UAV n.
- $D_{(n,m)}$ is the separating distance between the two UAVs n and m.
- $R_{(n,m)}$ is the rewarding indicator of UAV m in regard to UAV n.
- $E_{(n,m)}$ is the energy required to transmit k bits of data from UAV m to UAV n.
- $V_{(n,m)}$ is the respective speed of UAV m in regard to UAV n.
- α, β, ϕ, and μ are a prefixed values set based on the network's conditions where

$$\alpha + \beta + \phi + \mu = 1 \tag{4.2}$$

α, ψ, and μ have a negative impact on the weighted cluster indicator. The more distant the UAVs are, the less is the desire that the UAVs are selected in the same cluster [25, 26]. Whenever the UAVs are in the same cluster, the delays of packet transmission are minimized, which leads to better routing schema performance. The same condition also applies to the velocity [27]. The smaller the relative velocity variance is, the higher the desire that the two UAVs to be in the same cluster. The energy also has a negative weight since it is desired to be of minimal expenditure in data transmission [28].

The UAVs' location is represented in a three-dimensional position; thus the separating distance between the two UAVs n and m is

$$D_{(n,m)}(t) = \sqrt{(x_n - x_m)^2 + (y_n - y_m)^2 + (z_n - z_m)^2} \tag{4.3}$$

The rewarding indicator is founded on the packets' delay. The network's maximum tolerated delay, t_{max}, is a threshold set depending on the data's time sensitivity. For example, due to the faster fluctuation of temperature, it has a lower threshold level as compared to the threshold set for the water level. The packets are considered forwarded if their delay is less than the threshold level; otherwise, they are considered dropped as their data is most probably obsolete by the time they are delivered [29].

$$\begin{cases} t_{(n,m)}) \leq t_{max} \; the\ packet\ is\ forwarded \\ Otherwise\ \ the\ packet\ is\ \ dropped \end{cases} \tag{4.4}$$

where:

- t_{max} is the threshold delay.

- $t_{(n,m)}$ is the packet's delay sent from sender n to receiver m.

Consider $y(t)$ to represent the packets sent by all nodes [30]:

$$y(t) = \sum_{n=1}^{M(t)} \sum_{m=1}^{M(t)} P \tag{4.5}$$

- n is the transmitter UAV.
- m is the receiver UAV where $n \neq m$.
- $M(t)$ is the set representing the network's UAVs.
- $P = 1$ represents a packet.

Consider $f(t)$ to represent the packets considered forwarded:

$$f(t) = \sum_{n=1}^{M(t)} \sum_{m=1}^{M(t)} F \tag{4.6}$$

- F is a constant value set to 1 when a packet is considered forwarded; otherwise, it is 0.

The rewarding indicator, which is the proportionality of packets forwarded to the total packets, is [31]

$$R_{(n,m)}(t) = \frac{f_{(n,m)}(t)}{y_{(n,m)}(t)} = \frac{\sum_{n=1}^{M(t)} \sum_{m=1}^{M(t)} F}{\sum_{n=1}^{M(t)} \sum_{m=1}^{M(t)} P} \tag{4.7}$$

The third parameter in the weighted formula is energy which is allowed to be at its highest level of density due to technology [32]. The remaining energy is calculated as

$$E_{(n)}(t) = \frac{E_0 - E_\tau}{E_0} \tag{4.8}$$

where:

- E_0 is the initial energy of UAV n.
- E_τ is the total energy consumption of UAV n which is calculated as

$$E_\tau = E_{TX} + E_{RX} + E_F \tag{4.9}$$

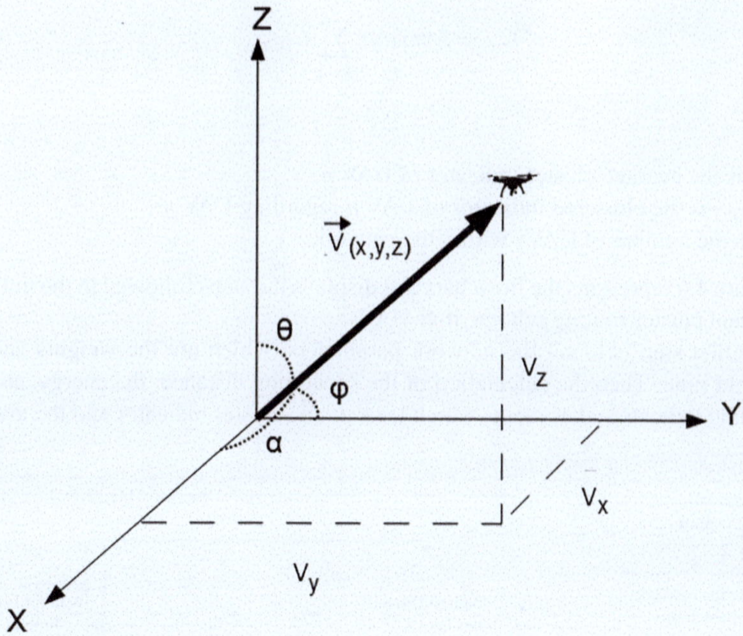

Fig. 4.5 UAV's velocity representation

where:

- E_{TX} is the energy spent for transmitting packets.
- E_{RX} is the energy spent for receiving packets.
- E_F is the energy spent for flying.

The relative velocity of UAV n in regard to UAV m is based on the vectorial difference between the two velocities [33, 34]. The UAV's speed vector represented in Fig. 4.5 can be split into the 3D vectorial components.

The magnitude of the relative velocity to be used in the weighted equation is calculated as [35]

$$V(t)_{(n,m)} = \begin{cases} V_{xn} - V_{xm} \\ V_{yn} - V_{ym} \\ V_{zn} - V_{zm} \end{cases} = \begin{cases} V_{UAVn} * cos\alpha' - V_{UAVm} * cos\alpha \\ V_{UAVn} * cos\phi' - V_{UAVm} * cos\phi \\ V_{UAVn} * cos\theta' - V_{UAVm} * cos\theta \end{cases} \tag{4.10}$$

Each UAV calculates its clustered indicator and broadcasts it to the neighboring nodes. At this stage, all nodes are ready to calculate the average cluster indicator that populates the routing tables in descending order [36].

$$C_n = Average \sum_{k=1}^{N} C_{(n,m)} \tag{4.11}$$

where:

- C_n is the average cluster indicator of UAV n.
- $C_{(n,m)}$ is the clustered indicator of UAV n regarding UAV m.
- N is the number of UAVs within the network.

Figure 4.6 represents the flowchart that displays the steps followed in the multiple redundant cluster routing scheme in S-UAVs.

The first step is to set the network parameters, which are the weights and the threshold time. Then the calculation of the separating distance, the energy, and the rewarding indicator takes place, which leads to the cluster indicator and the average

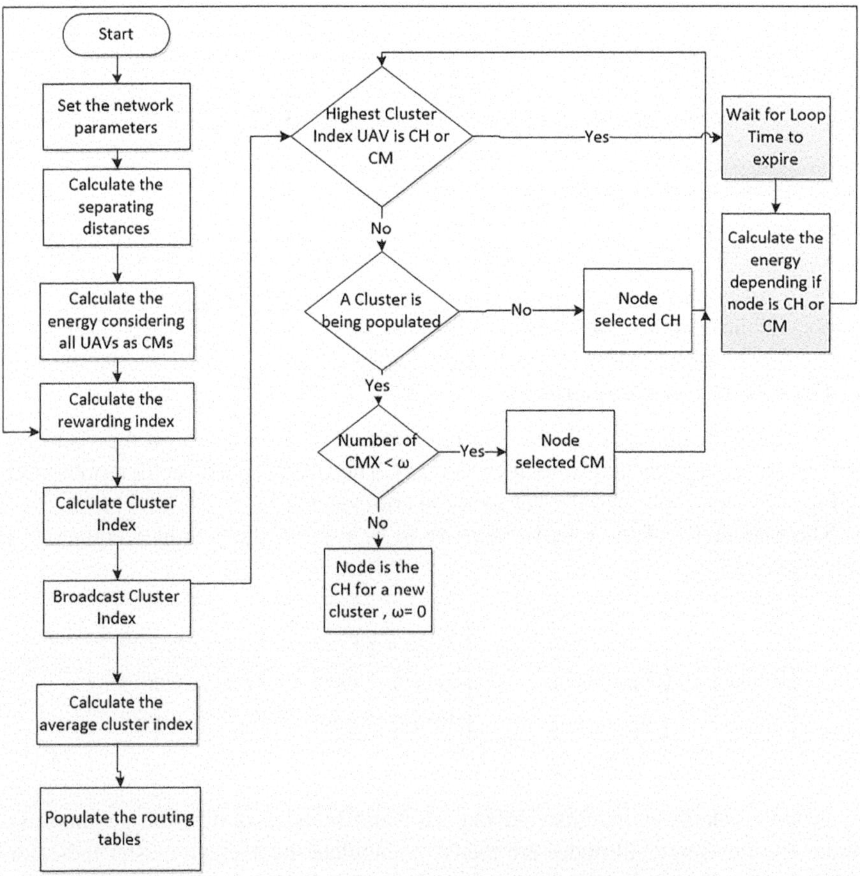

Fig. 4.6 Flowchart

cluster indicator. After the routing tables are populated and ordered high to low based on the average cluster indicator, the classification of the UAVs as CH or CM starts. The UAV with the maximal cluster indicator will be chosen to be the CH for the first cluster. The following ω UAVs with the maximal cluster indicator will be chosen automatically as CMs for the first cluster. The UAV of order $\omega + 2$ will then be chosen to be the CH for the second cluster. The selection prevails until all the UAVs are chosen to be CH or CMs. Every node has the consecutive node to be a redundant CH. Thus, the redundant CH for the first CH is the first CM. The first CM has a redundant CH which is the CM following it. The redundant CH will handle all the routing responsibilities the CH was handling whenever the CH is nonfunctional. If the redundant CH is nonfunctional as well, then the second redundant CH will take over its responsibilities. After the expiration of a predefined timer, the parameters are recalculated, and the cluster protocol repeats.

4.6 Summary

This chapter discussed a detailed routing scheme for S-UAVs. The multiple redundant routing scheme decreases the probability of disconnected networks resulting from crisis scenarios. In a clustering scheme, the CH plays a major role in routing data outside the cluster. Therefore, the risk of data loss occurs whenever the CH is nonfunctional. The redundant CH for every CH or CM will immediately act as CH in case of nonfunctional primary CH. The clusters are formed according to the cluster indicator, which is calculated and founded on a weighted indicator consisting of four parameters: the separation, the rewarding indicator, the energy, and the velocity.

References

1. Andreou, A, Mavromoustakis, C. X., Batalla, J. M., Markakis, E. K., Mastorakis, G., & Pallis, E. (2023). In *Secure Two-Way communications between UAVs and control center in IoV 5G communication*. IEEE Transactions on Intelligent Transportation Systems.
2. Kaleem, Z., Yousaf, M., Qamar, A., Ahmad, A., Duong, T. Q., Choi, W., & Jamalipour, A. (2019). UAV-empowered disaster-resilient edge architecture for delay-sensitive communication. *IEEE Network, 33*(6), 124–132.
3. Al-Emadi, S., & Al-Mohannadr, A. (2020). Towards enhancement of network communication architectures and routing protocols for FANETs: A survey. In *3rd international conference on advanced communication technologies and networking (CommNet)*.
4. Andreou, A., Mavromoustakis, C. X., Batalla, J. M., Markakis, E. K., & Mastorakis, G. (2022). UAV-Assisted RSUs for V2X connectivity using Voronoi diagrams in 6G infrastructures. IN *2022 IEEE 27th international workshop on computer aided modeling and design of communication links and networks CAMAD*.
5. Agoston, R. (2018). Water related disaster management supported by drone applications. *World Journal of Engineering and Technology, 6*(2), 116–126.
6. Riaz, M. N. (2018). Clustering algorithms of wireless sensor networks: A survey. *International Journal of Wireless and Microwave Technologies, 4*, 40–53.

7. Khayat, G., Mavromoustakis, C. X., Mastorakis, G., Batalla, J. M., & Pallis, E. (2022). Swarm UAV network constraints in damaged infrastructures. In *IEEE International Conference on Communications*.
8. Khelifi, M., & Butun, I. (2022). Swarm Unmanned Aerial Vehicles (SUAVs): A comprehensive analysis of localization, recent aspects, and future trends. *Journal of Sensors, 2022*(1), 8600674.
9. Khayat, G., Mavromoustakis, C. X., Batalla, J. M., Song, H. H., & Mastorakis, G. (2023). On the weighted cluster S-UAV scheme using latency-oriented trust. *IEEE Access,11*, 56310–56323.
10. Lav, G., Raj, J., & Gabor, V. (2015). Survey of important issues in UAV communication networks. *Journal of IEEE Communications Surveys and Tutorials, 18*(2), 1123–1152.
11. Gu, K., Mao, Z., Qi, M., & Duan, X. (2020). Finding subgroups of UAV swarms using a trajectory clustering method. In *Journal of physics: Conference series, ICCBDAI* (Vol. 1757(1), p. 012131). IOP Publishing.
12. Khayat, G., Mavromoustakis, C. X., Pitsillides, A., Batalla, J. M., Markakis, E. K., & Andreou, A. (2022). Enhanced redundant scheme based on weighted cluster-head selection for critical 6G infrastructures. In *IEEE Globecom Workshops: Workshop on Emerging Topics in 6G Communications*.
13. Yifan, S., Zhichao, M., Hai, W., Yuqing, J., Ning, Z. (2019). Research on UAV cluster routing strategy based on distributed SDN. In *19th International conference on communication technology (ICCT)* (pp. 1269–1274).
14. Asghar, K. M., Alamgir, S., Mansoor, Q. I., & Ullah, K. I. (2017). Flying ad-hoc networks (FANETs): A review of communication architectures, and routing protocols. In *17 First international conference on latest trends in electrical engineering and computing technologies (INTELLECT)* (pp. 1–9).
15. Khayat, G., Mavromoustakis, C. X., Mastorakis, G., Batalla, J. M., & Maalouf, H. (2021). Damaged critical infrastructure for VANETs. In *Intelligent Wireless Communications*. The Institution of Engineering and Technology
16. Gheisari, M., Abbasi, A. A., Sayari, Z., Rizvi, Q., Asheralieva, A., Banu, S., Awaysheh, F. M., Shah, S. B. H., & Raza, K. A. (2020). A survey on clustering algorithms in wireless sensor networks: Challenges, research, and trends. International Computer Symposium (ICS).
17. Cooper, C., Franklin, D., Ros, M., Safaei, F., & Abolhasan, M. (2017). A comparative survey of VANET clustering techniques. *IEEE Communication Surveys and Tutorials, 19*(1), 657–681.
18. Kaur, S., & Grewal, V. (2016). Wireless sensor networks recent trends and research issues. *Indian Journal of Science and Technology, 9*. https://doi.org/10.17485/ijst/2016/v9i48/106856.
19. Khayat, G., Mavromoustakis, C. X., Mastorakis, G., Maalouf, H., & Batalla, J. M. (2021). VASNET routing protocol in crisis scenario based on carrier vehicle. In *Intelligent technologies for internet of vehicles, in series internet of things, book*. Springer Nature Switzerland AG. https://doi.org/10.1007/978-3-030-76493-7.
20. Thakur, T. (2016). An access control protocol for wireless sensor network using double trapdoor chameleon hash function. *Journal of Sensors, 2016*(1), 1210938.
21. Khayat, G., Mavromoustakis, C. X., Mastorakis, G., Batalla, J. M., Maalouf, H., Mumtaz, S., & Pallis, E. (2020). Successful delivery in VANETs with damaged infrastructures based on double cluster head selection. In *IEEE 25th international workshop on computer aided modelling and design of communication links and networks*.
22. Alawad, W., Halima, N. B., & Aziz, L. (2023). *An unmanned aerial vehicle (UAV) system for disaster and crisis management in smart cities*. Electronics.
23. Shi, M., Zhang, X., Chen, J., & Cheng, H. (2023). UAV cluster-assisted task offloading for emergent disaster scenarios. *Applied Sciences, 13*(8), 4724.
24. Khayat, G., Mavromoustakis, C. X., Mastorakis, G., Maalouf, H., & Batalla, J. M. (2020). Intelligent vehicular networking protocols. In *Convergence of artificial intelligence and the internet of things in series internet of things, book*. Springer Nature Switzerland AG. https://doi.org/10.1007/978-3-030-44907-0.

25. Xia, X., Yan, Y., Li, Z., Meng, D., Xia, L., & Chen, C. (2022). A survey of UAV clustering algorithm. In *24th International conference on advanced communication technology* (pp. 191–196). https://doi.org/10.23919/ICACT53585.2022.9728826.
26. Andreou, A., Mavromoustakis, C. X., Batalla, J. M., Markakis, E. K., Mastorakis, G., & Mumtaz, S. (2023). UAV trajectory optimisation in smart cities using modified A* algorithm combined with haversine and vincenty formulas. *IEEE Transactions on Vehicular Technology, 72*(8), (pp. 1–13).
27. Arafat, M. Y., & Moh, S. (2019). Comparison of clustering algorithms based on weighted clustering metrics for unmanned aerial vehicle networks. In *International conference on electronics, information and communication.*
28. Khayat, G., Mavromoustakis, C. X., Mastorakis, G., Batalla, J. M., & Pallis, E. (2022). Weighted cluster routing protocol with redundant cluster head for damaged WSN. In *2022 IEEE 7th international energy conference (ENERGYCON)* (pp. 1–7). IEEE.
29. Abeywickrama, H. V., Jayawickrama, B. A., He, Y., & Dutkiewicz, E. (2018). Comprehensive energy consumption model for unmanned aerial vehicles, based on empirical studies of battery performance. *IEEE Access, 6*, 58383–58394. https://doi.org/10.1109/ACCESS.2018.2875040.
30. Batalla, J. M., Mavromoustakis, C. X., Mastorakis, G., Markakis, E., Pallis, E., Wichary, T., Krawiec, P., & Lekston, P. (2021). On analyzing routing selection for aerial autonomous vehicles connected to mobile network. Sensors **21**(2), 339.
31. Andreou, A., Mavromoustakis, C. X., Mastorakis, G., Batalla, J. M., & Pallis, E. (2022). Energy conservation by using the integration of distributed energy system in smart vehicles. In *EEE 7th International Energy Conference ENERGYCON.*
32. Khayat, G., Mavromoustakis, C. X., Mastorakis, G., Batalla, J. M., & Pallis, E. (2022). Redundant clustered scheme based on weighted cluster head selection for damaged S-UAV. In *IEEE Global Communications Conference.*
33. Abeywickrama, H. V., Jayawickrama, B. A., He, Y., & Dutkiewicz, E. (2018). Comprehensive Energy Consumption Model for Unmanned Aerial Vehicles, Based on Empirical Studies of Battery Performance. *IEEE Access, 6*, (pp. 58383–58394).
34. Khayat, G., Mavromoustakis, C. X., Mastorakis, G., Batalla, J. M., Maalouf, H., & Pallis, E. (2020). VANET clustering based on weighted trusted cluster head selection. In *16th International wireless communications and mobile computing conference.*
35. Song, H., Hu, S., Guo, Q., & Jiang, W. (2022). Relative positioning method for UAVs based on multi-source information fusion. In *Mathematical Problems in Engineering, Hindawi*
36. Khayat, G., Mavromoustakis, C. X., Pitsillides, A., Batalla, J. M., & Markakis, E. K. (2022). Enhanced redundant weighted clustered scheme for damaged S-UAV. In *IEEE International Conference on Communications.*

Chapter 5
The Evaluation of Key Performance Indicators for Medical and Digital Technologies in Healthcare

Magdalini Chatzikou

5.1 Introduction

Health care is one of the major success stories of our times. Medical science has improved rapidly, raising life expectancy around the world, but as longevity increases, health care systems face growing demand for their services, rising costs and a workforce that is struggling to meet the needs of its patients [1, 2]. Building on automation, artificial intelligence (AI) has the potential to revolutionize health care and help address some of the challenges set out above. AI can lead to better care outcomes and improve the productivity and efficiency of care delivery. It can also improve the day-to-day life of health care practitioners, letting them spend more time looking after patients and in so doing, raise productivity and improve retention. It can even get life-saving treatments to market faster. At the same time, questions have been raised about the impact AI could have on patients, practitioners and health systems and about its potential risks; there are ethical debates around how AI and the data that underpins it should be used [3, 4].

The objective of the chapter is to provide a holistic analysis/view of the importance of KPIs, their application in the health care sector, mainly in the field of the use of artificial intelligence technologies. This chapter explores first a description of what elements theoretically contribute to performance management and secondly, considerations in the application in different sectors and from large to smaller layers of organization and technologies.

Project performance can be measured using KPIs to evaluate all projects' outcomes, determined by strategic need or opportunity and associated objectives. The value of KPIs is that in standardizing a measure, comparative studies can be

M. Chatzikou (✉)
Pharmecons Easy Access Ltd., York, UK
e-mail: magda.chatzikou@pharmecons.com

© The Author(s), under exclusive license to Springer Nature Switzerland AG 2024

A. Bourdena et al. (eds.), *Intelligent Technologies for Healthcare Business Applications*, Signals and Communication Technology,
https://doi.org/10.1007/978-3-031-58527-2_5

made, when a comparator is used. Different combinations of KPI may be selected according to stakeholders' interests (perspective), typically decision makers. Each KPI may be a relatively direct reflection of the value of an outcome or use one of multiple choices of tool or instrument, such as questionnaires, to estimate a proxy value for that KPI. The current report covers the outcomes measurement of all involved stakeholders of the health care sector which are the following:

1. Policy makers (Ministry of health, hospital management, EU health care officials).
2. Physicians and health care professionals involved in medical decision-making process.
3. Patients, caregivers, and patient advocacy groups.
4. Academic society.

The identification of the health care-related KPIs was based on a thorough literature review to be able to capture the perspective of all stakeholders of the health care sector, covering the important outcomes pillars of:

- The health care systems which are medical, productivity, and economic.
- The patients and caregivers, which are patient-reported outcomes and patient-reported experience measures.

A challenge in the identification of KPIs for AI technologies lies in the diversification of technologies involved, where diverse outcomes required a variety of instruments for one or more KPIs for each specific technology. Additionally, multiple types of outcome, disease area, stakeholder, countries, and study designs added to the complexity of finding a common theme upon which to evaluate the different projects and their technologies. Ultimately, the economic evaluation enabled a level of comparison among different endpoints, while recognizing projects with different objectives, service recipients, and settings are less suitable for comparison than projects which include their own internal comparators.

5.2 The Role of Key Performance Indicators (KPIs) in Health Care

The quality movement concept, i.e. the management of quality improvement, has spread widely during the last decades from manufacturing to service, health care, non-profit organizations, and educational institutions [5]. In health care, the concept of quality has become an increasingly important factor both for patients' well-being and economic survival [6] as well as among authorities, policymakers, managers, physicians, and patients [7] using several quality management approaches, such as evidence-based medicine (EBM), total quality management (TQM), improvement science, professional development, and patient empowerment [7]. Raven et al. (2012) posited that understanding good quality of care and how it can be measured is critical to improving health services [8].

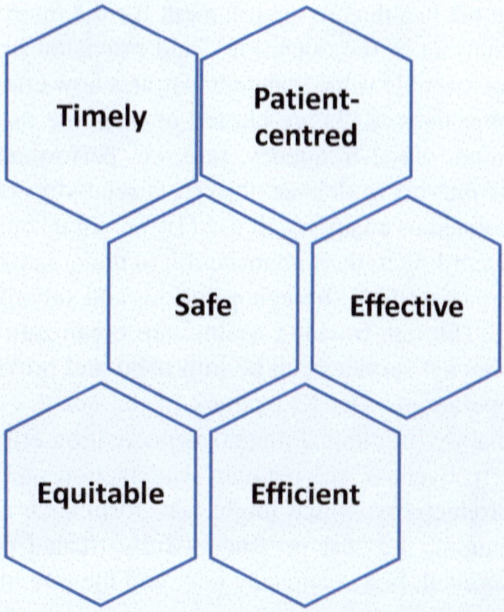

Fig. 5.1 Characteristics of high-quality care

Still, defining the facets of health and quality management for health care improvement is an ongoing challenge due to individual differences and the complex relationship between health services and health outcomes [9]. The Institute of Medicine (IoM) defines quality in health care as "*the degree to which health services for individuals and populations increase the likelihood of desired health outcomes and are consistent with current professional practice*." Building on this definition, the IoM presented six characteristics of high-quality care [9] (Fig. 5.1).

High quality care must be:

1. *Safe*: Avoiding injuries to patients from the care that is intended to help them.
2. *Effective*: Providing services based on scientific knowledge to all who could benefit and refraining from providing services to those not likely to benefit (avoiding underuse and overuse).
3. *Patient-centred*: Providing care that is respectful of, and responsive to, individual patient preferences, needs, and values and ensuring that patient values guide all clinical decisions.
4. *Timely*: Reducing waits and sometimes harmful delays for both those who receive and those who give care.
5. *Efficient*: Avoiding waste, in particular waste of equipment, supplies, ideas, and energy.
6. *Equitable*: Providing care that does not vary in quality because of personal characteristics such as gender, ethnicity, geographic location, and socioeconomic status.

The goal of any health care provider is to offer an optimal level of services to their clients. Understanding the efficiency and effectiveness of organizational operations is vital to finding areas to improve the provision of services. KPIs are important in the health care environment for the interpretation of the result/objective setting, analysis of the operations, and provision of evidence of effectiveness. A KPI is a measurable value that demonstrates how effectively an organization is achieving key objectives. KPIs are classes of outcome used to measure outcome size, direction, trend, class, frequency, rate, i.e. performance or preference levels for outcomes of interest to deliver objectives related to performance management (PM). PM is defined as an approach used by an organization to optimize or mitigate its activities according to their contribution to the organization's purpose, the later detailed in an organization's strategic priorities and subordinate objectives.

Through tracking health care organization's performance, the level of the provisional services can be improved and provide a greater understanding of hospital operations. The KPI pillars in the health care setting are quadruplicate, covering mainly (a) clinical/diagnosis/prevention effectiveness, (b) hospital/operational/cost effectiveness, (c) patients' satisfaction and quality of life improvement, and (d) productivity, which might take form such as the number of patients reviewed per annum, the cost per successfully treated patient, the cost per incremental years survival, bed occupancy rate, and the rate of non-scheduled recurrent patient visits to a hospital.

Figure 5.2 shows the role of KPIs in performance management, which is depicted as an iterative cycle of considerations. The cycle comprises statement of extant need/opportunity, definition of a project's objectives, measures of performance and service recipients, i.e. patients with the relevant condition. Furthermore, services options available to recipients, outcomes to be measured, analysis to be undertaken, and review of outcomes against objectives and need/opportunity should be defined and undertaken. Collectively this permits reflection on the value of outcomes and whether anything may additionally, likely significantly mitigate extant need or contribute to achieving extant opportunity. In such an ecosystem of inputs, outputs, and outcome, a change anywhere may have ramifications through the cycle, not only on that stage's activity.

The traditional measures of productivity, i.e. efficiency, output/input, and quality—adequacy of output and input—in health care and the service sector are natural considerations of performance management, but in order to be considered patient centric, patient contributions [10] and involvement [11] are considered necessary to establish high quality health care.

5.3 Measuring the Effectiveness of Medical Interventions

European longevity improvements are predicted to raise the >65-year-old population from 19% in 2015 to 30% by 2050, requiring planning for the care requirements of the future [12]. Health care interventions and comparators are used to determine each treatment strategy's effectiveness and cost. The extra effect per extra unit cost associated with intervention minus comparator costs and effects determines cost-effectiveness. Measures of effect are typically a clinician's most significant

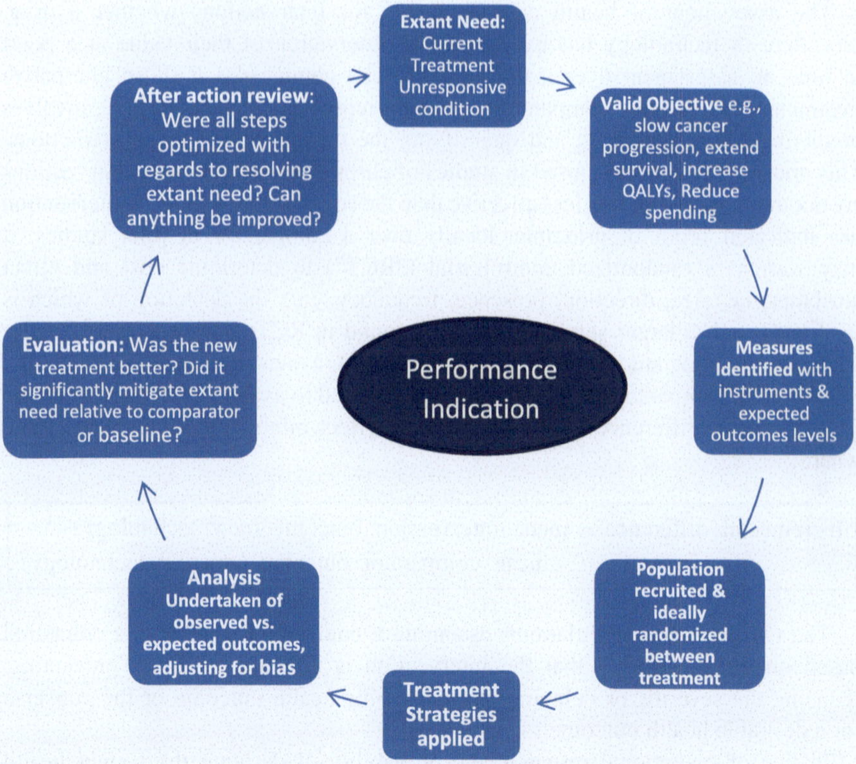

Fig. 5.2 KPIs in an operational/study ecosystem of inputs and outputs

measures to manage a disease, e.g. blood pressure to manage cardiovascular disease, but may vary depending on the nature of the intervention.

Research into interventions, permitting at least the maintenance of public health, needs to be evaluated using rigorous scientific and management methods. Public health interventions should try to optimize the delivery of both efficiency and effectiveness to avoid being usurped by opportunity cost considerations, i.e. the next best alternative method of using funding, such as usual care. Thus, evaluation designs must recognize and integrate the requirements of funding agents, ensure that intervention benefits can be accurately measured and conveyed, and ensure that areas for improvement are identified as needed, against extant opportunity or need. There are minimum requirements which every health care system should meet equitably: access to quality services for acute and chronic health needs; effective health promotion and disease prevention services; and appropriate response to new threats as they emerge (emerging infectious diseases, growing burden of non-communicable diseases and injuries, and the health effects of global environmental changes) [13].

The assessment of health care outcomes for interventions whether a drug, procedure or technology has evolved from observation of their value at a point in time, to assessment over a time course. The comparison with an alternative treatment strategy (the "comparator"), usually representing standard care, involves predicting future outcomes and quantifying the uncertainty of these predictions. This approach is generally used in studies of chronic diseases, where interventions are not more expensive and less effective than the comparator. Where an intervention has indicated proof of principle, ideally over a comparator in pilot studies, it may warrant a randomized control trial ("RCT") to determine cost and effect attributes, i.e. size, direction, presence, frequency, etc., the detection of which is facilitated with a larger sample population found in RCTs, rather than in smaller studies, e.g. pilot studies. The relative merit of a new treatment strategy, the intervention, compared to the comparator, is referred to as the incremental outcome or incremental difference of the intervention effect minus the comparator effect, where:

Incremental difference = mean intervention outcome (new technology) − mean comparator outcome (existing technology)

The two treatment populations, assuming a comparator is used, are compared based on the probability that the intervention is effective in either preventing, reducing the severity, or delaying an undesirable health outcome or the converse for a desirable health outcome.

In lieu of operational research, the probability of deriving the sought health outcome usually is based only on the clinical efficacy of the intervention.

Studies without a comparator may be used to demonstrate technological success rather than incremental clinical effect as without a comparator, there are limited ways to determine whether a population treated with an intervention has a higher or lower outcome. However, in some cases, historical studies have used usual care as the comparator. Synthetic and External Control Arms might be an option.

5.4 Why Measuring Health Care Outcomes Is Important

Quality measurement can be a costly and time-consuming activity. Accordingly, judicious selection of indicators contributing to the aggregate understanding of health care quality is imperative. If indicator development is to be systematic, targeting areas where the need is greatest, needs must be identified and classified by type of measure. Several indicators should be identified and classified:

- *Domain* to which they apply (hospital-wide, surgical, and non-surgical clinical specialties and departments).
- *Aspects of care provision* (structural, process improvement, and outcome).

- *Dimensions of quality* (safety, effectiveness, efficiency, timeliness, patient-centeredness, and equity). This information was then used to identify gaps in current measurement [14].

Health outcome estimates inform:

- Funding decisions for new treatment when compared to the best alternative treatment.
- Safety—recording serious events, e.g. death or disablement from an intervention or adverse events, which may only become apparent with longer use.
- Public accountability by conveying treatment strategy outcomes and recording the justification for funding decisions.
- The creation of a spirit of competitiveness and application whereby a research body may create a better or alternatively applied product, service, or process than other companies.

All these applications of measurement of health outcomes seek to improve or maintain the health of patients.

Estimation of outcomes (and incremental outcomes) is possible through a wide diversity of tools and approaches. Five classes have been identified outcomes relevant to health care—oriented projects seeking to determine their value to the health care system. For example, local measures, perhaps sponsored by a clinician, may be especially clinically informative. However, their use alone—without a comparator—often involves small samples or short studies, making it difficult to judge the incremental benefit and the "generalizability" of a treatment. This means it is challenging to determine whether the same treatment will exhibit the same effect in a different setting for the same condition, considering risk factors and the distribution of effects. In other words, an intervention without evidence to support generalizability, because of the dissimilarity of measures and outcomes, can prevent an intervention's use from being supported, where direct comparisons are necessary, in which usual care would most likely be the default.

5.5 Important Outcomes for Health Care Systems

Health care systems seek health improvement in outcomes at a sustainable cost or the maximum of outcome for an acceptable level of cost or extra cost. In both cases, the patient would benefit from maximization of value, where the level of value may be defined as a ratio of additional or incremental effect to the additional cost incurred from using a new treatment compared to that of a comparator. The reciprocal of this ratio, that is, the ratio of incremental cost/incremental effect, is known as the incremental cost-effectiveness ratio ("ICER"). Intervention ICERs are one of the considerations health technology agencies use in deciding on whether a new treatment represents value for money. New treatment ICERs falling below an ICER threshold, also referred to as a willingness to pay ("WTP") threshold, which is the level of extra cost per extra unit effect a funder will pay for a new intervention, are judged of sufficient value to be recommended for use, all elements being equal [15].

For health care system, health care outcomes inform decision makers with an estimate of the cost-effectiveness of a new treatment permitting them to derive a judgement of worth or value from the treatment's relative performance, where a comparator or baseline is included, informing them of a relative or temporal change in value, i.e. performance change from a different treatment or simply with the passage of time. Such information along with cost or economic effect helps a decision maker determine the worth or value of undertaking a new activity, e.g. permitting a new intervention onto health care systems' funding scheme. Value-based care, which is defined by Teisberg et al. (2020) as "the measured improvement in a person's health outcomes for the cost of achieving that improvement," is the holistic patient-centred approach that health care systems should follow [16]. Understanding outcomes is central in providing value and represents an opportunity for redefining patient care. Value is created by improving the outcomes of patients with a particular clinical condition over the full cycle of care, which normally involves multiple specialties and care sites. To be successful, a key aspect of value-based care is working as teams (integrated practice units) centred around the patient's clinical condition. As medicine has become more specialized and more complex, multidisciplinary communication and trust among the care team are paramount in providing value to patients.

5.6 Linking Outcomes with Key Performance Indicators in Health Care

5.6.1 Clinical Effectiveness and Safety

Clinical effectiveness could be considered the motivating force behind a study as unsurprisingly clinicians seek to administer either better or less adverse (side effects/adverse events) treatment, which are effective, efficient, and safe. Patients have broadly similar hopes although likely with less interest in Pareto gains, e.g. less willing to live with side effects such as a raised probability of cancer of the jaw for bone remineralization especially where the gains may have wide margins of uncertainty or be realized only in small subpopulation. Thus, measurement of the size of clinical effect, uncertainty (standard error), its cost, time scale, and any adverse events is of interest.

The clinical outcomes may include any outcome a clinician considers of use in the management of patient's condition. These may include the accuracy of a test, survival length, mean time between recurrence or progression to a qualitatively distinct worse/better state of health, e.g. disease free or diagnosed states of a disease, accuracy of diagnostic tools, minimization of variation between repeat events, identification and assessment of presence/absence/levels of risk factors, and their significance in predicting outcome, or simply saving time on the administration associated with a process, e.g. reviewing diagnostic video to determine the appropriate clinical approach. The size of the effect is measured over the duration of treatment for the treatment strategy, and it is typically compared with a control or comparator, e.g. usual care when used as in a randomized controlled trial.

A patient's health journey can be conceived as a continuum throughout their life, described either by complex algorithms that capture varying patterns of health inputs and outcomes associated with a condition, or as a transition through various discrete states of health. These states may cover the period from entry to a trial or diagnosis to the end of an observation period, i.e. a trial and extrapolated to the expected cessation of change in effect, e.g. at death or recovery from an infection, surgery, or a sprained ankle. In the discrete states approach, known as a state transition model [17], e.g. for cancer, a patient may be said to transition from progression free survival to a progressed state to death. There may be variations in the route. While for infections, at their simplest level, a model may be composed of the states: susceptible, infected, and recovered. Model variations could include exposed and reinfected states with various possible routes between states. Model parsimony is a useful discipline, enforcing hypothetical clarity on what elements constitute significant states, a necessity for model construction. Costs, quality of life, and risk rates for clinical effects within states and rates of transition between states with some other considerations allow, through the assignment of input parameters, to state an extrapolation of the model outcomes, identified in a trial. This process permits estimation of the level of long-term inputs, outcomes, and probability of cost-effectiveness through stochastic parametric variation.

Clinical effectiveness may track any activity thought to lend itself to an improvement in patient outcomes, although traditionally these activities and associated outcomes have tended to comprise diagnoses, measures or estimates of mortality, prognoses, and biochemical, electrophysiological, or other observed markers of the process of a functioning body. Likewise, the measurement and reporting of adverse events is important so that areas needing further research are identified. The essence of the measurement is to get an estimate of how well or poorly a process works as a proxy for how a patient is faring. Typically, this would be compared to existing process or treatment, e.g. usual care as the comparator to allow removal of background effects where an intervention was applied concurrent with a comparator or provide an alternative treatment strategy consideration where the two treatment strategies were each applied alone on a split sample population.

Aside from traditional interventions, additional services may also assist both patient and staff and these may require different outcomes to be measured. For example, compare the "treatment" strategies of receptionist usual care or an AI appointment scheduling algorithm, used, for illustrative purposes, around a busy hospital reception/administration desk, managing incoming and exiting day-care appointment patients and their digital notes from different departments. These two treatment strategy approaches may show differences in the speed of booking an appointment, the number of patients they can handle per day, the patient and staff experience through the intervention vs. comparator, and the fit to multiple and potentially departmentally varying priorities for resources and clinical areas with some parameters independent and others interacting; in short, it is a complex task, for which a suitably well programmed AI algorithm may be ideally suited to constant demand.

Other departments may have different outcome needs. For example, in a department using tissue structure to identify malignancies or pathology; factors such as accuracy, productivity, reproducibility, and patient survival and/or quality of life may show varied outcomes between intervention and comparator. For instance, the comparator (usual care performed by a clinician) or the intervention (an AI algorithm analyzing fused tissue imagery with other forms of data, such as genotypic) may help improve accuracy, increase the number of correctly diagnosed cases among all potential disease cases seen by the clinic, and reduce the number of incorrect diagnoses among people presenting without the disease. Mapping tissue samples and subsequent AI imagery analysis may permit more efficient analysis in the future, i.e. more analysis per unit time. Furthermore, minimized variation between expected and observed outcomes across serial analysis would permit improvements in accuracy, with potentially further benefits as dose refinement, fewer side effects/better safety, better treatment outcome and quality of life expectations in patients. However, the recent COVID pandemic has also highlighted the risks of a just in time marketplace with limited internal resilience. Of the two treatment strategies, the traditional approach ensures a supply of competent future surgeons, although whether their numbers alone would meet the needs of expanding ageing population is another matter.

5.6.2 Patient-Centred Approaches

In medicine, patient-centred approaches are used where the consequences of conditions can be better understood from an experiential, subjective experience, rather than a theoretical perspective of experience [22, 23]. For example, for dysarthria patients, affected by weak or poorly controlled speech muscles, a speech-language pathologist may be the best assessor of impairment risk factors related to velopharyngeal dysfunction and their contribution to dysarthria. Yet the patient is best suited to assess impact on psychosocial factors such as their participation in various professional, social, or personal activities [18]. Therefore, both clinical-effectiveness and PRO measures are needed to identify likely treatments outcomes for both clinical and quality of life improvement.

5.6.3 Patient Reported Outcomes Measures (PROMs)

PROMs are tools formulated as a series of health-related questions to evaluate individual patient health status such as when comparing different treatment strategies for their impact on patient health states [18]. PROMs are self-reported instruments and consequently are a direct reflection of the patient's assessment of their capacity to experience or undertake the subject of a PROM's questions, rather than an interpretation of patient reflections by a third party, e.g. a clinician or carer, unless the patient is unable to respond, then the carer may answer on behalf of the patient. PROMs ask patients to answer a typically limited number of questions, where the patient selects a level of experience most closely reflecting their current health status at the time of answering. The level reflects the patient's lesser to greater difficulty conducting or experiencing the subject of the question. The summed answers, subtracted from 1, yield the health status, e.g. quality of life, and when treatment duration is weighted by QoL, quality of life weighted years also known quality adjusted life years ("QALYs") are estimated. QALYs are a measure combining both the level and duration of quality of life for a patient. Accordingly, PROMs allow impact assessment of various treatment strategies on patient health outcomes to be assessed by patients and over time, on patients [18].

PROMs facilitate patient self-assessment of the impact of a treatment across different domains of their life from a capability perspective, i.e. the degree of a patient's ability to conduct that activity.

PROMs primary use is to measure patient's quality of life in qualitative terms. They are used in cost-effectiveness evaluations to determine health economic outcomes, i.e. QoL during treatment with different treatment strategies over time. When utility measures are used, the evaluation is referred to as a cost utility analysis [19]. A utility measure reflects individual preference for different health outcomes, e.g. life and death, measured on an interval scale with 0 reflecting death and 1 full health. During the years, QoL has become the basic metric for the reimbursement decision-making process in medicine, both pharmaceuticals and medical technologies [20, 21].

5.6.3.1 PROMs in Economic Analysis

In cost-effectiveness or cost-utility analysis, incremental cost-effectiveness ratio ("ICER") is estimated using the cost difference as a numerator divided by the effect difference as denominator. The effect is typically measured in both clinical effectiveness measures and with PROMs, normally as QALYs in a CUA. However, a variation of theme exists where if, no primary outcome difference or QALY difference is noted, a cost minimization strategy might be undertaken to identify the treatment with the lowest cost, i.e. why pay more if there are no further clinical or health economic consequences, unless there were significantly different safety or adverse events or side effects with one treatment over another.

5.6.3.2 Types of PROM

There are many sorts of PROM which may be categorized (University of Oxford PROM Group, accessed 2021) as follows:

- *Condition-specific*, e.g. the Rotator Cuff-Quality of Life (RC-QOL), cancer-specific EORTC-QLQ-C30.
- *Population-specific*, e.g. Child Health and Illness Profile–Child Edition (CHP-CE), Child Health Utility-9 Dimension (CHU-9D).
- *Dimension-specific*, e.g. Hospital Anxiety and Depression Scale (HADS).
- *Generic/general population*, e.g. SF-36, EQ5D, HUI.
- *Individualized*, e.g. Patient Generated Index.
- *Summary items*, e.g. UK General Lifestyle Survey questions about accidents.
- *Utility measures*, e.g. EuroQol, Health utilities index (HUI), SF6D.

For example, for a condition-specific PROM, the European Organisation for Research and Treatment of Cancer has created instruments, e.g. EORTC-QLQ-C30 Quality of Life of Cancer Patients [24]. With EORTC, patients select between not at all, a little, quite a bit, very much for the questionnaire's domains. Using cut-offs in the EORTC-QLQ-C30 outcome, another study was able to identify patients with unmet needs, helpful for clinical management [25–27].

In addition to a PROM being categorized as one form or another of the preceding list, multiple PROMs may be used to determine where or whether a patient is (most) affected by some treatment strategy above another. For example, for atopic dermatitis (AD) and chronic hand eczema (CHE), the condition specific PROMs Dermatology Life Quality Index, Pruritus/Itch Numeric Rating Scale, Patient-Oriented Eczema Measure and Quality of Life in Hand Eczema Questionnaire appear frequently in the literature [28], even at the risk of some overlap [29, 30].

Alternatively, generic PROMs could be used or additionally PROMs such as EQ-5D [31, 32], WHOQOL [33] and HUI [21] are all utility measures which measure QoL in the general population. Utility measures measure the quality of life, permitting comparison across diseases, e.g. Health Utilities Index (HUI) [21]. HUI is formatted as HUI-2 with 24,000 unique health states or HUI-3 with 972, 000 unique health states. HUI measures sensation, mobility, pain, cognition, ambulation and emotion. It can be used to calculate QALYs. Short Form 6 Dimensions (SF6D), a truncated version of SF36, is suitable for deriving QoL [34, 35]. Rather than SF36, which is unsuitable alone for creating a value set because it does not allow trade-offs between different dimensions of the questionnaire, SF6D has an algorithm to create a continuous measure of health and was tested against a large sample of the UK population [35].

There has been a proliferation of measures of quality of life and health status over the last two decades. In 2000, 1275 separate measures existed, and the production of new measures was considerably growing [36]. As such, there is a need for generic, comparable measures. Among this variety of measures, previous studies have highlighted three instruments important for measuring PROMs: the SF-36® [34], PROMIS 10 [26, 37] and EQ-5D [31]. All three instruments provide a means of describing (generating a "profile" of) health. The SF-36® applies an algorithm to patients' responses to individual questionnaire items and scales to produce two summary scores: one for physical health and one for mental health. The EQ-5D uses a visual analogue scale to elicit from patients a single score for their overall health. The PROMIS 10 does not yield an overall score but gives physical health and mental health component scores. Extensive research has been done on the validity, reliability, reproducibility and utility of health status surveys when applied to general audiences and sub-groups based on age, sex, nationality and disease entity. The EQ-5D and SF-36® have both been used in large surveys of the general public—population norms are available for both that may have relevance in "benchmarking" performance. Both generic measures—EQ-5D and SF-36®—have validated translations of their instruments available in a range of languages. The PROMIS instrument, being much newer, has a limited evidence base. Table 5.1 presents the comparison of the three most widely used generic PROM instruments.

The SF-36 is a widely used generic measure of health status. Of 36 items 35 are grouped into eight scales that address health constructs considered to be important to most health care situations: physical functioning, role limitations (physical problems), bodily pain, general health, vitality, social functioning, role limitations (emotional problems) and mental health. One item assesses the perception of changes in health but is not used to compute scale scores. The SF-36v1® was developed in 1990 during the Medical Outcomes Study (MOS) to measure generic health concepts relevant across age, disease and treatment groups. It is available in 161 languages [34]. The EQ-5D has two components: EQ-5D Visual Analogue Score asks patients how good or bad [their] health is today, on a scale of 0 (worst) to 100 (best). The second component, the EQ-5D index score, asks patients to indicate their current health status in dimensions of mobility, ability to undertake self-care, ability to undertake usual activities, pain/discomfort and anxiety/depression. It was developed in 1990 and is available in 170 languages. The PROMIS Global Health questionnaire was developed by the National Institutes of Health in 2009. The questionnaire includes a 10-question survey that assesses generic health-related quality of life compared with population norms. PROMIS 10 gives a summary indicator of health status by assessing five domains: physical function, fatigue, pain, emotional distress and social health. Nine of 10 questions are answered using 5-point Likert scales, and the tenth question is answered using a numerical rating scale.

5.6.4 Patient Reported Experiences Measures (PREMs)

Health systems are searching for ways to make their services more responsive to patients and the public. Often there is a perceived need to respond to consumer pressure and to make health care more like other consumer experiences, which has advantages and disadvantages. In order for a health system to be able to identify consumer/patients' experiences, there is a need for patient engagement. The patient is encouraged to take an active role as a key player in protecting their health, choosing appropriate treatments for episodes of ill health and managing chronic disease.

Table 5.1 Comparison of the three generic PROMs instruments

PROM instrument	Domains measured	No. of questions	Discrimination between domains and pt. types and populations	Validation	Translation
SF-36	Nine domains: Physical functioning (PF) (10), role limitation-physical (RP) (4), bodily Pain (BP) (2), general health (GH) (5), vitality (VT) (4), social functioning (SF) (2), role limitation-emotional (RE) (3), mental health (MH) (5) and health transition (1)	36	Able to detect differences between groups defined by age, sex, socio-economic status, geographical region and clinical conditions	Validated across a range of conditions, settings and languages	170 languages
EQ-5D	Four domains: Anxiety/depression (1), mobility (1), pain/discomfort (1), self-care (1) and usual activities (1)	5	Underperforms in the pain/discomfort dimension	Validated in a diverse patient population in several countries, including patient groups with chronic conditions (cardiovascular disease, respiratory disease, depression, diabetes, liver disease, personality disorders, arthritis, stroke)	170 languages
PROMIS Global 10	Five domains: Physical function, fatigue, pain, emotional distress and social health	10	N/A	Newer than the previous two measures. Validated for some conditions and patient groups	8 languages

Source: Measuring Generic Patient Reported Outcome Measures for Health System Improvement, OECD, 2017. OECD Workshop on Generic PROMs

Table 5.2 The distinct role of patients in their health care

Patients can play a distinct role in their health care by:
Understanding the causes of disease and the factors that influence health
Self-diagnosing and treating minor self-limiting conditions
Selecting the most appropriate treatment for acute conditions, in partnership with health professionals
Managing treatments and taking medications appropriately
Monitoring symptoms and the effects of treatment
Being aware of safety issues and reporting them
Learning to manage the symptoms of chronic disease
Adopting healthy behaviour, to prevent the occurrence or recurrence of disease

Considerable evidence suggests that patient engagement has been proved to improve patient's satisfaction with a positive impact on their clinical and economic aspects. The distinct role of patients in health care is presented in Table 5.2.

Recognizing their role and seeking to strengthen, it is fundamental to securing a more patient-centred approach to health care delivery. It also provides the essential underpinning for strategies that aim to reduce health inequalities and improve health for all.

PREMs seek to determine how patients find the quality of their care from the patient's perspective. Similar to PROs, patient experience is also measured using surveys or questionnaires. These can be administered in various ways. A number of approaches and questions have been developed. Questions can be tailored to a certain setting, e.g. primary care, home, hospital, long-term care or assess a specific aspect of care (e.g. continuity, autonomy, quality of information provision). PREMs, developed from a patient marking a 0–100 rating scale "thermometer" according to their satisfaction with the subject of the question, e.g. quality of today's service, fulfilment of needs, etc., have gone on to generate more granular instruments which seek to deconstruct the aggregate ratings scale score or broaden the range of questions, e.g. how patients have found service accessibility, communication, continuity and confidence. These data are now used to inform development of health services and treatments [38].

When collecting and using patient-reported data, various factors influence the outcomes of care as reported by patients, including behaviour, adherence, age and comorbidities. But readmission and mortality are subject to the same confounding variables. Like any outcome data that are used for benchmarking, confounders for patient-reported indicators should usually be adjusted to enable meaningful comparisons [39]. All data, whether patient-reported or not, have limitations and should be interpreted with the necessary caution [40].

PREMs include myriad specific condition/treatment/population instruments. Alternative to patient considerations, user reported experience measures ("UREMs") might be considered to determine treatment preference from different stakeholder groups, e.g. clinicians/nurses/other hospital staff/carer, to answer questions relating to how easy the use of new treatment strategy was, how easy it was to use aspect "abc," would you recommend the use of treatment strategy "a" or "b" to colleagues. Once again, answers to such questions help inform the development of better instruments.

5.6.4.1 PREMs Evaluation Methods

PREMs come in a variety of forms depending on the objective, the disease area, the patient manifestation and the technology, which is going to be assessed. In the simplest form, a PREM might be used to answer how good was your treatment or experience today? It could be answered by the user marking a line across a 0–100 visual analogue (thermometer-like) scale or Visual Analogue Scale (VAS) to determine a user's satisfaction with the treatment, where 100 represents absolute satisfaction and no satisfaction, as illustrated in Fig. 5.3 below. The patient is asked to indicate the level of satisfaction from the health care service she/he used by drawing a line through the 0–100 thermometer scale. The lower the mark, the less satisfied patient and vice versa. A mark at the bottom indicates absolute dissatisfaction and at the top absolute satisfaction.

Regarding PROMs, a generic measure to measure quality of life is Likert Scale, which is also used for patient experience measures, as described below.

The Likert scale is a form of a mode analysis that involves progressively strengthening ordinal categories of response to allow estimation of the frequency of responses over a continuum across respondents. This is done through the categorization of "bins" in response to questions, such as, "How satisfied were you with today's service?" [41–43]. The bins split a data series into not necessarily equally sized, but non-overlapping intervals to measure frequency over discrete ranges. For example, on a 2-point scale for the question, "How satisfied were you with the Likert scale explanation?"

Not at all Fully

The bins are clearly non-overlapping. As the number of bins increases, maintaining discrete distinction could become a challenge, e.g. over the last year, how often did you feel your clinical problems were completely met:

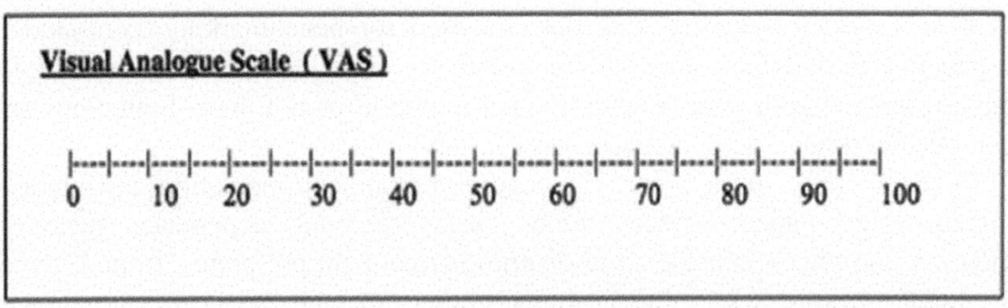

Fig. 5.3 A visual analogue scale for assessing patient reported experience of treatment

never, rarely, now and then, sometimes, frequently, always

where the difference between now and then and rarely or sometimes is debatable, which could create different responses and so unreliability if a study were repeated. Accordingly, deleting ambiguous bins, i.e. "now and then" to produce fewer but more reliable and easily distinguishable interpretations, would create a better instrument, e.g. if you asked to rank from least to most frequent, the following terms, what would be the answer?

never, rarely, sometimes, frequently, always

In this case, rarely is easily understood as less frequent than sometimes and sometimes less frequent than frequently, with never being the least frequent.

Indeed, infinite division of categories approaches reversion to a continuum, where integration of the area under the curve would define a quantitative response value to a single question, but with less intuitive interpretability than a limited number of ordinal category bins exploring qualitative progression, defeating the purpose of a categorization.

Likert scales can also be constructed to measure:

- Strength of agreement.
- Frequency of occurrence.
- Pre-event quality expectation.
- Post-event quality ranking.
- Importance.
- Likelihood.

VAS or Likert scales might be used to gather patient satisfaction, for example, where there is a low or mixed reading age [41]. However, single-item scales have previously been reported as lacking reliability and so validity [45]. Accordingly, more sophisticated instruments, disease or treatment specific should at least be considered. There are many disease specific PREMs, which are like PROMs.

PREMs represent an alternative perspective of how well a treatment seemed today, from the patient or alternative user's (carer or clinician) perspective. Some examples of PREM questionnaires are presented with a short description below:

- *PSQ-18*: The Patient Satisfaction Questionnaire Short Form a Likert scale patient satisfaction questionnaire short form (PSQ-18) uses seven domains of question, namely, general satisfaction, technical quality, interpersonal manner, communication, financial aspects, time spent with doctor and accessibility and convenience [46].
- *ENDOPREM*: Patient Experience of GI Endoscopy Questionnaire in both Routine Clinical Care and Research Studies: five domains: Anxiety, Expectations, Choice and control, Communication and Information, and Embarrassment and Dignity [47].

- *PSNCQQ*: Patient Satisfaction with Nursing Care Quality Questionnaire: 12 domains: nursing and daily care, ancillary staff and hospital environment, medical care, information, admissions, discharge and billing, overall quality of care and services, recommendations and intentions, overall quality of care during the hospital stay, overall quality of nursing care, intention to recommend the hospital to family and friends, and overall health outcomes [48].

Alternative to patient considerations, User Reported Experience Measures (UREMs) might be considered to determine treatment preference from different stakeholder groups, e.g. patient/clinicians/carer. There appears to be no consensus on a particular PREM or group of PREMs as dominating use. Accordingly, pilot leaders must make their own choices or whether they need to address user or patient satisfaction or experience.

A few examples of User Satisfaction Experience Measures are described below:

- *SUTAQ*: Service User Technology Acceptability Questionnaire: Digital system assessment by end users. Questionnaire domains: perceived benefit, privacy and discomfort, care personnel concerns, Kit as substitution and satisfaction [49].
- *SUS*: System Usability Scale: Ease of use or functional operation of technology (or lack thereof) software, hardware, mobile devices and other technological applications. Questionnaire domains: Effectiveness, efficiency and satisfaction [50].
- *UEQ*: User Experience Questionnaire. Questionnaire domains: attractiveness: perspicuity, efficiency, dependability, stimulation and novelty using a new technology [51].

5.7 Hospital Efficiency/Productivity Measures

Health care efficiency is a growing issue in most European countries where health care expenditure is rapidly increasing. Therefore, accurate productivity metrics are essential to avoid sub-optimization within the health care system. A major feature of health-care systems is substantial variation in hospital productivity. Hospital productivity varies widely across countries. The presence of such variation suggests potential areas for improvement, which can substantially lower health care costs.

This trend has resulted in the proliferation of quality indicators to measure performance and outcomes. Indicators may be used to monitor the quality of care in a single institution or across the health care system, to promote quality improvement activities, to make comparisons over time between institutions (Benchmarking) or to assist consumers to choose health-care providers [52].

For health production processes of any complexity, there are usually several stages in the transformation of resources to outcomes, and much of the confusion in discussing efficiency arises because commentators are discussing different parts of that process. To illustrate, Fig. 5.4 represents a typical (but simplified) process

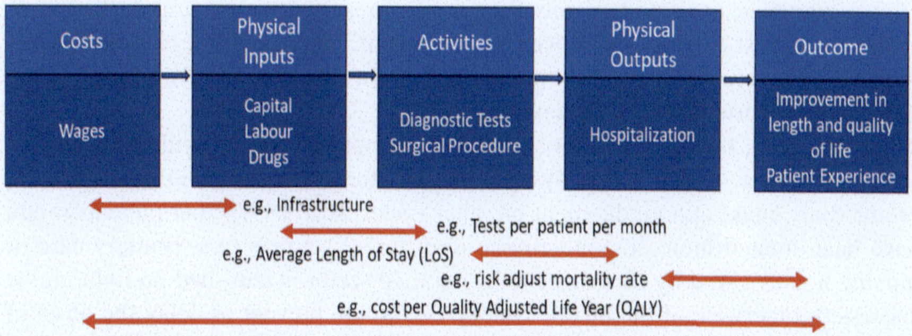

Fig. 5.4 The production process in hospital care

associated with the treatment of hospital patients. The overarching concern is with cost-effectiveness, which summarizes the transformation of costs (on the left-hand side) into valued health outcomes (the right-hand side). However, the data demands of a full system cost-effectiveness analysis are often prohibitive, and the results of such endeavours may in any case not provide policymakers with relevant information on the causes of inefficiency, or where to make improvements. To take remedial action, decision makers require more detailed diagnostic indicators of just part of the transformation process.

Physical outputs are created by aggregating activities for a particular service user. In a hospital setting, this usually refers to single episodes of patient care, an aggregation of many actions such as tests, procedures, nursing care and physician consultations. There is great scope for waste in this process, for example, in the form of duplicate or unnecessary diagnostic tests, use of branded rather than generic drugs, or unnecessarily long length of stay. Much depends on how the internal processes of the hospital are organized to maximize outputs using the given inputs. The well-known metric of length of stay, which indicates the number of bed days expended per case, falls into this category. The final stage of the health system production process is the quality of the outputs produced. Even when they employ the same physical inputs, activities or physical outputs, there is great scope for variation in effectiveness among providers. The notion of quality in health care has several connotations, including the clinical outcomes achieved (usually measured in terms of the gain in the length and quality of life) and the patient experience (a multidimensional concept). So, for example, even though two hospitals produce identical numbers of hip replacements, because of variations in clinical practice and competence, the value they confer on patients (in the form of length and quality of life and patient experience) can vary considerably. Quality-adjusted output is usually referred to as the outcome of care in the literature. Quality of care has become a central concern of policymakers, and its measurement, while contentious, is usually essential if a comprehensive picture of efficiency is to be secured. Note that the unit costs metric usually links costs to physical outputs. The numerous partial efficiency indicators that have been developed seek to shed some light on the reasons for variations in unit costs. Some metrics, such as the labour productivity or length of stay examples, are based on only partial measures of inputs or outputs. Some are capable to adjust external influences on attainment, others are not. None addresses the production process in its entirety, that is, the cost-effectiveness with which costly inputs are converted into valued outputs.

Furthermore, this example looks only at the hospital sector, without reference to other aspects of the health system. It, therefore, focuses mainly on hospital productivity, making no judgement on other issues, such as whether patients might have been treated more cost-effectively in different settings (e.g. primary care or nursing homes). And by focusing on the curative sector, it can shed no light on the success or otherwise of the health system's efforts to prevent or delay the onset of disease. A further aspect of whole system performance that is ignored is the impact of hospital performance on other sectors within the health system. For example, it may be the case that apparently high levels of efficiency in the average length of stay are being secured at the expense of heavy workloads for rehabilitative and primary care services, which may or may not be efficient from a whole system perspective.

Each organization, like a hospital or health centre, consumes a series of physical resources, referred to as inputs, often measured in terms of total costs. The organization then transforms those inputs into a series of valued outputs. Although measuring the aggregate value of inputs in terms of total costs is relatively uncontroversial, the valuation of aggregate outputs in the health sector depends on the importance placed on different health system outputs, such as health improvement and quality of life.

Almost all efficiency analysis relies on comparisons, so it is important to ensure that the entities being compared are similar. A great deal of efficiency analysis is concerned with securing such comparability. If organizational entities are operating in different circumstances, perhaps due to the marked differences in populations cared for or the patients being treated, some sort of adjustment will be needed to ensure that comparisons are made appropriately.

5.8 Economic Outcomes

Economics assesses the optimal use of resources to produce beneficial outcome for society. Cost analysis for various treatments is a useful component of outcome analysis to allow the weighting of other outcomes against unit cost or the inverse, cost per unit effect [53]. Costs may be categorized as capital (amortized or one-off) and resources which are recurrent costs. While all costs will need a unit cost record by tier, recurrent costs will also need a volume per unit time. Accordingly, economic evaluation of health care treatment options assesses among other outcomes cost, a common component of health care economic evaluations. Other outcomes include clinical effectiveness and health economic outcomes such as PROMs including utility measures such as "QALYs." As demand typically exceeds supply for health care, health care suppliers seek value for money. Accordingly, economic evaluations use opportunity cost to identify the best value option out of a choice of the intervention and the next best alternative treatment, the comparator, typically usual care, and the current treatment [54].

5.9 Combining Cost and Effect

In health economics, the cost alone does not translate the value of a specific treatment or technology without considering the effect of the specific technology. The combination of the lower cost and higher beneficial effect outcomes is the desired composition for the decision-making process. Yet, if each outcome falls on a different treatment option, a determination is still needed between options, with a consistent approach, i.e. without reverting to personnel preference which can create a varied health care accessibility landscape for treatments across a country. The answer lies in using a ratio of incremental cost divided by incremental effect where the intervention's outcomes are used after subtraction of the comparator's equivalent outcomes, e.g. intervention cost-comparator cost divided by intervention effect minus comparator effect [54]. This creates the incremental cost-effectiveness ratio ("ICER"), which may be written as indicated below:

$$\text{ICER} = \frac{\text{Cost of intervention–cost of comparator}}{\text{Effect of intervention–effect of comparator}}$$

where the effect may be expressed in clinical effect or health economic terms, i.e. PROMs such as quality-adjusted life years (QALYs) or more typically, both.

The economic analysis should provide an estimate of the treatment strategies costs over different time periods, e.g. over the course of the study, per treatment event and per annum. The economic analysis should be an estimate of the regular day to day operational cost for treatment of a patient with both treatment strategies and the incremental difference between the two (intervention minus comparator over the course of the study, with duration of each treatment stated).

For economic outcome, an analysis of direct medical costs, direct non-medical costs, indirect non-medical costs, symptom impact and adverse event costs should be measured per patient per unit time, with the unit being the duration of each treatment strategy. One-off and recurrent costs should be assessed for unit cost and resource quantity. Cost can be estimated from broadly two perspectives.

- The payer's or National Health System.
- The patient's or society's perspective.

For the later, one must add the cost of carers unremunerated time and the patient's time off when sick [54].

The NHS provider perspective includes treatment costs such as medicine costs, administration and monitoring, other health service resource use costs associated with the managing the disease (e.g. GP visits, hospital admissions) and costs of managing adverse events caused by treatment. It does not include patients' costs of obtaining care such as transportation, over-the-counter purchases, co-payments or time off work. Yet, it is up to technology pilots if they wish to gather more data, e.g. on productivity losses arising from patients' inability to work, charged according to their policy at either a common minimum rate or the national average wage to be able to present the social perspective.

The cost to health payer whether government department or insurer for each treatment strategy equates to:

$$\text{Departmental Cost} = \text{n patients} \times \text{mean patient cost per treatment strategy}$$

Costs are separated into three categories which are further analysed below: (a) direct medical costs, (b) direct non-medical costs and (c) indirect non-medical costs.

- Direct medical costs can include hospitalization (short- and long-term), outpatient follow-up, residential and day care, pharmaceutical interventions and laboratory testing. Costs of treatment adverse events should also be noted by severity.
- Direct non-medical costs include transport costs to and from hospital, e.g. non-emergency ambulance for non-motile patients and paid carer giver time.
- Indirect non-medical costs include patient and unpaid carer time off work, charged either at a country's minimum wage or social security payments.

And likewise, the quality-of-life profile and QALYs generated from each treatment over the course of the study should be noted [54].

For the economic analysis of AI technologies, an analysis of direct medical costs, direct non-medical costs, indirect non-medical costs, symptom impact and adverse event costs will be performed. The resource utilization should be measured per patient per unit time, following the micro-costing methodology, including the number and type of major resources of the patient needs. The product of unit cost and volume is used to determine the overall cost of each treatment strategy, noting recurrent costs quantity. Incremental outcomes from intervention and comparator may be calculated for clinical, health economic and economic outcomes whereby economic incremental outcome would be the sum of costs across treatment duration for each treatment strategy with comparator subtracted from intervention's cost. The equations are presented below:

1. $$\text{Incremental Cost} = \text{Cost of intervention (new AI technology)} - \text{cost of comparator (current technology)}$$
2. $$\text{Incremental Effect} = \text{Effect of intervention (new AI technology)} - \text{Effect of comparator (current technology)}$$

References

1. Dilsizian, S. E., & Siegel, E. L. (2014). Artificial intelligence in medicine and cardiac imaging: Harnessing big data and advanced computing to provide personalized medical diagnosis and treatment. *Current Cardiology Reports, 16*(1), 441. https://doi.org/10.1007/s11886-013-0441-8
2. Jha, S., & Topol, E. J. (2016). Adapting to Artificial Intelligence: Radiologists and pathologists as information specialists. *JAMA, 316*(22), 2353–2354. https://doi.org/10.1001/jama.2016.17438
3. Lee, C. S., Nagy, P. G., Weaver, S. J., et al. (2013). Cognitive and system factors contributing to diagnostic errors in radiology. *AJR. American Journal of Roentgenology, 201*(3), 611–617. https://doi.org/10.2214/AJR.12.10375
4. Neill, D. B. (2013). Using artificial intelligence to improve hospital inpatient care. *IEEE Intelligent Systems, 28*, 92–95. https://doi.org/10.1109/MIS.2013.51
5. Cole, R. E., & Scott, W. R. (2000). *The quality movement & organization theory*. Sage.
6. Institute of Medicine (US). (2001). *Committee on Quality of Health Care in America, Crossing the quality chasm: A new health system for the 21st century*. National Academies Press (US). https://doi.org/10.17226/10027
7. Grol, R. (2001). Improving the quality of medical care: Building bridges among professional pride, payer profit, and patient satisfaction. *JAMA, 286*(20), 2578–2585. https://doi.org/10.1001/jama.286.20.2578
8. Raven, J. H., Tolhurst, R. J., Tang, S., & van den Broek, N. (2012). What is quality in maternal and neonatal health care? *Midwifery, 28*(5), e676–e683. https://doi.org/10.1016/j.midw.2011.09.003
9. Institute of Medicine (US) Committee to Design a Strategy for Quality Review and Assurance in Medicare. (1990). In K. N. Lohr (Ed.), *Medicare: A strategy for quality assurance* (Vol. 1). National Academies Press (US). https://doi.org/10.17226/1547
10. Nordgren, L. (2009). Value creation in health care services – Developing service productivity: Experiences from Sweden. *International Journal of Public Sector Management, 22*, 114–127.
11. Longtin, Y., Sax, H., Leape, L. L., Sheridan, S. E., Donaldson, L., & Pittet, D. (2010). Patient participation: Current knowledge and applicability to patient safety. *Mayo Clinic Proceedings, 85*(1), 53–62. https://doi.org/10.4065/mcp.2009.0248
12. EC. (2014). *The 2015 ageing report – Underlying assumptions and projection methodologies* (European Economy, 8/2014). European Commission.
13. Singh, O., & Kumar, S. (2012). Measuring effectiveness of health program intervention in the field. *Intelligent Information Management, 4*(5), 194–206. https://doi.org/10.4236/iim.2012.45029
14. Ramalho, A., Castro, P., Gonçalves-Pinho, M., Teixeira, J., Santos, J. V., Viana, J., Lobo, M., Santos, P., & Freitas, A. (2019). Primary health care quality indicators: An umbrella review. *PLoS One, 14*(8), e0220888. https://doi.org/10.1371/journal.pone.0220888
15. Fenwick, E., Marshall, D. A., Levy, A. R., et al. (2006). Using and interpreting cost-effectiveness acceptability curves: An example using data from a trial of management strategies for atrial fibrillation. *BMC Health Services Research, 6*, 52. https://doi.org/10.1186/1472-6963-6-52
16. Teisberg, E., Wallace, S., & O'Hara, S. (2020). Defining and implementing value-based health care: A strategic framework. *Academic Medicine: Journal of the Association of American Medical Colleges, 95*(5), 682–685. https://doi.org/10.1097/ACM.0000000000003122l9
17. Street, R. L., Elwyn, G., & Epstein, R. M. (2012). Patient preferences and healthcare outcomes: An ecological perspective. *Expert Review of Pharmacoeconomics & Outcomes Research, 12*(2), 167–180. https://doi.org/10.1586/erp.12.3
18. Yorkston, K., & Baylor, C. (2019). Tutorial – Patient-reported outcomes measures: An introduction for clinicians. *Perspectives of the ASHA Special Interest Groups, 4*(1), 8–15. https://pubs.asha.org/doi/abs/10.1044/2018_PERS-ST-2018-0001

19. Torrance, G. W., Thomas, W. H., & Sackett, D. L. (1972). A utility maximization model for evaluation of health care programs. *Health Services Research, 7*(2), 118–133.
20. McCabe, C. J., Stevens, K. J., & Brazier, J. E. (2005). Utility scores for the Health Utilities Index Mark 2: An empirical assessment of alternative mapping functions. *Medical Care, 43*(6), 627–635. https://doi.org/10.1097/01.mlr.0000163666.00471.8e
21. Furlong, W. J., Feeny, D. H., Torrance, G. W., & Barr, R. D. (2001). The Health Utilities Index (HUI) system for assessing health-related quality of life in clinical studies. *Annals of Medicine, 33*(5), 375–384. https://doi.org/10.3109/07853890109002092
22. Eadie, T. L., Otero, D., Cox, S., Johnson, J., Baylor, C. R., Yorkston, K. M., & Doyle, P. C. (2016). The relationship between communicative participation and postlaryngectomy speech outcomes. *Head & Neck, 38*(1), E1955–61. https://doi.org/10.1002/hed.24353
23. Francis, D. O. (2014). Patient-centered outcomes research in voice. *SIG 3 Perspectives on Voice and Voice Disorders, 24*(1), 21–31. https://doi.org/10.1044/vvd24.1.21
24. Petersen, M. A., Groenvold, M., Aaronson, N. K., Chie, W. C., Conroy, T., Costantini, A., Fayers, P., Helbostad, J., Holzner, B., Kaasa, S., Singer, S., Velikova, G., Young, T., & EORTC Quality of Life Group. (2010). Development of computerised adaptive testing (CAT) for the EORTC QLQ-C30 dimensions – General approach and initial results for physical functioning. *European Journal of Cancer, 46*(8), 1352–1358. https://doi.org/10.1016/j.ejca.2010.02.011
25. Snyder, A., Makarov, V., Merghoub, T., et al. (2014). Genetic basis for clinical response to CTLA-4 blockade in melanoma. *The New England Journal of Medicine, 371*(23), 2189. https://www.nejm.org/doi/full/10.1056/NEJMoa1406498
26. Amtmann, D., Cook, K. F., Johnson, K. L., & Cella, D. (2011). The PROMIS initiative: Involvement of rehabilitation stakeholders in development and examples of applications in rehabilitation research. *Archives of Physical Medicine and Rehabilitation, 92*(10), S12–S19. https://doi.org/10.1016/j.apmr.2011.04.025
27. Cella, D., Gershon, R., Lai, J. S., & Choi, S. (2007). The future of outcomes measurement: Item banking, tailored short-forms, and computerized adaptive assessment. *Quality of Life Research, 16*(1), 133–141. https://doi.org/10.1007/s11136-007-9204-6
28. Barrett, A., Hahn-Pedersen, J., Kragh, N., Evans, E., & Gnanasakthy, A. (2019). Patient-reported outcome measures in atopic dermatitis and chronic hand eczema in adults. *The Patient, 12*(5), 445–459. https://doi.org/10.1007/s40271-19-00373-y
29. Cook, K. F., Monahan, P. O., & McHorney, C. A. (2003). Delicate balance between theory and practice: Health status assessment and item response theory. *Medical Care, 41*(5), 571–574. https://doi.org/10.1097/01.MLR.0000064780.30399.A4
30. Valderas, J. M., Kotzeva, A., Espallargues, M., Guyatt, G., Ferrans, C. E., Halyard, M. Y., Revicki, D. A., Symonds, T., Parada, A., & Alonso, J. (2008). The impact of measuring patient-reported outcomes in clinical practice: A systematic review of the literature. *Quality of Life Research, 17*(2), 179–193. https://doi.org/10.1007/s11136-007-9295-0. Epub 2008 Jan 4.
31. EuroQol Group. (1990). EuroQol – A new facility for the measurement of health-related quality of life. *Health Policy, 16*(3), 199–208. https://doi.org/10.1016/0168-8510(90)90421-9
32. Dolan, P. (1997). Modeling valuations for EuroQol health states. *Medical Care, 35*(11), 1095–1108. https://doi.org/10.1097/00005650-199711000-00002
33. World Health Organization. Division of Mental Health and Prevention of Substance Abuse. (1997). *WHOQOL: measuring quality of life*. World Health Organization. https://apps.who.int/iris/handle/10665/63482
34. Ware, J. E., Jr., & Sherbourne, C. D. (1992). The MOS 36-item short-form health survey (SF-36). I. Conceptual framework and item selection. *Medical Care, 30*(6), 473–483.
35. Brazier, J., Roberts, J., & Deverill, M. (2002). The estimation of a preference-based measure of health from the SF-36. *Journal of Health Economics, 21*(2), 271–292. https://doi.org/10.1016/s0167-6296(01)00130-8
36. Garratt, A., Schmidt, L., Mackintosh, A., & Fitzpatrick, R. (2002). Quality of life measurement: bibliographic study of patient assessed health outcome measures. *BMJ, 324*(7351), 1417. https://doi.org/10.1136/bmj.324.7351.1417

37. Cella, D., Yount, S., Rothrock, N., Gershon, R., Cook, K., Reeve, B., et al. (2007). The Patient-Reported Outcomes Measurement Information System (PROMIS): Progress of an NIH Roadmap cooperative group during its first two years. *Medical Care, 45*(1), S3–S11. https://doi.org/10.1097/01.mlr.0000258615.42478.55
38. Doty, M., et al. (2017). *Mirror*: International comparison reflects flaws and opportunities for better U.S. *Health Care*. https://doi.org/10.15868/socialsector.27698
39. Nuttall, D., Parkin, D., & Devlin, N. (2015). Inter-provider comparison of patient reported outcomes: Developing and adjustment to account for differences in patient case mix. *Health Economics, 24*(1), 41–54. https://doi.org/10.1002/hec.2999
40. Calvert, M., O'Connor, D., & Basch, E. (2019). Harnessing the patient voice in real-world evidence: The essential role of patient-reported outcomes. *Nature Reviews Drug Discovery*. https://doi.org/10.1038/d41573-019-00088-7
41. Likert, R. (1932). A technique for the measurement of attitudes. *Archives of Psychology, 22*(140), 55.
42. Norman, G. (2010). Likert scales, levels of measurement and the "laws" of statistics. *Advances in Health Sciences Education: Theory and Practice, 15*(5), 625–632. https://doi.org/10.1007/s10459-010-9222-y. Epub 2010 Feb 10.
43. Sullivan, G. M., & Artino, A. R., Jr. (2013). Analyzing and interpreting data from likert-type scales. *Journal of Graduate Medical Education, 5*(4), 541–542. https://doi.org/10.4300/jgme-5-4-18
44. McLeod, S. A. (2019). *Likert scale definition, examples and analysis*. Simply Psychology. https://www.simplypsychology.org/likert-scale.html
45. Ayearst, L. E., Flett, G. L., & Hewitt, P. L. (2012). Where is multidimensional perfectionism in DSM-5? A question posed to the DSM-5 personality and personality disorders work group. *Personality Disorders: Theory, Research, and Treatment, 3*(4), 458–469. https://doi.org/10.1037/a0026354
46. Thayaparan, A. J., & Mahdi, E. (2013). The Patient Satisfaction Questionnaire Short Form (PSQ-18) as an adaptable, reliable, and validated tool for use in various settings. *Medical Education Online, 18*, 21747. https://doi.org/10.3402/meo.v18i0.21747
47. Neilson, L. J., Patterson, J., von Wagner, C., et al. (2020). *Frontline Gastroenterology, 11*, 209–217. https://doi.org/10.1136/flgastro-2019-101321
48. Laschinger, H. S., McGillis, L., Pedersen, C., & Almost, J. (2005). A psychometric analysis of the patient satisfaction with nursing care quality questionnaire. *Journal of Nursing Care Quality, 20*(3), 220–230.
49. Torbjørnsen, A., Småstuen, M. C., Jenum, A. K., Årsand, E., & Ribu, L. (2018). The service user technology acceptability questionnaire: Psychometric evaluation of the Norwegian version. *JMIR Human Factors, 5*(4), e10255. https://doi.org/10.2196/10255
50. Brook, J. (2013). SUS: A retrospective. *Journal of Usability Studies, 8*(2), 29–40. JUS Journal Template (uxpajournal.org)
51. Hinderks, A., Schrepp, M., Domínguez Mayo, M. J., Escalona, M. J., & Thomaschewski, J. (2019). Developing a UX KPI based on the user experience questionnaire. *Computer Standards & Interfaces, 65*, 38–44. https://doi.org/10.1016/j.csi.2019.01.007
52. Copnell, B., Hagger, V., Wilson, S. G., Evans, S. M., Sprivulis, P. C., & Cameron, P. A. (2009). Measuring the quality of hospital care: An inventory of indicators. *Internal Medicine Journal, 39*(6), 352–360. https://doi.org/10.1111/j.1445-5994.2009.01961.x
53. Aluko, P., Graybill, E., Craig, D., Henderson, C., Drummond, M., Wilson, E. C. F., Robalino, S., Vale, L., & on behalf of the Campbell and Cochrane Economics Methods Group. (2021). Chapter 20: Economic evidence. In J. P. T. Higgins, J. Thomas, J. Chandler, M. Cumpston, T. Li, M. J. Page, & V. A. Welch (Eds.), *Cochrane handbook for systematic reviews of interventions version 6.2 (updated February 2021)*. Cochrane. Available from www.training.cochrane.org/handbook
54. Drummond, M. F., Sculpher, M. J., Torrance, G. W., O'Brien, B. J., & Stoddart, G. L. (2005). *Methods for the economic evaluation of health care programme* (3rd ed.). Oxford University Press.

Chapter 6
Survey Design and Methodology of a Universal Cybersecurity Toolkit and a Thread Architecture for Intelligent Healthcare Business Applications

Athina Bourdena, Evangelos K. Markakis, Michael Kontoulis, Sotiris Pelekis, Ariadni Michalitsi-Psarrou, Anna Georgiadou, Georgios Doukas, Christos Ntanos, Irini Dimou, Markos Kourgiantakis, George Mastorakis, Evangelos Pallis, Constandinos X. Mavromoustakis, and Andreas Andreou

6.1 Introduction

The European Commission has placed digital at the core of its strategy, by setting the Digital Single Market as one of its 10 priorities. The aim is to open up digital opportunities for people and business and to make the EU's single market fit for the digital age [1]. The healthcare market is a major player for this transformation: the incorporation of Information and Communications Technologies (ICT), digitalisation and data exchange (including health records and data) are profoundly changing the way (and the dynamics) healthcare services provide for citizens at the national and pan-European levels: hospitals and care centres handle, store and exchange large amounts of sensitive patient data; medical devices (e.g. medication infusion systems, pacemakers) collecting personal health details are becoming more sophisticated and connected, allowing remote visualisation and the automatic

A. Bourdena (✉) · I. Dimou · M. Kourgiantakis
Department of Business Administration & Tourism, Hellenic Mediterranean University, Heraklion, Iraklion, Greece
e-mail: bourdena@hmu.gr; irdimou@hmu.gr; mkourg@hmu.gr

E. K. Markakis
Department of Electrical and Computer Engineering, Hellenic Mediterranean University, Heraklion, Crete, Greece
e-mail: markakis@pasiphae.eu

M. Kontoulis · S. Pelekis · A. Michalitsi-Psarrou · A. Georgiadou · G. Doukas · C. Ntanos
Decision Support Systems Laboratory, National Technical University of Athens, Zografou, Greece
e-mail: mkontoulis@epu.ntua.gr; spelekis@epu.ntua.gr; amichal@epu.ntua.gr; ageorgiadou@epu.ntua.gr; gdoukas@epu.ntua.gr; cntanos@epu.ntua.gr

© The Author(s), under exclusive license to Springer Nature Switzerland AG 2024

A. Bourdena et al. (eds.), *Intelligent Technologies for Healthcare Business Applications*, Signals and Communication Technology,
https://doi.org/10.1007/978-3-031-58527-2_6

incorporation of data in personal health records; even wearables and IoT devices, such as activity trackers, watches incorporating heart rate sensors, smart home sensors, albeit not rated as medical devices, may produce data that is directly or indirectly relevant for the purposes of assessing a patient's health and wellness status (thus sensitive data).

Among many benefits, providers and other stakeholders are using digital health in their efforts to reduce inefficiencies, improve access, reduce costs, increase quality, and make medicine more personalised for patients [2]. As patients, consumers use digital health to better manage and monitor their health and wellness-related activities [3]. However, this rich and promising ecosystem, when more open and accessible, also brings new risks and vulnerabilities regarding cyber threats and incidents.

Additionally, the universal use of a variety of communication devices and enabling devices such as tablets, phones, wearables has created a new audience ignorant to the dangers existing in this connected world. Furthermore, the types of applications and sensitive information used and maintained on such devices have increased exponentially over recent years. It is not uncommon for a device [4] to uphold info of patient, individual patient datagrams, patient photographs and variety of other sensitive info secured by a four numbers password [5] that can be "cracked" in less than 20 s [6] or the relatively small size of these devices make such devices increasingly susceptible to loss and/or theft. Moreover, these agnostic users feel comfortable with technology not understanding the risks and the value of the info [7] they control.

In this respect, hospitals and care centres are prime targets for cyber criminals, especially concerning data theft (electronic medical records could be worth up to $USD 1000 [8, 9]), denial-of-service (e.g. DDoS attacks) and ransomware (the labelled WannaCry caused the "biggest ransomware attack in history" with 57,000 infections in 99 countries [10], which included several hospitals). Only in 2014, according to the U.S. Department of Health and Human Services Office for Civil Rights, almost 1.6 million people had their medical information stolen from healthcare providers. Relative analysis predicts more than 25 million people [9] will have their medical and/or personal information stolen from their healthcare

G. Mastorakis
Department of Management Science and Technology, Hellenic Mediterranean University, Agios Nikolaos, Crete, Greece
e-mail: gmastorakis@hmu.gr

E. Pallis
Department of Industrial Design and Production Engineering, School of Engineering, University of West Attica, Athens, Greece
e-mail: epallis@uniwa.gr

C. X. Mavromoustakis · A. Andreou
Department of Computer Science, University of Nicosia and University of Nicosia Research Foundation, Nicosia, Cyprus
e-mail: mavromoustakis.c@unic.ac.cy; andreou.andreas@unic.ac.cy

provider's digitised records between 2015 and 2019 [11]. Aside from not having cybersecurity as part of their core concerns, healthcare institutions typically operate on legacy hardware or software with unpatched vulnerabilities ripe for exploitation, including operating systems and also medical devices' firmware [12]. Still, cyber attackers may also exploit the many vulnerabilities of the increasing healthcare ecosystem brought by smartphones, apps, smart devices (in hospitals, care centres or at a patient's home).

- 80% of European companies have experienced at least one cybersecurity incident in 2016
- In 2013 Target suffered a breach losing 110 M customer's data and 40 million credit cards. In 2014 Home Depot suffered a similar attack.
- Community Health Systems suffered a breach having 4.5 M patient records stolen.
- NHS also suffered attacks.

In particular, medical data breaches have been estimated to cost the healthcare industry about $6 billion. The Ponemon study reported that malware attacks caused security breaches in 78% of healthcare organisations. Cyber-attacks are up 125% since 2010 and are the leading cause of health data security breaches [13].

What Healthcare Organizations Can Learn From the Latest Cyberattack? WannaCry, the largest ransomware attack in history, was discovered on May 12 in the UK and swiftly spread to an estimated 57,000 computers. The virus proliferated quickly and within days, hit more than 200,000 victims from 150 countries, disrupting healthcare systems, banks, schools and major businesses. According to Europol, the European law enforcement agency, FedEx, Nissan, electronics maker Hitachi, Spanish telecom company Telefónica and the United Kingdom's National Health Service (NHS) were among the victims. The recently introduced SECurity as a Service (SECaaS) model offers a novel security solution for cloud-services' users. This paradigm grants a variety of advances in security services such as Authentication as a Service (AaaS) and Encryption as a Service (ENCaaS) to Cloud Infrastructure costumers [14].

Subsequently, the maturity of cloud computing [15], with its abundancy of IT resources and its connected security policies databases, allows for the seamless realisation of resource-demanding solutions such as SECaaS. Nonetheless, several security aspects such as vulnerability assessment of existing and newly added devices as well as real-time alerting and mitigation of security threats are not addressed, rendering those solutions unable to cope with the state-of-the-art cybersecurity threats [16]. This can result in major loss of reputation and revenue, for large organisations such as healthcare institutions, where their widespread heterogeneous infrastructure is almost impossible to maintain and administer, rendering them prone to cyber-attacks [17]. Moreover, companies' security posture should constantly adapt to the ever-evolving cyber-security risks imposed by multiple sources. However, traditional penetration testing is still very much a point-in-time assessment, dealing with specific tasks. And on top of that, most of the commercial solutions cannot deal with new sophisticated advanced attacks such as zero-hour exploits and advanced persistent threats that have triggered unknown threads. Attackers and malicious code move fast, making preparation and quick attack intervention and remediation vitally important. Finally, cloud computing by design cannot deliver services in real-time. Thus, deployment of latency-crucial services in the cloud proves to be inefficient. On the other hand, the advancements in edge computing (EC) [18, 19] allow for the efficient deployment and delivery of minimum-latency services. Therefore, a health and care tailored Cyber Security vulnerability assessment toolkit, able to proactively assess and mitigate cyber-security threats known or unknown, imposed by devices and services within a corporate ecosystem, is missing.

6.2 Purpose, Scope and Architecture of a Universal Cyber Security Toolkit

SPHINX project [20] aims to introduce a health tailored Universal Cyber Security Toolkit, thus enhancing the cyber protection of health and care IT Ecosystem and ensuring the patient data privacy and integrity. SPHINX toolkit provides an automated zero-touch device and service verification toolkit that can be easily adapted or embedded into existing medical, clinical or health infrastructures, whereas a user/admin will be able to choose from a number of available security services through SPHINX cyber security toolkit. The SPHINX toolkit enables service providers to specify complete services and sell or advertise these through a secure and easy to use interface.

In other words, SPHINX specifically focuses on the research, design, development and pilot prototyping of framework solutions that address the following threat forms: (i) cyber terrorism directly involving radicalisation and illegitimate groups, aiming to bridge the gap between social, policy research and security practices; (ii) threats to public critical infrastructures of health care actors that are traditionally involved in real-world tasks. The concept of cyber-espionage and trust building between entities will also be considered in this case. (iii) Threats to ecosystems of connected devices via IoT applications where low-level network research will be introduced and via specially designated testbeds. To provide for the sustainability and adaptability of the SPHINX solution, an advanced testbed will be set up and operated during and after the project course, demonstrating the advanced concepts of network level (protocol layer) advanced cybersecurity known or unknown threats detections and deference.

In this respect, this chapter presents the SPHINX detailed planning of pilot operations. The pilot operations plan describes the activities to be performed, the roles and responsibilities, organisational structures, assets, security processes and logistics processes in all the four pilot sites, as well as the evaluation framework to be applied for the assessment and validation of the SPHINX toolkit.

Healthcare organisations (e.g. hospitals, care centres) from different countries became targets of cyber-attacks (e.g. data theft, denial-of-service, ransomware) due to the high value of health records in the black market and the growth of the attack surface of those healthcare organisations due to the introduction of the digitisation of processes, eHealth and mHealth technologies, the Internet of Medical Things (IoMT) and the need to exchange healthcare data among healthcare organisations to support healthcare delivery.

As shown in Fig. 6.1, the SPHINX toolkit delivers advanced cybersecurity protection to four healthcare organisations, acting as reference pilot sites in three countries: Greece, Romania and Portugal. It protects the exchange of medical data between healthcare providers through its components and improves cyber protection of the infrastructure of healthcare organisations. It also ensures the patients' data privacy and integrity, by identifying modern and advanced cyber threats and by preventing or reducing the occurrence of cyber-attacks. According to *SPHINX Architecture*, the major building blocks that comprise the SPHINX toolkit and its advanced cybersecurity capabilities for the healthcare sector are the Device Verification and Certification, the Automated Cyber Security Risk Assessment, the Decision Support System and Interactive Dashboards, the Cyber Security Toolbox, the Third-

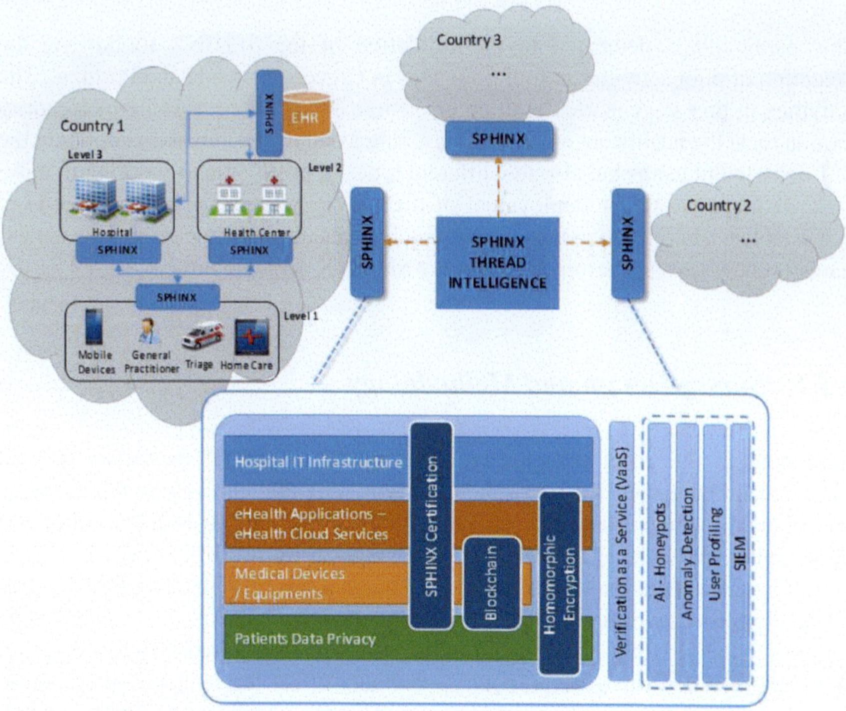

Fig. 6.1 Description of the SPHINX concept

party APIs and the Common Integration Platform. Specific SPHINX tools will be dedicated to specific elements of the ICT ecosystem, such as protocol analysis, detection of anomalous behaviour, security events, intrusion detection, vulnerability assessment and honeypots. Through the Common Integration Platform, the SPHINX toolkit enables each SPHINX tool to be deployed independently and enables the interaction of third-party healthcare solution providers with SPHINX's tools.

SPHINX users are able to interact with the multiple services and functions of the SPHINX toolkit in an intuitive and user-friendly way, through Interactive Dashboards. In the Interactive Dashboard, users receive alerts about cyber security threats or attacks and associated reports, containing recommendations on appropriate response actions following a detected cyber-attack and where the cyber-attack happened. Aside from the interactive dashboard, the SPHINX toolkit provides a personalised data security management tool that allows users to setup the tools required by the ICT ecosystem. The SPHINX toolkit even allows users to run and validate simulated application scenarios and use cases in a safe and isolated testing environment.

6.3 The Cybersecurity Awareness Status of Pilot Sites

This paragraph is dedicated to the validation of the SPHINX toolkit via the execution of pilot activities in four pilot sites in Greece, Romania and Portugal. The activities in this stage started with an effort to establish the level of cybersecurity awareness at the healthcare organisations acting as pilot sites, involving not only the ICT department teams but also the different types of professionals working in those organisations, before the deployment of the SPHINX toolkit. The objective is to first establish a baseline and then to adequately evaluate the cybersecurity awareness status of the pilot sites before and after the SPHINX deployment.

6.3.1 Survey Design and Methodology

According to the 2018 statistics on the proportion of ICT specialists in total employment published by Eurostat, it is observed that the relevant percentage for Portugal, Romania and Greece (the countries hosting the SPHINX pilots) is significantly below the EU-28 average percentage, as illustrated in Fig. 6.2.

Taking into account the aforementioned report, it is the SPHINX partners' objective to establish the level of cybersecurity awareness in the healthcare organisations involved in the SPHINX pilots and to explore whether the limitation in ICT employment and resources, in general, could potentially affect the vulnerability of those organisations to cybersecurity-related threats. To this end, two surveys were created:

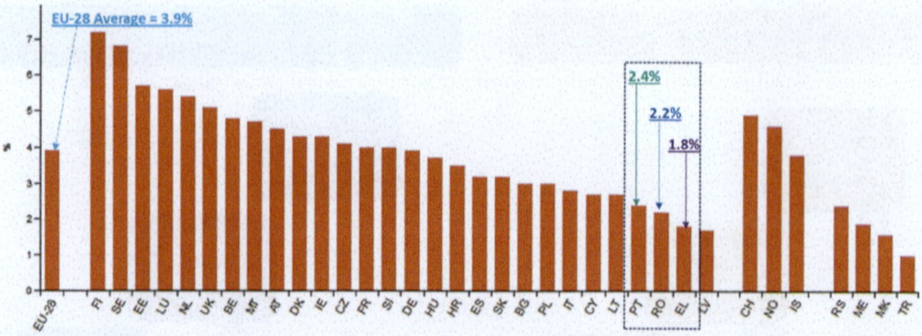

Fig. 6.2 Proportion of ICT specialists in total employment

the first is targeted to the ICT departments and the second one is focused on the non-ICT employees (medical, auxiliary, laboratory and administrative personnel).

The ICT questionnaires present five parts: the first part refers to demographics (i.e. years of experience, served population, type of healthcare organisation and total number of employees); the second part deals with questions related to ICT daily activities, such as the number of performed cybersecurity trainings, the cybersecurity budget allocation, the ICT percentage employment and the presence of Cybersecurity departments; the third section focuses on the employed login and networking policies and users' external accesses; the fourth section includes questions on existing cybersecurity practices; and the fifth section contains questions security incidents and the *time to respond*. On the other hand, the non-ICT questionnaire comprises questions on demographics, status of the employment, performed training on the General Data Protection Regulation (GDPR), the capacity to identify cyberattacks and the familiarity with security processes and precautions.

Figures 6.3 and 6.4 present the two employees' categories targeted in the questionnaires and the procedures followed to distribute the questionnaires and collect the results. After having the questionnaires translated to the Greek, Romanian and Portuguese languages, invitations were sent to the employees of the three SPHINX end-user partners, requesting them to voluntarily participate in the anonymous surveys online. The requests for participation were shared through the organisation's formal procedures (DYPE5 and HESE) or through social networks (e.g. Facebook) for the POLARIS case, and Google forms were used to make the questionnaires accessible online. The project embraced about 11.000 healthcare professionals (9000 in Greece, 1700 in Portugal and 218 in Romania) and approximately 69 ICT employees (60 in Greece, 7 in Portugal and 2 in Romania). It is noted that DYPE5 sent the invitations to 13 supervised hospitals and 60 supervised primary care units. The survey was conducted between September and November 2019.

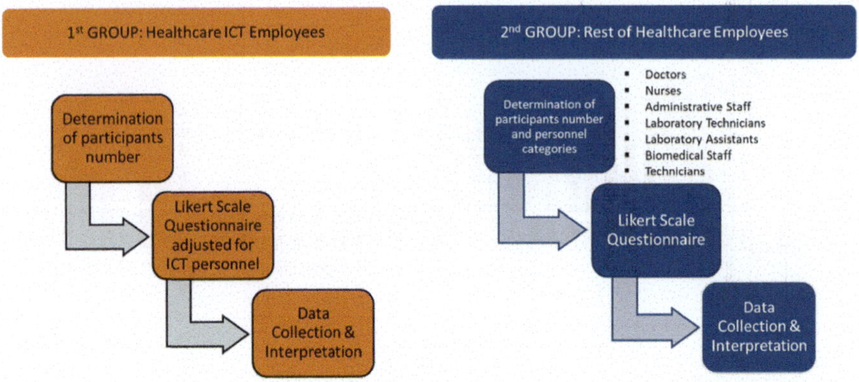

Fig. 6.3 Target group determination and survey design

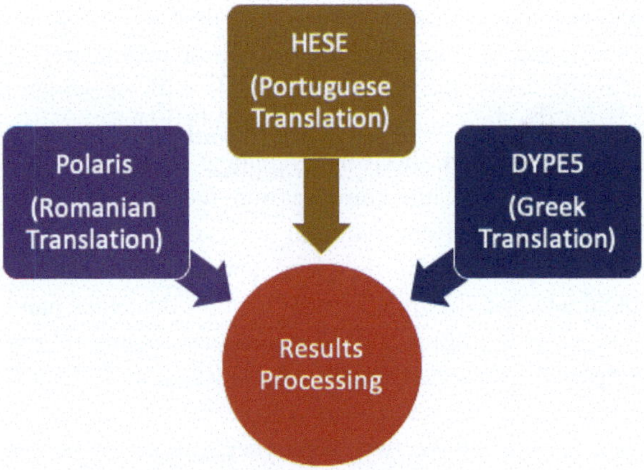

Fig. 6.4 Questionnaires translation process and results processing

6.3.2 Questionnaires Results and the Analysis of the Cybersecurity Awareness Status

6.3.2.1 The ICT Questionnaire

A total of 37 answers were received for the ICT questionnaire, resulting in a 53.6% response rate. The questionnaire's demographic results are shown in Table 6.1.

The evaluation of the ICT questionnaire responses revealed that the proportion of ICT employees in total employment is below 1% for all pilot sites, a percentage that is also below the countries' average as depicted on Fig. 6.2. 46% of the ICT employees reported that, in average, 100 K Euros had been spent to procure ICT equipment during the last 2 years (less than 5% from this amount was allocated to cybersecurity appliances, software or hardware). All ICT departments

Table 6.1 Demographics of ICT Questionnaire responses

	DYPE5	HESE	POLARIS
Number of answers	$n = 28$ (100%)	$n = 7$ (100%)	$n = 2$ (100%)
Gender			
Male	18 (64.3%)	6 (85.7%)	2 (100%)
Female	10 (35.7%)	1 (14.3%)	–
Age			
20–39	9 (32.1%)	2 (28.6%)	–
40–60	19 (67.9%)	5 (71.4%)	2 (100%)
60+	–	–	–
Education			
Secondary education	4 (14.3%)	3 (42.9%)	–
Vocational training institute	1 (3.6%)	1 (14.3%)	–
Bachelor's degree	16 (57.1%)	1 (14.3%)	1 (50%)
MSc	6 (21.4%)	2 (28.6%)	1 (50%)
PhD	1 (3.6%)	–	–
Years of experience			
0–5	4 (14.3%)	–	–
6–10	3 (10.7%)	1 (14.3%)	–
More than 10	21 (75%)	6 (85.7%)	2 (100%)
Position			
ICT staff	21 (75%)	6 (85.7%)	1 (50%)
ICT manager	4 (14.3%)	1 (14.3%)	1 (50%)
ICT director	3 (10.7%)	–	–
Healthcare organisation			
Hospital	25 (89.3%)	7 (100%)	2 (100%)
Clinic	–	–	–
Health authority	3 (10.7%)	–	–
Organisation range			
National	–	–	–
Regional	3 (10.7%)	7 (100%)	–
Local	25 (89.3%)	–	2 (100%)
Serving area population			
Population < 100 k	8 (28.5%)	–	–
Population 100 k–300 k	15 (53.6%)	1 (14.3%)	–
Population > 300 k	5 (17.9%)	6 (85.7%)	2 (100%)
Employees in the organisation			
Employees <100	5 (17.9%)	–	–
Employees 100–300	5 (17.9%)	–	2 (100%)
Employees 301–600	1 (3.6%)	–	–
Employees 601–1000	8 (28.5%)	–	–
Employees >1000	9 (32.1%)	7 (100%)	–

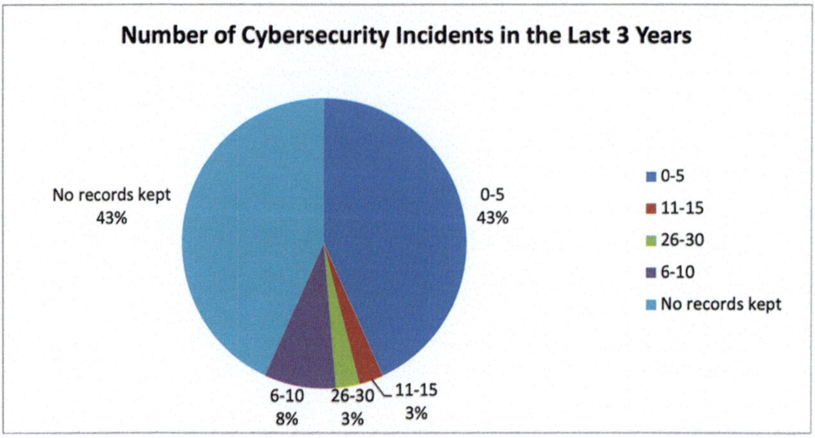

Fig. 6.5 Cybersecurity incidents in the last 3 years

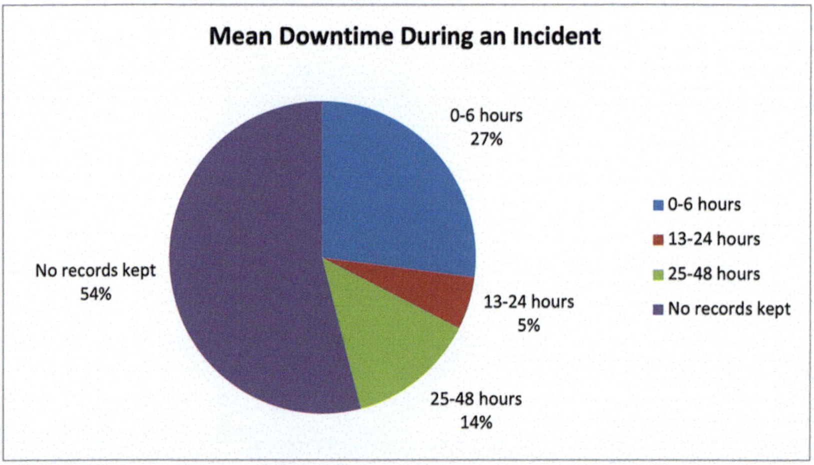

Fig. 6.6 Mean downtime during an incident

had firewalls and antivirus software installed in their organisations, but official cybersecurity plans were not in place and the incident reporting system is basically absent. Moreover, a separate cybersecurity unit does not exist in the end-users' organisations. The ICT departments do not regularly keep log files of cybersecurity-related events or login actions and cybersecurity-related key performance indicators (KPIs) are not measured. Indeed, almost 50% of ICT employees (aggregated responses) replied that no records are kept for cybersecurity attacks (Fig. 6.5).

The absence of incident logging reported by almost 50% of the ICT employees is shown in Fig. 6.6:

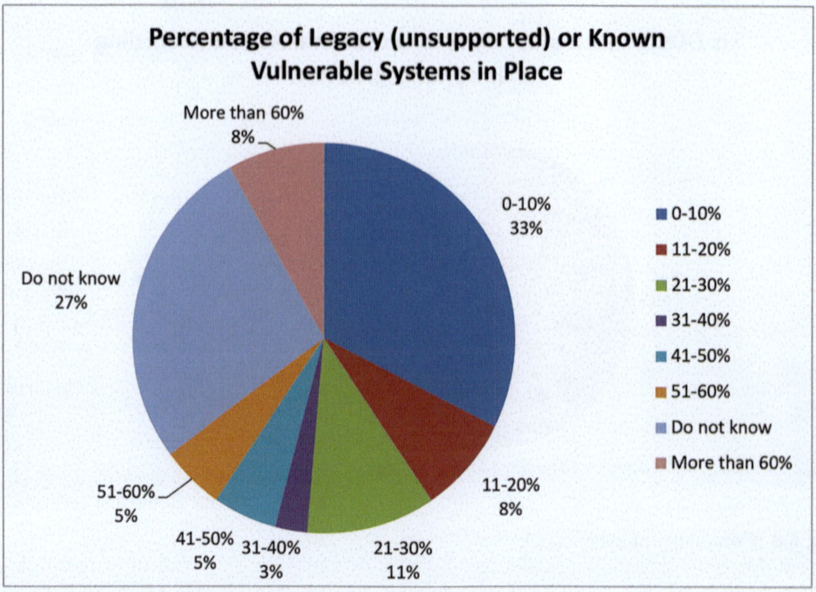

Fig. 6.7 Legacy, unsupported and known vulnerable systems in place

An additional relevant fact from a cybersecurity perspective relates to the daily use of legacy and vulnerable devices by the healthcare organisation, namely, workstations or machines with Windows XP or Windows Embedded operating systems. Although such equipment adds to the vulnerability of the healthcare organisations' ICT infrastructures, these legacy systems cannot be decommissioned since most of them are medical equipment (Fig. 6.7).

Notwithstanding, the questionnaire also revealed that there is a moderate level of cybersecurity awareness and knowledge among ICT employees, mostly because ICT departments are under-staffed, do not execute the required training, do not perform penetration tests and do not have an official cybersecurity policy. It is also noted that the ICT Departments' work is hampered by the absence of methods, tools and cybersecurity procedures. As a result, training to raise the level of cybersecurity awareness is deemed highly important.

Another significant finding is that ICT employees are not aware of the national legislation in force. For example, half of the respondents answered that they do not know whether Distributed Denial of Service (DDOS) attacks are considered criminal actions (Fig. 6.8).

Importantly, the questionnaire's responses imply that cybersecurity tests should be organised, for example, by the national Computer Security Incident Response Teams (CSIRTs), in order to assess the current cybersecurity and protection levels against cyber threats and attacks of healthcare organisations (Fig. 6.9).

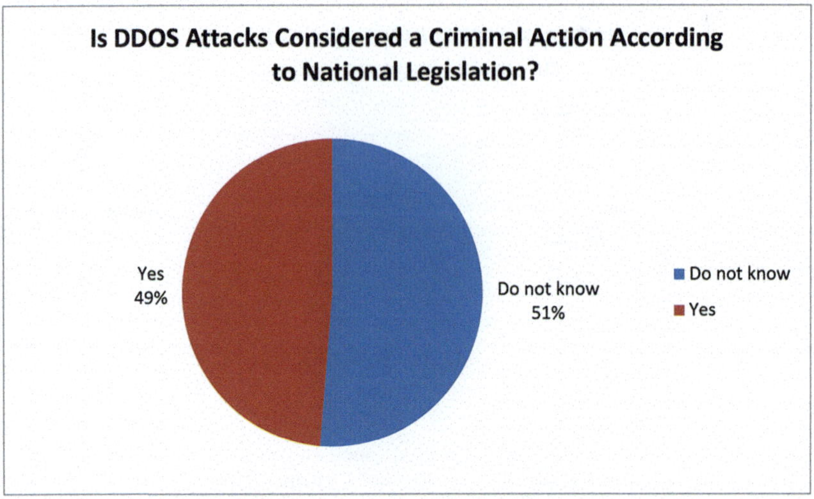

Fig. 6.8 Criminality of cyber attacks

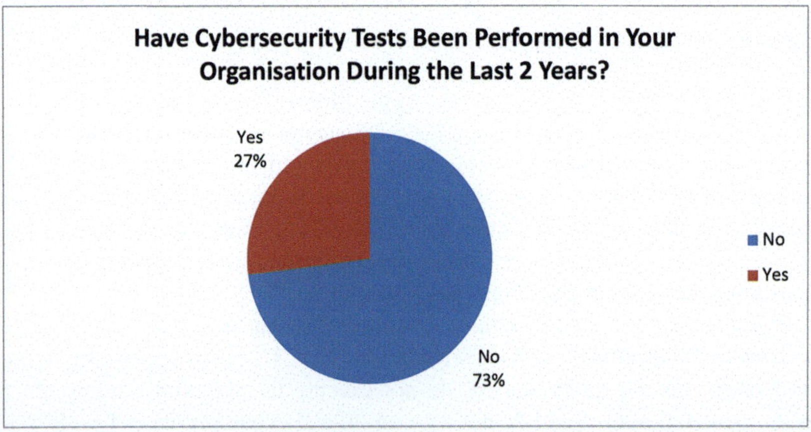

Fig. 6.9 Frequency of cybersecurity tests

6.3.2.2 The Non-ICT Questionnaire

A total of 699 answers were received for the non-ICT questionnaire, resulting in a 6.71% response rate. The limited number of responses considering the non-ICT professionals' universe is explained by the reduced time healthcare professionals have to allocate to voluntary external assignments (non-official duty). The questionnaire's demographic results are shown in Table 6.2.

The majority of healthcare employees (Doctors, Nurses, Auxiliary, Laboratory, administrative personnel and technical personnel) answered that the organisation

Table 6.2 Demographics of non-ICT questionnaire responses

	DYPE5	HESE	POLARIS
Number of answers	$n = 449$ (100%)	$n = 124$ (100%)	$n = 126$ (100%)
Gender			
Male	112 (25%)	46 (37.09%)	21 (16.67%)
Female	337 (75%)	78 (62.91%)	105 (83.33%)
Age			
21–30	33 (7.3%)	10 (8.06%)	19 (15.08%)
31–40	91 (20.3%)	36 (29.04%)	28 (22.22%)
41–50	171 (38.1%)	45 (36.30%)	66 (52.38%)
51–60	134 (29.8%)	20 (16.12%)	10 (7.93%)
>61	20 (4.5%)	13 (10.48%)	3 (2.38%)
Education			
Secondary education	63 (14.0%)	42 (33.87%)	9 (7.14%)
Vocational training institute	32 (7.1%)	10 (8.06%)	10 (7.93%)
Bachelor's degree	247 (55.0%)	5 (4.03%)	68 (53.97%)
MSc	94 (20.9%)	66 (53.23%)	29 (23.01%)
PhD	13 (3.0%)	1 (0.81%)	10 (7.93%)
Position			
Doctor	88 (19.6%)	88 (19.6%)	37 (29.35%)
Nurse	156 (34.7%)	156 (34.7%)	57 (45.23%)
Auxiliary personnel	5 (1.1%)	5 (1.1%)	1 (0.79%)
Lab. personnel	33 (7.4%)	33 (7.4%)	3 (2.38%)
Administrative personnel	127 (28.3%)	127 (28.3%)	23 (18.26%)
Technical personnel	9 (2.0%)	9 (2.0%)	2 (1.59%)
Other	31 (6.9%)	31 (6.9%)	3 (2.38%)

does not have a cybersecurity department, which is in line with the answers of the ICT professionals. Another factor affecting the organisations' cybersecurity protection is the fact that more than 50% of the respondents were not aware of information security policies, albeit they could understand when a computer was hacked or infected and knew whom to contact. This revealed that respondents were not confident about their cybersecurity awareness level (Fig. 6.10).

More than 50% of the non-ICT professionals answered that their computers had not been infected, while 60% verified whether an anti-virus was installed on their computer and knew how to recognise the presence of such an installation. Approximately 60% of them responded that they trusted the person or company that sent an email with an attachment, so they usually proceeded with opening it. Strangely, they also reported that more than 50% of them did not know what an email fraud was or how to identify it. Furthermore, 75% did not know what a social engineering attack is, nor could they recognise a cybersecurity event. The following figure depicts the behaviour of non-ICT personnel when operating email communications, and a direct conclusion is that the majority of email users check the identity of the senders of the electronic messages (Fig. 6.11).

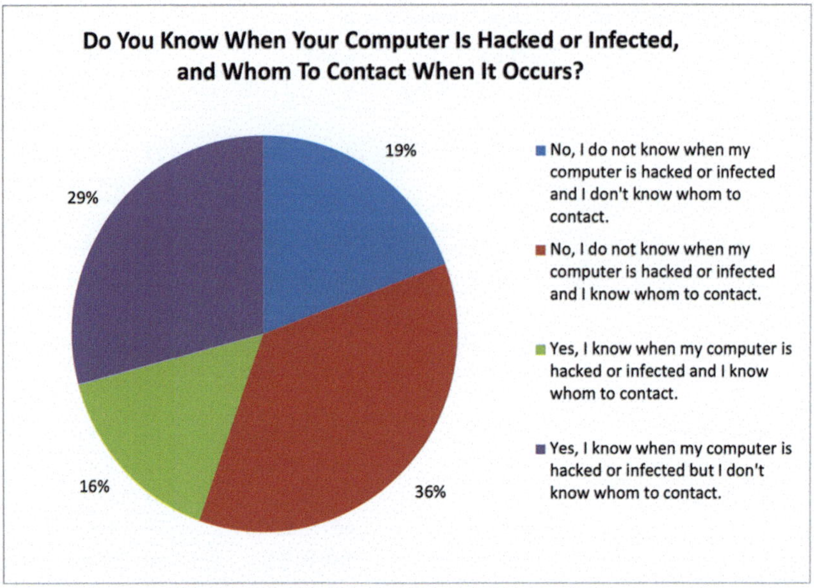

Fig. 6.10 Recognition of hacked or infected computers

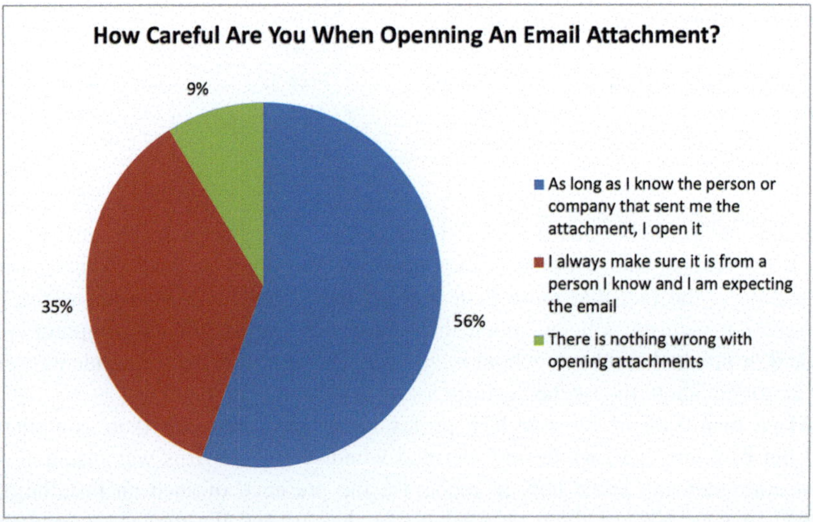

Fig. 6.11 Behaviour concerning email communication

About a fifth of non-ICT employees recognised that they use their own personal devices to store or transfer confidential hospital information, with 16% of non-ICT employees having downloaded and installed software on their computer at work and

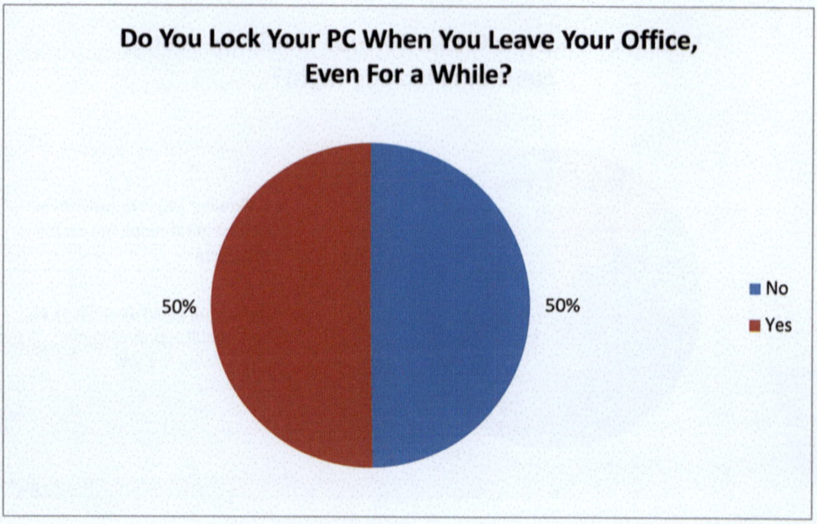

Fig. 6.12 Computer locking habits

30% of them having given their password to colleagues. Notably, half of them do not usually lock their computers when leaving the office (Fig. 6.12).

The questionnaire responses also revealed that more than 60% of non-ICT professionals have not been officially informed or trained on the GDPR to minimise personal data breaches or cybersecurity incidents, even though more than 65% of the respondents acknowledged that their duties involve access to patient data (75% of them were aware that there is valuable information on the computers they work on), which is considered confidential and sensitive information.

Overall, the non-ICT healthcare professionals considered positive the impact of adopting security policies in their daily activities (Fig. 6.13).

Table 6.3 summarises the findings regarding the cyber behaviour and security comprehension level of non-ICT healthcare employees. Indicatively, 25% disagreed that there was a sufficient level of cybersecurity training in the organisation, whereas 27% did not answer; similarly, 23% stated that they could not recognise a cybersecurity problem or incident if one should happen, though 42% did not answer.

The responses obtained on the recognition of security issues or incidents allow to determine that the behaviour and level of cybersecurity awareness of non-ICT healthcare professionals represent a significant risk factor to the healthcare organisations' cybersecurity. Importantly, 75% of respondents consider that organisational security policies would help improve their own work. Consequently, it is the conclusion of the SPHINX partners that cybersecurity policies should be enforced in the healthcare organisations involved in the SPHINX pilots, assisted with regular cybersecurity awareness training campaigns to disseminate information on the GDPR. The cybersecurity awareness training activities are deemed an effective tool to propagate the adequate cybersecurity policies and measures throughout

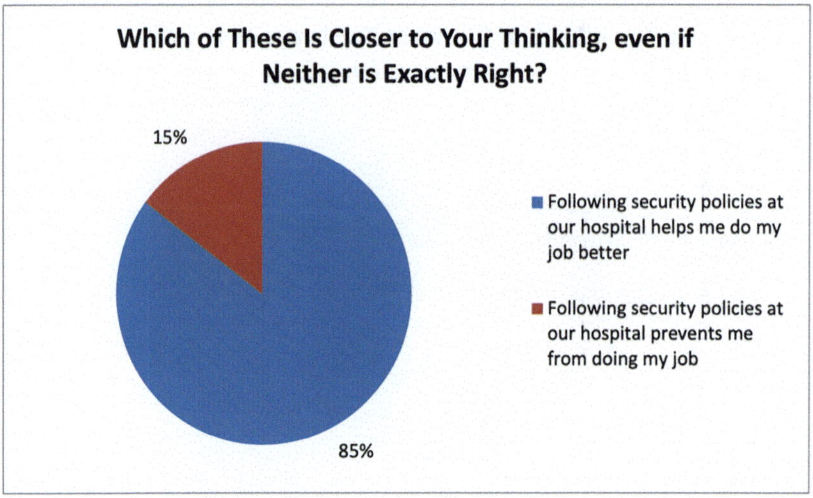

Fig. 6.13 Impact of security policies in daily work activities

the organisations. Further, it is the SPHINX Consortium's expectation that the analysis here presented may potentially assist the formulation of specific guidelines and actions to be adopted by and applied in those organisations, to cope with cybersecurity issues.

6.4 Summary

Overall, the proposed chapter outlines the development, implementation and validation of a comprehensive cybersecurity toolkit for healthcare institutions. This toolkit aims to enhance the security of medical facilities by automating vulnerability assessments and providing a range of security services to address potential cyber threats effectively. The approach is validated through real-world scenarios and pilot site deployments, ensuring its practicality and effectiveness in safeguarding healthcare environments.

Table 6.3 Digital behaviour and security comprehension level of healthcare employees (positive answers)

Question	Doctor	Nurse	Auxiliary personnel	Laboratory personnel	Administrative personnel	Technical personnel	Other
Do you know when your computer is hacked or infected, and whom to contact when it occurs?	40.8%	42.2%	33.3%	30.2%	42.8%	38.9%	40.5%
Have you ever found a virus or Trojan on your computer at work?	20.4%	23.9%	11.1%	16.3%	20.9%	33.3%	9.5%
Is anti-virus currently installed on your computer?	63.3%	59.6%	44.4%	46.5%	70.6%	66.7%	54.8%
How careful are you when you open an attachment in email?	38.1%	35.7%	27.8%	37.2%	39.3%	33.3%	40.5%
Do you know what a social-engineering attack is?	25.2%	25.7%	22.2%	30.2%	31.3%	33.3%	11.9%
Do you know what an email scam is and how to identify one?	27.2%	17.0%	22.2%	23.3%	22.9%	44.4%	14.3%
My computer has no value to hackers, they do not target me.	17.0%	23.5%	44.4%	25.6%	23.4%	22.2%	33.3%
Can you use your own personal devices, such as your mobile phone or USB sticks or CD/DVD discs to store or transfer confidential hospital information?	24.5%	17.0%	22.2%	23.3%	21.9%	33.3%	23.8%
Have you downloaded and installed software on your computer at work?	25.2%	10.9%	27.8%	18.6%	18.4%	38.9%	11.9%
Have you given your password to your colleagues or your manager, when you were asked for it?	21.8%	27.0%	38.9%	14.0%	42.3%	16.7%	50.0%
I feel I have been sufficiently trained in security at our hospital.	19.7%	25.2%	11.1%	25.6%	23.9%	16.7%	19.0%
I am confident that I could recognise a security issue or incident if I saw one.	38.1%	39.6%	16.7%	34.9%	41.3%	33.3%	35.7%
Do you lock your PC when you leave your office even for a while?	55.8%	50.9%	44.4%	46.5%	53.7%	72.2%	52.4%

Acknowledgments This research work was funded by the Sphinx Project "A universal Cyber-security Toolkit for Healthcare Sector," which has received funding from the European Union's Horizon 2020 research and innovation programme under grant agreement No 826183.

References

1. Cini, M., & Czulno, P. (2022). Digital single market and the EU competition regime: An explanation of policy change. *Journal of European Integration, 44*(1), 41–57.
2. Cutler, D., et al. (2012). Reducing administrative costs and improving the health care system. *The New England Journal of Medicine, 367*, 1875–1878. https://doi.org/10.1056/NEJMp1209711
3. https://www.fda.gov/MedicalDevices/DigitalHealth/default.htm
4. Vawdrey, D. K., Wilcox, L. G., Collins, S. A., Bakken, S., Feiner, S., Boyer, A., & Restaino, S. W. (2011). A tablet computer application for patients to participate in their hospital care. In *AMIA annual symposium proceedings* (p. 1428). American Medical Informatics Association.
5. Medlin, B. D., Corley, K., & Adriana Romaniello, B. (2011). Passwords selected by hospital employees: An investigative study. *IJACSA Editorial.*
6. https://www.popsci.com/technology/article/2012-09/infographic-day-fastest-way-crack-4-digit-pin-number
7. http://pwc.blogs.com/health_matters/2016/05/the-value-of-patient-data.html
8. https://www.forbes.com/sites/mariyayao/2017/04/14/your-electronic-medical-records-can-be-worth-1000-to-hackers/#76d7fd3750cf
9. https://ocrportal.hhs.gov/ocr/breach/breach_report.jsf
10. https://www.telegraph.co.uk/news/2017/05/12/nhs-hit-major-cyber-attack-hackers-demanding-ransom/
11. http://medidfraud.org/wp-content/uploads/2015/02/2014_Medical_ID_Theft_Study1.pdf
12. https://www.cyberisk.biz/healthcare-cyber-attacks-hospitals-critical-unit-cyber-threat/
13. Frazier, T. G., Walker, M. H., Kumari, A., & Thompson, C. M. (2013). Opportunities and constraints to hazard mitigation planning. *Applied Geography, 40*, 52–60.
14. Zkik, K., Tebaa, M., Tachihante, T., & Orhanou, G. (2017). A new authentication and homomorphic encryption as a service model for preserving privacy in clouds. *Journal of Computer Science, 13*(12), 702–717. https://doi.org/10.3844/jcssp.2017.702.717
15. Mavromoustakis, C. X., Mastorakis, G., & Dobre, C. (Eds.). (2017). *Advances in mobile cloud computing and big data in the 5G era*. Springer.
16. Andreas, A., Mavromoustakis, C. X., Mastorakis, G., Do, D. T., Batalla, J. M., Pallis, E., & Markakis, E. K. (2021). Towards an optimized security approach to IoT devices with confidential healthcare data exchange. *Multimedia Tools and Applications, 80*, 31435–31449.
17. Markakis, E., Nikoloudakis, Y., Mastorakis, G., Mavromoustakis, C. X., Pallis, E., Sideris, A., et al. (2019). Acceleration at the edge for supporting SMEs security: The FORTIKA paradigm. *IEEE Communications Magazine, 57*(2), 41–47.
18. Andreou, A., Mavromoustakis, C. X., Batalla, J. M., Markakis, E., Mastorakis, G., & Chatzimisios, P. (2023). Evaluating urban environments for the integration of cutting-edge technologies enhances smart cities' evolution. In *ICC 2023-IEEE international conference on communications* (pp. 3327–3332). IEEE.
19. Karras, K., Pallis, E., Mastorakis, G., Nikoloudakis, Y., Batalla, J. M., Mavromoustakis, C. X., & Markakis, E. (2020). A hardware acceleration platform for AI-based inference at the edge. *Circuits, Systems, and Signal Processing, 39*, 1059–1070.
20. https://sphinx-project.eu/

Chapter 7
Personas of Older Adults in Social and Health Context

Zdenek Meier, Kristyna Gabova, Radka Zidkova, and Peter Tavel

7.1 Introduction

The population is growing and living standards are rising. From a global perspective, it is important to remember that between 1960 and 2011, the world's population grew from 3 billion to 7 billion. This is a rate that is unlikely to be repeated [52]. As the population grows and its demographic distribution increases, certain phenomena take on greater contours and urgency. One such phenomenon is population ageing, including increasing life expectancy. Population ageing is one of the most important demographic trends of the twenty-first century and is a problem that affects all aspects of our society, from the economy and healthcare to social structure and culture. In particular, it is increasing the burden on social and health services and is becoming an important policy and sustainability issue.

One of the main reasons for the ageing population is the increasing life expectancy. A few centuries ago, it was common for people to live only a few decades. Disease, poor living conditions and limited access to medical and social care meant that many people died at a young age. However, over the last century, advances in medicine, nutrition and social welfare have dramatically increased life expectancy. In 2000, according to World Health Organization [90], the global life expectancy at birth was 66.79 (males 64.42 and females 69.27) and in 2019 it increased to 73.31 (males 70.85 and females 75.87). Moreover, average life expectancy is higher in Europe. In 2000, the European life expectancy at birth was 72.51 (males 68.44 and females 76.44), and in 2019 it increased to 78.24 (males

Z. Meier · K. Gabova · R. Zidkova (✉) · P. Tavel
Olomouc University Social Health Institute (OUSHI), Palacky University, Olomouc, Czech Republic
e-mail: zdenek.meier@oushi.upol.cz; kristyna.gabova@oushi.upol.cz; radka.zidkova@oushi.upol.cz; peter.tavel@oushi.upol.cz

© The Author(s), under exclusive license to Springer Nature Switzerland AG 2024
A. Bourdena et al. (eds.), *Intelligent Technologies for Healthcare Business Applications*, Signals and Communication Technology,
https://doi.org/10.1007/978-3-031-58527-2_7

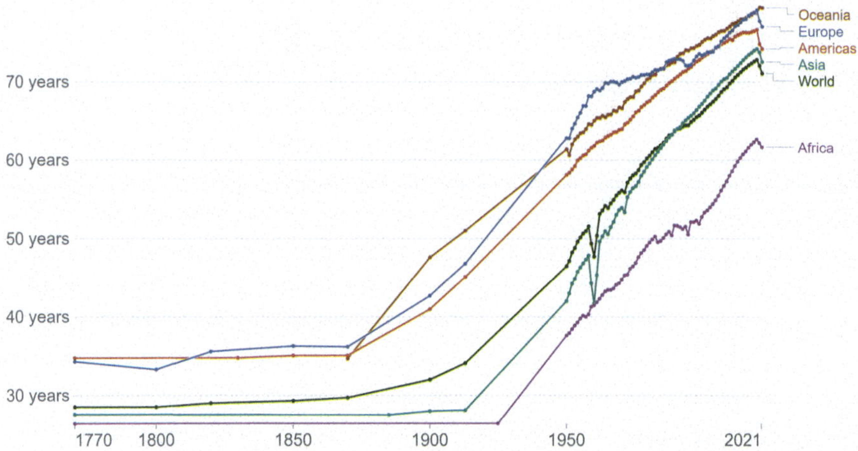

Fig. 7.1 Life expectancy from 1770 to 2021. The total number of years a newborn is expected to live [71]

75.09 and females 81.29), with the highest being in Spain in 2019, where it was 83.2 years (Fig. 7.1).

The increasing life expectancy is also linked to the growing number of people aged 60 and over in the world population. In 2019, there were one billion people aged 60+, and this number will increase to 1.4 billion by 2030 and 2.1 billion by 2050 [89]. This increase is unprecedented and will accelerate in the coming decades. An important related issue is that the increase in the number of older people is also changing the old-age dependency ratio (the number of people aged 65 and over per 100 people of working age, defined as people aged 20 to 64). Data from the Organisation for Economic Co-operation and Development (OECD) show that in the European Union, the old-age dependency ratio was 32.3 in 2020 and will be 55.4 in 2050. In the USA, the old-age dependency ratio was 28.4 in 2020 and is expected to rise to 40.4 in 2050. In Italy, the country with the fastest ageing population in the EU, the old-age dependency ratio is 39.5 and is estimated to rise to 74.4 in 2050 [64].

Figure 7.2 shows that the decline in the number of children and the significant increase in the number of older people worldwide. In North America and Europe, the 65+ population is already far outstripping the growth of the working age population. At the same time, Europe, with its advanced health system and wide range of prevention programmes, is one of the fastest ageing in the world. In Europe, older citizens represented 20.90% of the population in 2021. In the same year, the highest proportion of people of pensionable age was in Italy, where they make up 23.67% of the total population. The older population is more likely to be female. All these facts point to the need to find solutions for social and health services in order to maintain the standard of these services and to address their financing (Fig. 7.3).

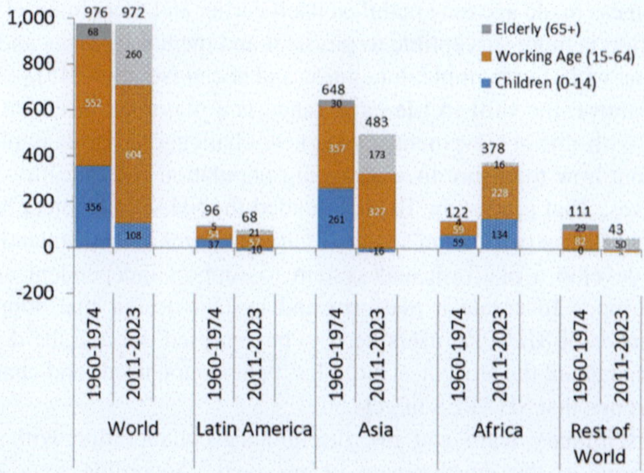

Fig. 7.2 The different age composition per billion growth in 1960–1974 and 2011–2023. (Source [52])

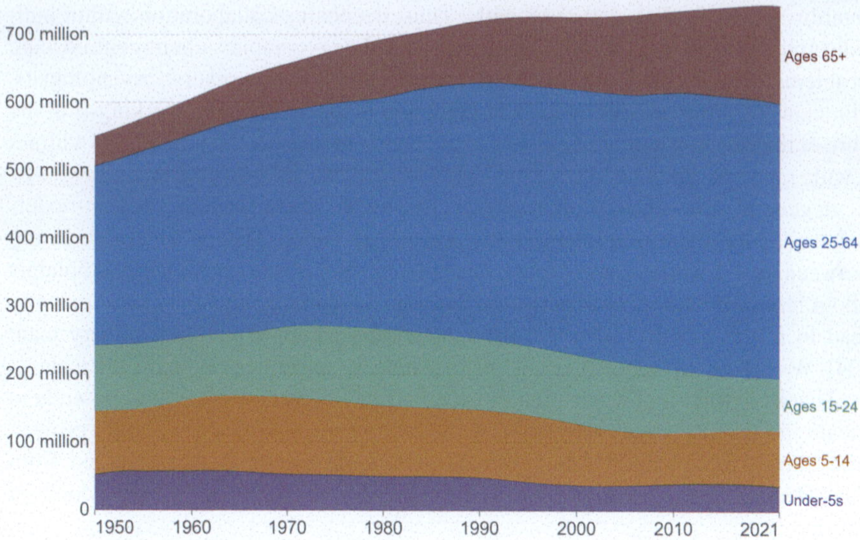

Fig. 7.3 Population by age group in Europe [71]

Older age can bring a number of complications in different areas of life. Health problems are common, exacerbating other difficulties in life and placing demands on social and health systems. Another of these problems can be loneliness in older adults, mainly due to poor physical mobility and shrinking social networks (death of friends) [66]. In relation to social work, for example, for the phenomenon of loneliness, it appears that if there is a limited number of social services for older people, loneliness in old age may manifest itself earlier and more intensely [60]. The older generation is more susceptible to physical and mental illnesses and combines these problems with, for example, loneliness and social isolation [45].

As noted above, the shift in life expectancy is a major achievement of human progress but with this achievement comes new challenges. For example, we face questions about how to ensure that an ageing population lives healthy, happy and productive lives. That is why the EU has funded the SHAPES project, which with the involvement of experts from many disciplines aims to understand ageing in Europe and develop a platform and system to support independent and healthy ageing in Europe. To create a platform and system design that supports older people, the needs of SHAPES users need to be analysed through the development of personas that detail the attributes, attitudes, behaviours, needs and characteristics of the user groups that SHAPES targets.

A multidisciplinary team and interdisciplinary collaboration with practitioners were crucial to the development of personas. According to a number of research findings, interdisciplinary collaboration is a key factor in achieving effective outcomes in a variety of areas. The results show that there is a strong belief in the importance of interdisciplinary collaboration in teams where strong interdisciplinary collaboration prevails. Thus, deepening collaboration within multidisciplinary teams is seen as essential to solving complex client-centred care problems [27]. In our case, the team consisted of social workers, psychologists, clinicians of different specialties and older adults themselves. Networking is at the core of the way this multidisciplinary team works, increasing the potential to address a wide range of client needs.

In general, however, this approach has its pitfalls. There is a lack of clear models for managing interdisciplinary work, despite the long history of collaboration between social workers and professionals from other disciplines [13]. Complaints about interprofessional boundaries between lower status groups may paradoxically lead to further conflict between different groups within a multidisciplinary team [24]. We tried to avoid these problems by carefully selecting people for the team.

Thanks to this careful selection of experts from different fields, it was possible to create the personas that were the essential and primary task of the whole project. The aim of this chapter is therefore to present the personas that emerged from the SHAPES research activities and offer insights into the lives of older people in Europe.

7.2 Methodology

The persona creation methodology in the SHAPES project combined a literature review and qualitative methods. There is no standardised approach for developing personas; they can either be crafted at the inception of a design process or emerge during the design and pilot phases [46]. While several studies highlight the empirical essence of persona creation [61, 75], some also acknowledge the significance of

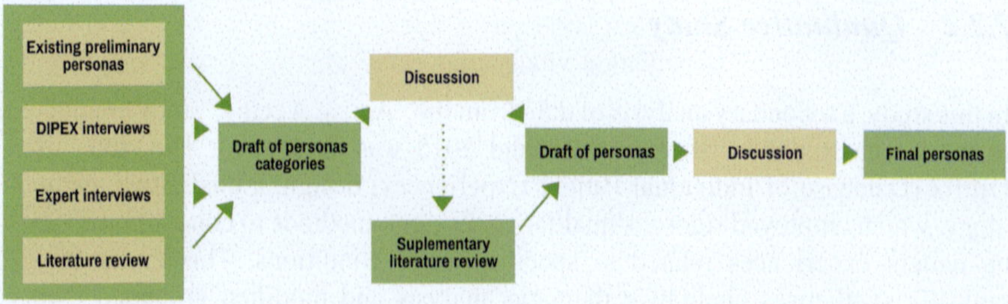

Fig. 7.4 Development of personas [83]

designers' insights and ad hoc assumptions [46]. The techniques used for persona development vary widely among studies. Some rely solely on qualitative methods, employing ethnographic techniques, interviews or focus groups [73]. In contrast, others utilise mixed methods [61, 95] or entirely quantitative approaches, often employing cluster analysis [46, 75].

The persona creation process in this study comprised four phases, as illustrated in Fig. 7.2.

The initial version of the persona categories aimed to identify preliminary persona types and was constructed using the following data sources:

1. Existing persona files developed for the project submission.
2. Data from a qualitative study on active ageing in the Czech Republic.
3. A literature review encompassing case studies and qualitative studies on various categories of older adults, considering health status and behavioural patterns.
4. Insights from expert interviews with four geriatricians and two social workers specialising in older adults.
5. Discussions with SHAPES experts and members who had extensive experience from ethnographic studies involving older adults (Fig. 7.4).

All data utilised in crafting the personas were anonymised, and the management of these non-personal data adhered completely to the Regulation on the free flow of non-personal data (FFD) [Regulation (EU) 2018/1807].

7.2.1 *Existing Preliminary Personas*

The preliminary personas were adopted from the previous project titled "Smart and Healthy Ageing through People Engaging in Supportive Systems," which defined the fundamental types of personas. These personas served as a basis for further research in this study.

7.2.2 *Qualitative Study*

In this study, a secondary analysis of data from the "Active Ageing" study conducted in the Czech Republic between 2014 and 2015 was performed. The study used DIPEx (Database of Individual Patient Experiences) design, a qualitative methodology, which employed rigorous qualitative research methods to conduct interviews on patient experiences related to specific health conditions. This methodology typically synthetises qualitative thematic analysis and modified grounded theory with narrative analysis [96]. Within the original study, 50 in-depth interviews were conducted with older adults aged 65 and above, exploring various significant aspects of ageing. The existing data were revisited and re-evaluated to gain new insights, perspectives or interpretations relevant to the research objectives. This approach allowed the valuable information collected during the original study to be leveraged for addressing specific research questions in the current investigation. The data were analysed using both thematic analysis and narrative analysis methodologies [26].

7.2.3 *Literature Review*

For the review, an integrative review approach was utilised [84], as it is valuable when the intention is not to encompass all articles ever published on the subject, but rather to find viewpoints to understand the topic [79].

The articles were searched on the Web of Science and Scopus databases. Recent (not older than 5 years) studies on various categories of older adults considering health status and behavioural patterns were included. By focusing the review, potentially relevant sources identified were reduced from 258 to fewer than 20 articles. The goal was to create a new under-standing of the topic through a form of synthesis [84]. The main ideas and themes from the literature were identified and analysed. As data were conceptualised at higher levels of abstraction, each source was reviewed to verify that the new conceptualisation was congruent with other sources [87]. A synthesis in the form of researcher's notes was written and shared with the research team to comprehensively portray the key topics of articles relevant to the identification of personas.

7.2.4 *Expert Interviews*

To complete the understanding of the topic, six experts were interviewed after being familiarised with preliminary findings. Interviews were carried out with four geriatricians from the Czech Republic, including one leading a major geriatric clinic, and two social workers and psychologist specialising in older adults. For the analysis of the topic, the open coding method and thematic analysis were used.

7.2.5 Finalisation of Personas

Initially, the most prevalent types based on health status and behavioural patterns were identified. The first draft of persona categories was prepared, followed by extensive team discussions. Subsequently, consultations were held with the expert team. After reviewing additional literature, draft personas were formulated based on these categories and circulated among team members for a second round of discussions. These discussions led to the finalisation of the personas and the addition of two others.

7.3 Personas

Before introducing the individual personas, it is necessary to first define what a persona is. A *persona*, also referred to as a 'user persona', represents a detailed description of a fictional individual (often a composite of real-life people). Its primary purpose is to convey the fundamental motivations, challenges and interests of a particular user segment [10, 74]. Personas include fictitious characters described in narrative form in order to help solve design questions. They assist designers in honing their focus on the main users, shedding light on their behavioural tendencies and specific needs [34, 35, 46]. Personas are widely used in system design organisations as a complement to individual or other user data and serve as foundational models for understanding how an individual might interact with a product or digital solution.

Within the SHAPES project, the task involved creating personas characterising older people. All natural processes, including the ageing process, are influenced by inherent variations. One of the challenges arises from these variations in the diverse characteristics of the personas. This implies that the personas differ in various aspects such as their health conditions, sensory and motor capabilities, levels of cognitive decline, healthcare needs, economic status, digital literacy, health literacy, affinity to ICT technologies and numerous other parameters. Certain degrees of these parameters might act as constraints, limiting the use of technology and the suitability of specific use cases for a given persona. For instance, assessing the suitability of a use case based solely on healthcare requirements is insufficient, as the persona in question may have inadequate sensory or motor skills, limited digital literacy or cognitive impairments hindering the use of specific technology. Determining the appropriate parameter to link use cases with personas becomes crucial. Focusing solely on one or a few aspects risks constitutive and explanatory reductionism. To address this, complex models of human subjects in different life stages are being developed. Hence, understanding variations in the needs, health conditions, sensory and motor abilities, cognitive decline, healthcare requirements, economic situations, digital literacy, health literacy, affinity to ICT technologies, etc., in personas representing older adults can draw inspiration from an available complex patient model.

7.3.1 *Categories (or Segments) Representing Personas*

Based on the conducted research, 12 personas of older adults were defined. The personas represent different facets of the ageing population, offering insights into their unique challenges and circumstances. From active, healthy older adults to those with chronic musculoskeletal disorders, neurodegenerative diseases and social isolation, each persona provides a distinct perspective. Additionally, there are personas highlighting the experiences of older adults dealing with alcohol or drug dependency, deafblindness and the impact of the COVID-19 pandemic on mental health. Informal caregivers for older adults with neurodegenerative disorders, formal caregivers in Nordic areas and refugees' perspectives further contribute to this diverse exploration of ageing. These personas serve as typical cases, shedding light on the varied realities faced by older adults and their caregivers in different contexts.

All of the personas listed below were presented in the report D2.7—SHAPES Personas and Use Cases. As musculoskeletal problems and various health problems are very often associated with old age, which is also confirmed by Global Burden of Disease (GBD) data [33], where musculoskeletal disorders and non-communicable diseases are among the most common causes of years lived with disabilities, we have dedicated more space to these personas (Persona 2 and Persona 3). In addition, as loneliness is a problem not only for older adults but also for the younger generation according to the EU report of June 2023 [8], and at the same time many scientific articles highlight the links between loneliness and mental and physical health, we decided to address this phenomenon in more detail in Persona 5 as well.

7.3.1.1 Active, Healthy Older Adults

The initial persona represents a unique subset of younger older adults, aged between 65 and 75, characterised by overall good health and an active lifestyle. Many of these individuals are retired, although some continue to work part-time or engage in semi-retirement. They enjoy travelling, pursuing diverse hobbies, and they maintain a fulfilling social life. Actively participating in community life through various volunteer activities is also significant for them.

While the concept of "active ageing" often emphasises physical activity, for many older adults, it encompasses autonomy, curiosity, enthusiasm and a zest for life [80]. Physical activity plays a crucial role in maintaining good health in older age and is influenced by the enjoyment of the specific exercise, the desire to stay in good shape and the social connections associated with the activity. The quality of the natural environment is a substantial factor influencing the level of physical activity among older adults. Accessible parks or forests, for example, encourage higher levels of physical activity [32, 50]. In this context, the first persona, represented by Ernst from Germany, is defined. Ernst belongs to a relatively rare group of physically active individuals compared to national averages. His active lifestyle contributes positively to his physical well-being. Additionally, his interest in digital health solutions allows him to monitor his health data. If shared with his general physician, this data can aid in regular health evaluations and preventive measures (Fig. 7.5).

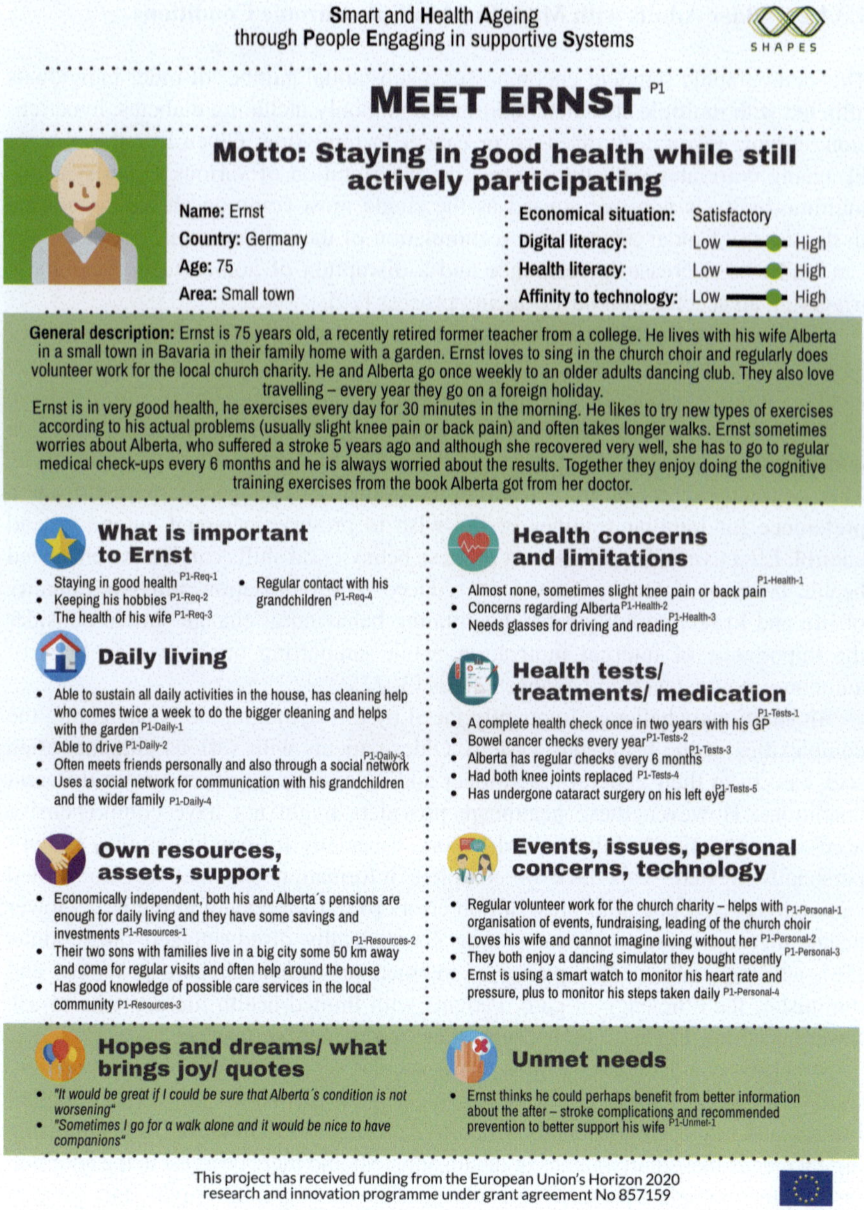

Fig. 7.5 Persona 1: Active, healthy older adults [83]

7.3.1.2 Older Adults with Mild, But Multiple Chronic Conditions

This demographic segment encompasses a substantial number of older individuals afflicted with multiple chronic conditions, commonly including diabetes, hypertension, chronic respiratory diseases, or cancer in remission. Given that the process of ageing correlates with the progressive deterioration of various organ systems, multimorbidity is now recognised as the single most common chronic condition in the group of older adults. The accumulation of these illnesses in advanced age can lead to a decrease in resilience and a disruption of homeostasis, potentially triggering an acceleration of the ageing process [29].

A substantial challenge within this older adult population is the necessity of adopting behavioural changes, often stressed by healthcare professionals. Such changes might include dietary improvements, quitting smoking or cutting down on alcohol consumption. These adults frequently grapple with the tension between understanding the need for change and the desire to maintain their usual lifestyle. This conflict can result in a form of resistance to change, stemming from a preference for familiar routines or the wish to preserve personal autonomy and control. Effective self-management of these behavioural shifts can lead to enhanced health, better symptom management, reduced rehospitalisation, improved quality of life and lower mortality rates. Facilitating behavioural change should consider the importance of internal motivation, while supporting one's own feelings of autonomy, competence and connectedness [3, 72].

An additional challenge frequently faced by this demographic is navigating the complexities of the healthcare system. Older patients with various ailments often seek care from their general practitioner and several specialists, each for different conditions. However, these healthcare providers might not have comprehensive access to the patient's full medical history, especially for conditions they haven't personally treated. This lack of complete information can lead to fragmented care delivery and potential prescription errors [63]. Compounding the issue, lower health literacy, more prevalent among economically disadvantaged older adults [56], adversely affects the quality of interactions with healthcare providers and diminishes the efficiency of care. Patients with limited health literacy tend to ask fewer questions, hindered by feelings of embarrassment or fear [1].

Roberto's character exemplifies this particular segment of the older population. In Italy, the advanced age group (65 and older) generally shows low levels of digital literacy and usage. Consequently, Roberto isn't inclined to monitor his health using digital means like smartwatches or health apps. Should there be a rise in the adoption of such technologies, Roberto and others in his demographic might start actively managing their health metrics and communicating them to their doctors. This could lead healthcare professionals to tailor diagnoses and treatments more effectively, utilise reminders for consistent medication usage and foster greater trust among these patients. Establishing a specialised government or health ministry website offering disease information and guidance can address the mistrust in online health resources, enabling health information to more effectively reach and be trusted by older patients. However, the implementation of modern technology for health monitoring among patients faces challenges, notably because a significant number of physicians (39.5%) are over 55 [64], indicating potential resistance to new technologies. In Italy, health risks are often linked to social habits like smoking, drinking and overeating, coupled with lower physical activity levels, as seen in Roberto's case. These factors contribute to the heightened risk of chronic diseases, especially cardiovascular diseases, which are the predominant cause of death in the region (Fig. 7.6).

7.3.1.3 Older Adults with Chronic Musculoskeletal Disorders

The third persona is Ayesha, a resident of the United Kingdom, with growing movement problems, which represents older adults with chronic musculoskeletal disorders. Mobility difficulties, typically arthrosis and vertebrogenic syndrome (back pain), are some of the most common problems of older adults. These conditions may negatively affect the ability to move around the home as well as outside, maintain independence and keep hobbies and often may lead to increased social isolation. In order to preserve the quality of life of this population, it is important to maintain their functional capacity for as long as possible [30].

An important element associated with this condition is the risk of falls, and even more critical, the fear of falls. This has been associated with many negative consequences such as limited movement, decreased muscle strength, higher risk of disability and threat of social isolation [77]. A fear of falls can also develop in people who have never experienced an actual fall, is a predictor of future falls and is also associated with functional decline [4].

Older adults with mobility problems are also more likely to experience difficulties with basic daily activities like dressing, combing one's hair, taking a shower or going to the toilet, and also more instrumental tasks such as preparing meals, shopping or lifting things. The inability to execute routine tasks may cause frustration and embarrassment [48]. Moreover, they may have to cope with many inconveniences and difficulties at home, such as stairs, narrow doorways, missing railings or other supports. A frequent strategy to overcome these threats is, for example, leaving several walking sticks in strategic places around the house or so-called "furniture cruising" or "furniture surfing": placing the furniture strategically, such so it can be grabbed for keeping balance [48]. Most common house adaptations are installing grab bars or special railings, using shower chairs, raised toilet seats, etc. [48]. Notable characteristics of the in-house and also outside-the-house movement are extended planning of each, even short, journey.

Whether an older person will cope with all these setbacks depends on many factors, one of the most essential being their resilience. This can be characterised as the ability to achieve good outcomes in spite of serious threats to adaptation or development [55], the capacity to bounce back following adversity or trauma [12] or simply finding a way to 'keep going' [70]. Resilience is associated with inner strength or resourcefulness and can be eroded after experiencing several difficult falls or other unpleasant or embarrassing situations (e.g., such as not being able to get out of the shower).

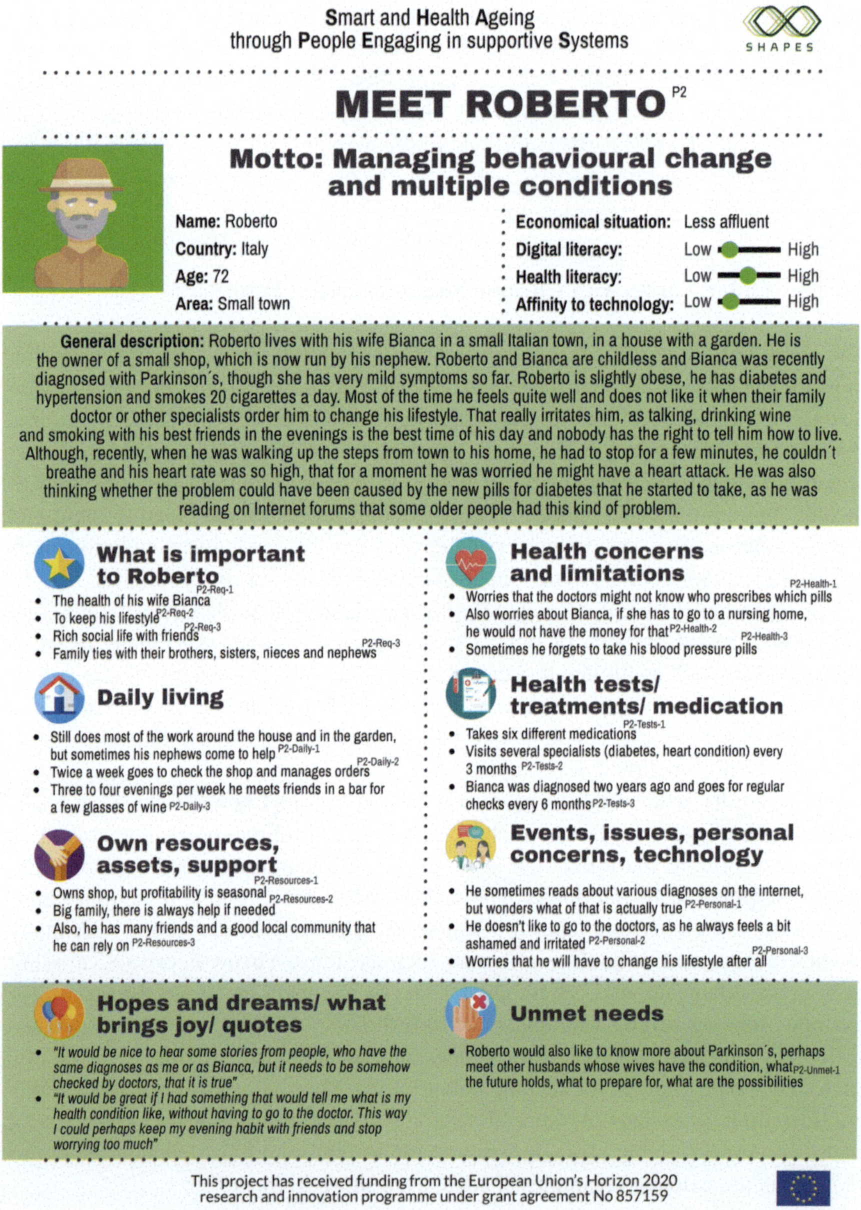

Fig. 7.6 Persona 2: Older adults with mild, but multiple chronic conditions [83]

Ayesha, a UK resident with severe mobility issues, lives with her family who assist her with daily activities. However, due to her limited movement and anxiety from previous falls, she faces escalating pain from osteoporosis. Language barriers restrict her access to medical advice, as she requires a translator. She is a client of a home care programme, but her requirements go beyond its offerings. She could greatly benefit from a nursing home offering continuous care and physiotherapy. However, the availability of such facilities is limited, and her specific language needs further complicate the situation (Fig. 7.7).

7.3.1.4 Older Adults with Neurodegenerative Diseases

The fourth persona, Isabel from Spain, focuses on Alzheimer's disease in its early to middle stage, addressing the challenges faced by older adults who still receive home care. Due to cognitive decline, individuals in this population often experience embarrassing situations, leading to feelings of shame and withdrawal. Fear of stigmatisation can further limit their social activity, resulting in loneliness and isolation. Despite memory deterioration, preserving their sense of identity is crucial for people with Alzheimer's. Sharing narratives, even if fragmented, helps them maintain their identity and social roles [82]. This form of narrative care [6, 69] has good results even in more severe phases of the illness [82].

Isabel is introduced, diagnosed with Alzheimer's dementia. Her condition is serious, with increasing memory loss and navigation difficulties; she often gets lost. Memory loss hampers her adherence to prescribed medication, worsening her health. While some aid is available, a significant gap exists. Isabel's son, Marco, takes on her caregiving responsibilities, experiencing caretaker stress syndrome. Marco feels the pressure of ensuring his mother's safety at home. More financial aid, frequent nurse visits, education and support groups for Marco, along with socialisation opportunities for Isabel, are needed to improve her care and well-being (Fig. 7.8).

7.3.1.5 Lonely and/or Socially Isolated Older Adults

The purpose of this persona is to draw attention to the problem of loneliness. Loneliness is an emotionally challenging condition, a psychological distress that occurs when a person perceives a mismatch with his or her social relationships, either in the sense that there are not enough of them or that they are not as good as he or she would like. It is important to remember that loneliness is a subjective experience and can vary between individuals. Some individuals may feel lonely even in company, while another individual may feel content even when alone [41].

Furthermore, it is important to mention that loneliness can be characterised as a phenomenon that exhibits geographical heterogeneity [49]. In older adults, social loneliness is associated with a number of factors. One of these is social dislocation, a situation in which individuals move away from their original place of residence,

Smart and **H**ealth **A**geing
through **P**eople **E**ngaging in supportive **S**ystems

SHAPES

MEET AYESHA [P3]

Motto: Limiting risk of falls while increasing self-sufficiency and mobility

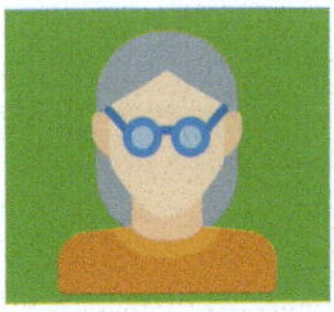

Name: Ayesha
Country: United Kingdom
Age: 79
Area: Outskirts of a big city

Economical situation: Low to moderate
Digital literacy: Low — High
Health literacy: Low — High
Affinity to technology: Low — High

General description: Ayesha is a widowed 79-year-old Iraqi woman and she suffers from severe osteoporosis. Ayesha lives with her son's family and their children in a two storey terraced house with a small garden. The family runs a small bistro, she used to help there but now she can´t due to her problems. Fortunately, her room is on the ground floor, as for a few years now she has had a big problem to climb up the stairs, even the five steps that are at the front door take her a long time to manage. She used to meet at the nearby café with other women from the muslim community but now cannot go, as she walks so slowly, that she is afraid to walk on the street - too many cars that cross the road feels like a nightmare. But if she happens to go out on some special occasion, she is very carefully in plotting the route: she thinks beforehand about where the benches are on the way, where there is a small wall to sit on, where there are the missing railings… Sometimes she spends much more time on planning the route than on the actual realization. Ayesha has also problems with movement around the house and after a few unpleasant falls she developed a fear of falls, so she is limiting her movement even more. They rearranged the furniture downstairs, so she has places to grab on and she also has walking sticks in almost every corner. But most of the day she just sits in the living room and watches TV or she sits on the chair in the kitchen. Besides walking Ayesha also experiences problems with smaller movements like combing her hair or putting on socks and two years ago she had a very unpleasant accident in the bathroom where she fell and could not get out of the bath. Since then she uses a bath chair. They talk Arabic at home and Ayesha doesn´t speak English too well, se when the rehabilitation nurse comes, the grandchildren always help to translate.

What is important to Ayesha

- Keeping social ties with the community and with her family [P3-Req-1]
- Limiting risk of falls [P3-Req-2]
- Staying self-sufficient [P3-Req-3]

Daily living

- She is able to do some light work around the house, but only on the ground floor [P3-Daily-1]
- Usually sits in her room or in the kitchen and watches TV [P3-Daily-2]

Own resources, assets, support

- The family offers big support, but that makes Ayesha often feel like she is a burden [P3-Resources-1]
- Loves cooking for the whole family but it is getting more and more difficult [P3-Resources-2]

Health concerns and limitations

- Limping, limited shoulder movement, severe back pain [P3-Health-1]
- Often relies on pain medication and worries she could become addicted [P3-Health-2]

Health tests/ treatments/ medication

- Rehabilitation helps, but the nurse comes only once in two weeks [P3-Tests-1]
- In case of a fall she often has to wait until somebody comes home and helps her [P3-Tests-2]

Events, issues, personal concerns, technology

- Mobility restrictions led gradually to more isolation [P3-Personal-1]
- She is often feeling lonely and would like to go out to see friends [P3-Personal-2]

Hopes and dreams/ what brings joy/ quotes

- *"It would be great if I could see my friends and hear all their news more often"*
- *"I would exercise on my own, but I don´t know if I am doing it right"*

Unmet needs

- Support of better movement, better coping of domestic tasks (cooking, etc.) [P3-Unmet-1]
- Some physiotherapy that she could follow on her own [P3-Unmet-2]
- Easier pain management, that would not require a personal visit to the doctor [P3-Unmet-3]
- Adapting some leisure activities so she can still participate [P3-Unmet-4]
- Spending more time with friends and her community [P3-Unmet-5]

This project has received funding from the European Union's Horizon 2020 research and innovation programme under grant agreement No 857159

Fig. 7.7 Persona 3: Older adults with chronic musculoskeletal disorder [83]

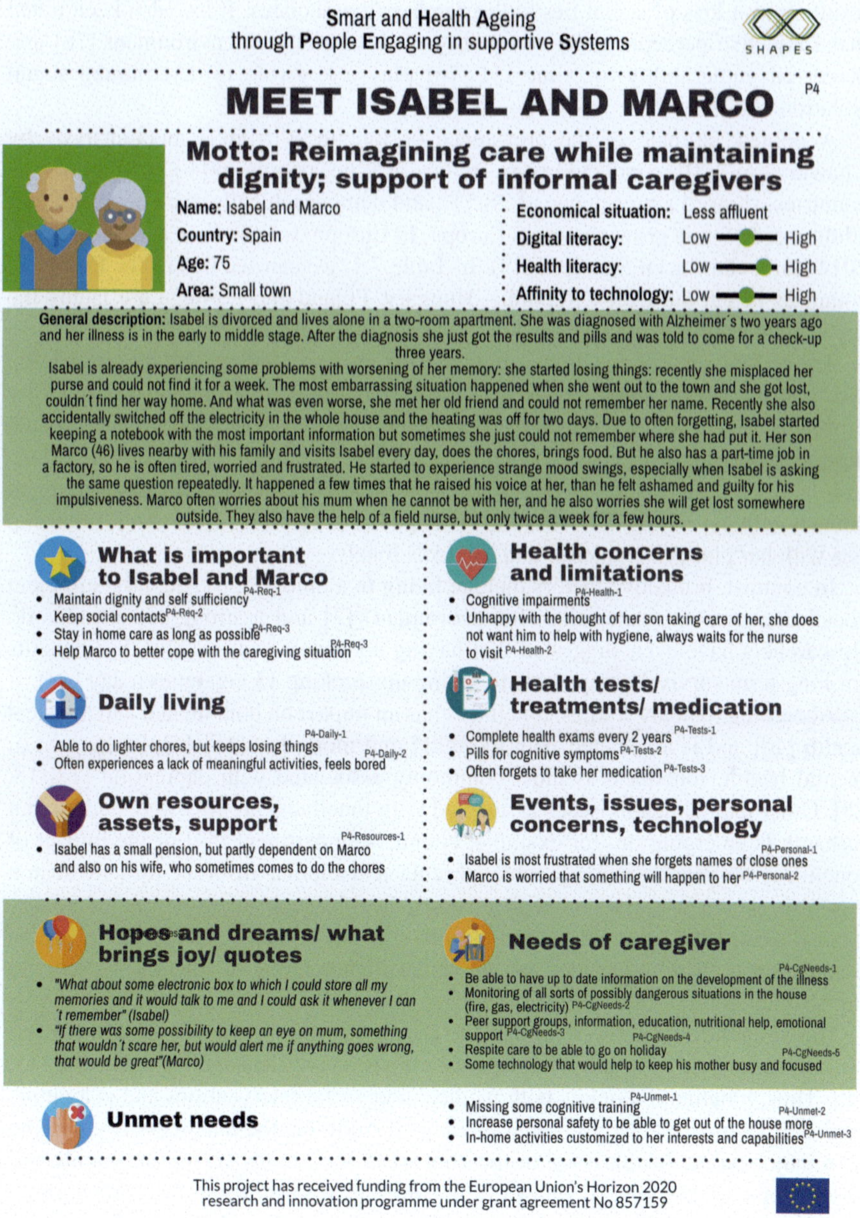

Fig. 7.8 Persona 4: Older adults with neurodegenerative diseases [83]

resulting in a loss of social ties with friends and associates. It has also been noted that subjective perceptions of the quality of the residential environment [76] and perceived vulnerability to crime [51, 76] play a key role in determining social isolation.

A pooled estimate of the prevalence of loneliness from a meta-analysis by Chawla et al. [20], conducted from studies of older people (60+) in high-income countries, showed a prevalence of 28.5%, and demographically, the cohort of older adults aged 65+ is growing across Europe. In Europe, we can look at data from the 2014 European Social Survey (ESS). In Table 7.1, we can see that of the European countries listed, the Czech Republic, Hungary, Poland and Portugal are facing the highest levels of loneliness (very lonely) at around 11% [93].

The risk factors for loneliness in adulthood are, e.g. widowhood, poorer health, less contact with friends, never having been married [67] or physical mobility problems and shrinking social networks (death of friends) [66]. A similar case is the description of another persona, Roisin (Ireland). Roisin moved from a small village to a large city. Here she has better access to medical care and has more frequent contact with her family. However, this change has severed long-standing friendship ties with her place of residence and she feels lonely.

In contrast, protective factors include living in a union [5, 31, 38, 54], sufficient social engagement (especially after retirement) [7] and a strong social network. Researchers have even suggested that having a strong social network has benefits for long-term survival comparable to giving up smoking 15 cigarettes a day [47].

According to many studies, loneliness has an impact on both mental and physical health [40] and is associated with mortality and morbidity [16, 44]. In the area of mental health, loneliness is most commonly associated with depression [17, 18, 28]. Other mental health issues associated with loneliness are less well studied, but research is emerging on, for example, cognitive impairment [53] or the impact of loneliness on psychosis [19], schizophrenia and bipolar disorder [86]. Research has also shown associations with physical health, such as stroke and coronary heart disease [85], and with various health risk behaviours ([2, 37] as well as an association with falls in older adults, where higher levels of loneliness predict a higher likelihood of falling [94].

Based on the above, it is reasonable to conclude the importance of loneliness as a social determinant of health with negative effects on physical and mental health [15, 68]. Thus, loneliness requires both medical and social interventions and is a public health problem, especially in older adults [7]. Additionally, loneliness is emerging as a major public health issue in the context of the rapidly increasing number of older people in developed countries [15]. Loneliness is also increasingly recognised as a significant health and social problem in the scientific world [81]. Understanding the mechanisms of loneliness serves as a basis for targeted interventions in this area [42].

We have addressed certain aspects of this problem through a different persona, Roisin (Fig. 7.9).

Table 7.1 Prevalence of loneliness in Europe [93]

Country	*How often felt lonely last week*				Frequently lonely (Most and all of the time)	Sample size (n)
	None or almost none of the time	Some of the time	Most of the time	All or almost all of the time		
Austria	73.42	20.59	4.20	1.79	5.99	1787
Belgium	74.04	19.57	3.85	2.55	6.39	1768
Switzerland	79.03	17.37	2.55	1.05	3.59	1531
Czechia	59.76	29.65	7.11	3.48	10.59	2125
Germany	79.92	16.75	2.44	0.89	3.32	3038
Denmark	83.03	13.89	1.74	1.34	3.07	1497
Estonia	65.91	26.24	5.74	2.11	7.85	2039
Spain	69.45	21.84	5.91	2.80	8.71	1928
Finland	81.18	15.79	1.49	1.54	3.02	2083
France	68.34	23.32	5.22	3.13	8.35	1917
UK	74.99	19.90	2.93	2.18	5.11	2251
Hungary	62.68	26.12	7.78	3.42	11.20	1696
Ireland	71.22	23.98	3.11	1.68	4.80	2377
Israel	71.62	21.26	5.51	1.61	7.11	2488
Lithuania	55.69	36.77	6.19	1.36	7.54	2214
Netherlands	81.87	15.37	1.88	0.89	2.76	1919
Norway	79.48	17.38	2.16	0.98	3.14	1433
Poland	73.39	14.78	8.20	3.63	11.83	1597
Portugal	64.79	24.60	5.06	5.54	10.60	1264
Sweden	72.71	22.37	2.96	1.96	4.92	1788
Slovenia	74.45	18.98	5.34	1.23	6.57	1217

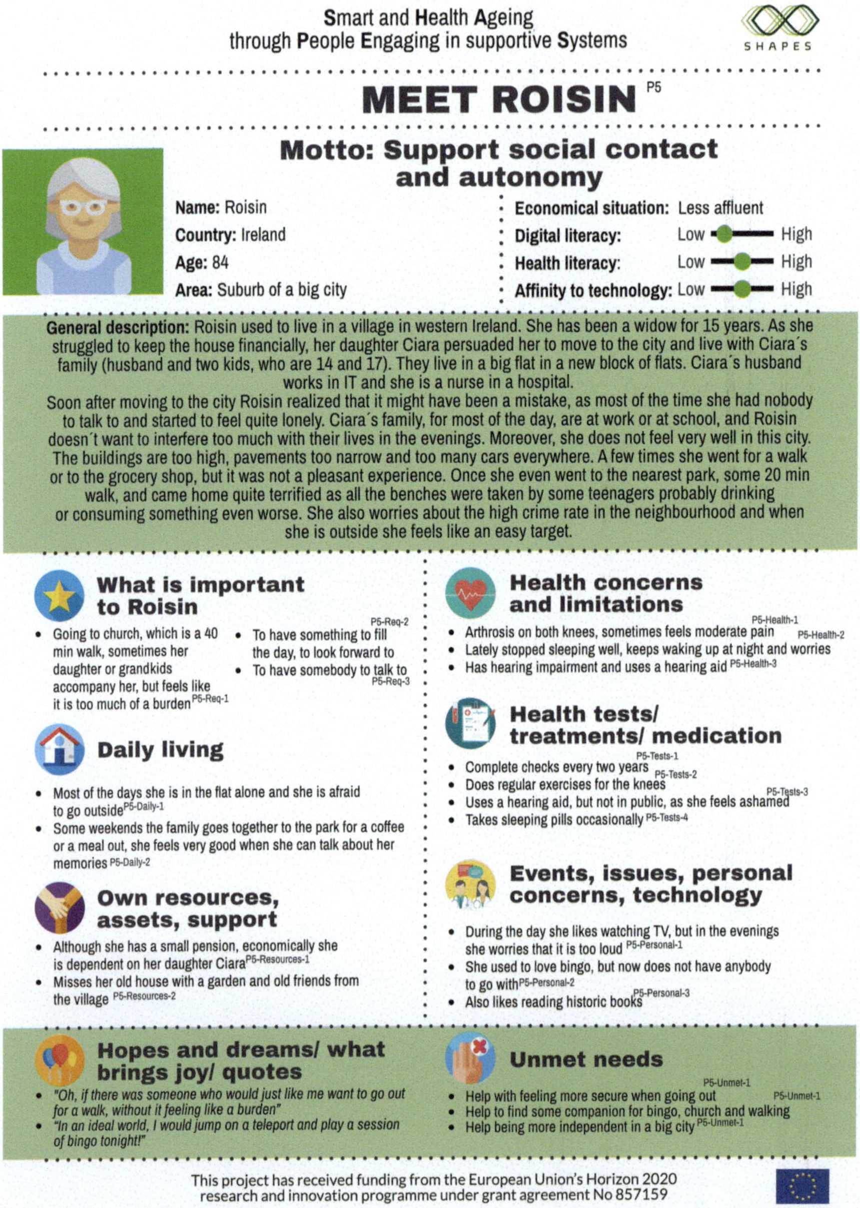

Fig. 7.9 Persona 5: Lonely and/or socially isolated older adults [83]

7.3.1.6 Older Adults with Alcohol or Drug Dependency and Severe Chronic Conditions Non-complying with Medical Recommendations

The challenge of alcohol and drug dependency extends to older adults, as highlighted by studies [14]. This problem becomes more significant when coupled with multiple chronic illnesses like diabetes, heart conditions or COPD. In this demographic, individuals often disregard doctors' advice, avoiding visits to their GPs. Instead, they tend to handle acute health crises by resorting to emergency services or visiting the emergency room, as indicated in research [21].

Persona six, Jarda from the Czech Republic, represents the complex issue of alcohol and drug dependency among older adults, a problem exacerbated when coupled with multiple chronic illnesses. This group often avoids doctor visits and relies on emergency services for healthcare, imposing a burden on the healthcare system. Addressing this challenge requires understanding their limited motivation for lifestyle changes, a reluctance to be told how to live and their desire to maintain autonomy. Harm reduction methods, focusing on enabling individuals to manage their health, rather than forcing change, could be a viable approach. Jarda's story illustrates the deep impact addiction has not only on the individual but also on their families, leading to complex emotional dilemmas and strained relationships. Distrust in medical experts, reluctance to take responsibility for health and avoidance of medical visits characterise this persona, reflecting wider issues in the Czech Republic's healthcare system. Improving doctor-patient communication, exploring digital healthcare options and increasing public spending on prevention could enhance healthcare utilisation and early detection of health problems, thus improving the quality of life for older adults like Jarda (Fig. 7.10).

7.3.1.7 Oldest and Frail

The seventh is represented by Helena from Slovakia. This persona focuses on the oldest old, typically defined as individuals over 85 years of age, and delves into the phenomenon of frailty syndrome, a natural consequence of age-related decline [22]. Frailty is prevalent in a significant portion of this population, characterised by sudden worsening of overall health, frequent falls, exhaustion, unexplained weight loss and acute confusion triggered by minor stressors [22]. It exhibits a dynamic nature, alternating between acute episodes and periods of normal functioning, often referred to as good days and bad days or frailer seasons [23]. Frailty leads to increased dependency on others and may necessitate relocation to institutionalised settings [36, 78].

While the majority of older individuals strongly prefer ageing in their own homes, decisions to move are often delayed until major incidents or health crises related to frailty occur. The process of deciding to move can be complex and demanding, often met with resentment if older adults feel pressured [78]. Sometimes, the decision is altruistically motivated, aiming to make the family happy or

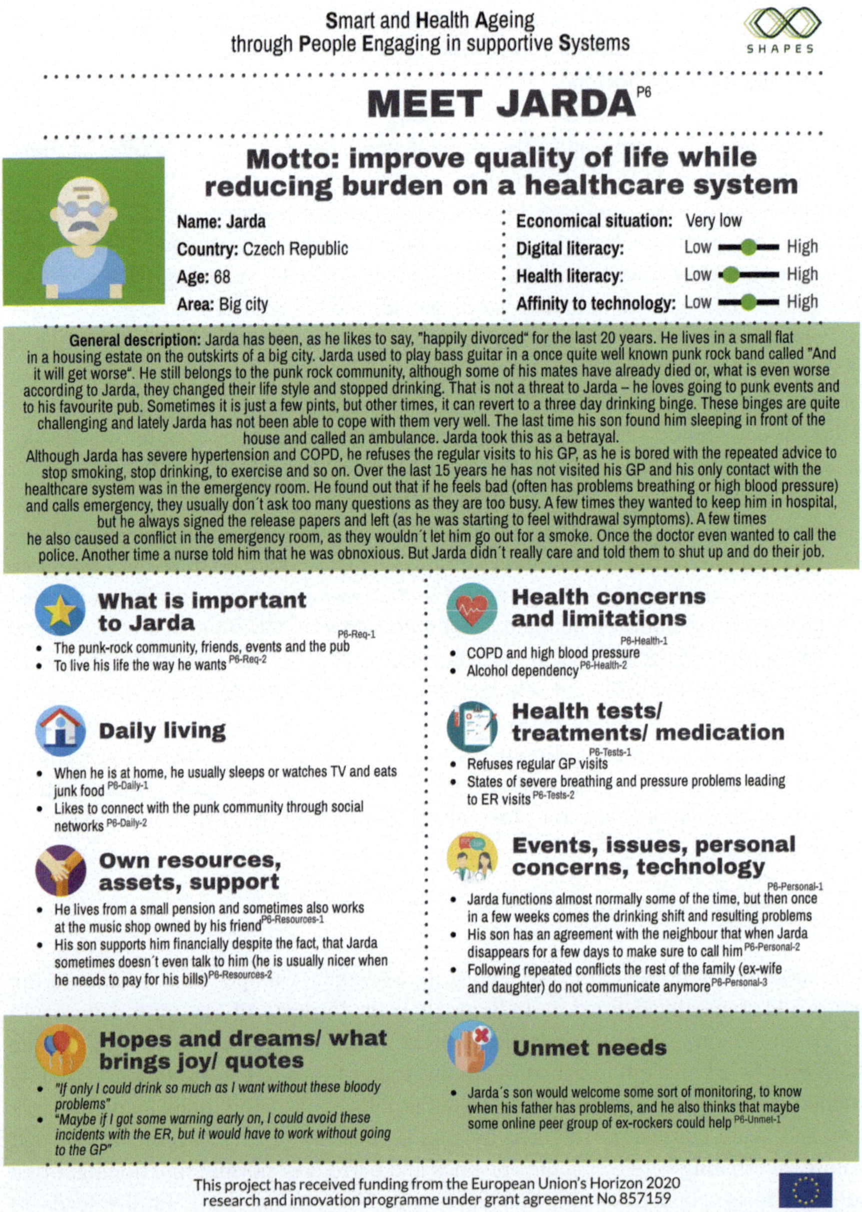

Fig. 7.10 Persona 6: Older adults with alcohol or drug dependency and severe chronic conditions non-complying with medical recommendations [83]

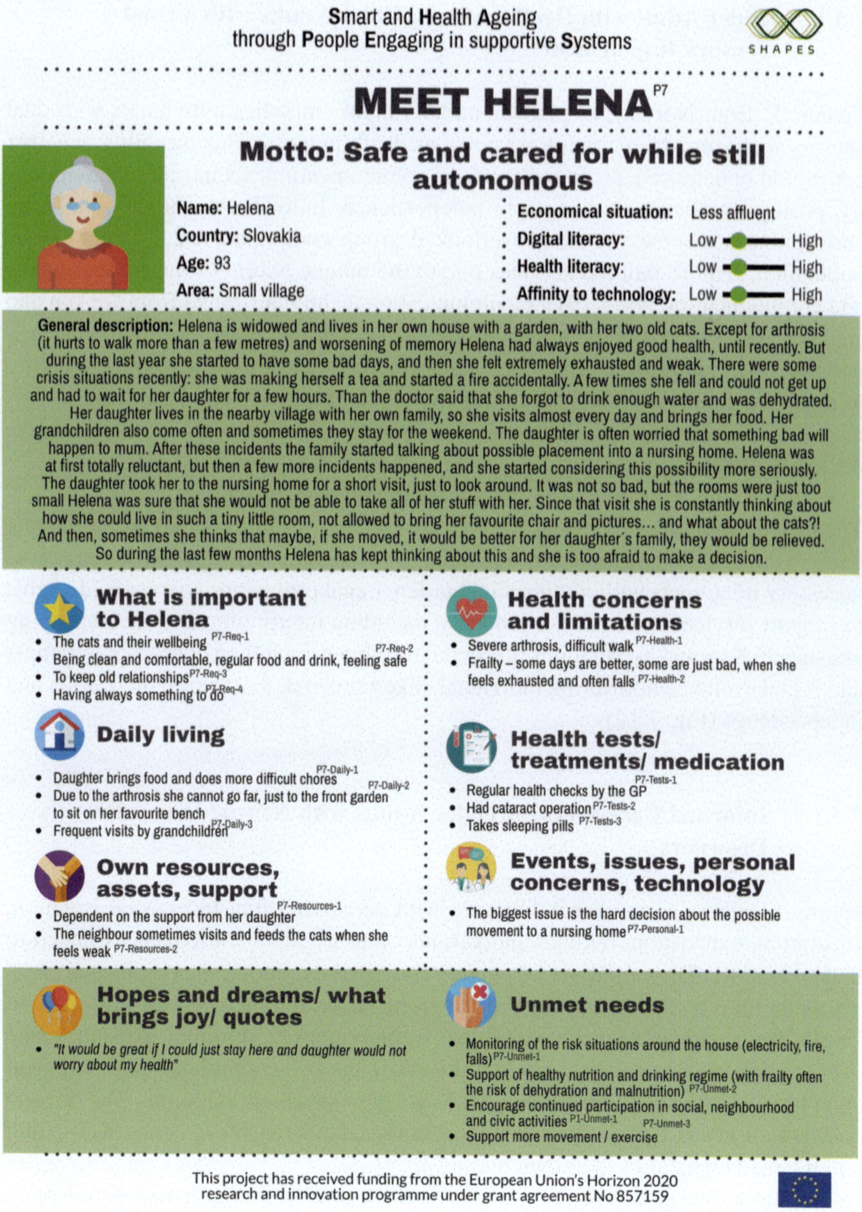

Fig. 7.11 Persona 7: Oldest and frail [83]

reduce the burden on informal caregivers [65]. Informal caregivers' motivations for institutionalising an older person usually revolve around safety concerns, whereas the older individual typically prioritises their autonomy [78] (Fig. 7.11).

7.3.1.8 Older Adult with Deafblindness (Older Adults with a Dual Sensory Impairment)

Frederick, from Norway, as persona number eight embodies individuals with dual sensory impairments, a condition known as deafblindness. This disability, whether congenital or acquired, profoundly affects communication, socialisation and mobility, posing significant challenges to independence. Individuals who are deafblind, constituting a diverse yet often overlooked group comprising 0.2% to 2% of the population, require tailored services due to the unique nature of their impairments and communication needs [91]. Communication techniques range from spoken and sign languages to tactile methods. Obstacles in communication, information access and mobility can result in emotional and social repercussions. They limit the ability to make informed decisions, curtail functional independence and hinder the performance of daily tasks [11]. There is a need for the development of more assistive devices to support communication, additional interpreter-guides and training for hearing and sighted people in communicating with persons with deafblindness [43]. The lack of appropriate services leads to dependency, limiting social and economic participation. In Norway, the robust healthcare system ensures Frederick can access necessary treatments without financial burden. Legal provisions guarantee his rights to support services and assistive products, including interpreting and accompanying assistance. National associations offer vital resources, including courses, newsletters and social events, empowering individuals like Frederick to enhance their skills and independence (Fig. 7.12).

7.3.1.9 Informal Caregivers for Older Adults with Neurodegenerative Disorders

Family members caring for individuals with dementia often face social isolation, frustration, exhaustion, burnout and various other negative consequences linked to their role [58]. The initial set of unmet requirements among these informal caregivers pertains to the caregiving process itself, including the need for information, breaks from caregiving responsibilities, formal support, informal assistance like peer support groups and assistance in handling the behavioural and psychological symptoms of the care recipients, such as aggression or agitation. The second category of needs is more personal, concerning the caregiver's mental well-being and the management of their own lives [57, 59].

To present this phenomenon, we introduce the ninth persona, Astrid–an informal caregiver from Belgium. This persona embodies the challenges and complexities faced by informal caregivers in the context of neurodegenerative diseases like dementia. Astrid has been caring for her mother, who was diagnosed with Alzheimer's 6 years ago. Despite the severe symptoms her mother experiences, Astrid is determined to provide care, yet struggles to balance her own needs with her caregiving responsibilities. The progression of dementia underscores the escalating costs of care, raising concerns about socioeconomic inequality. Informal caregivers

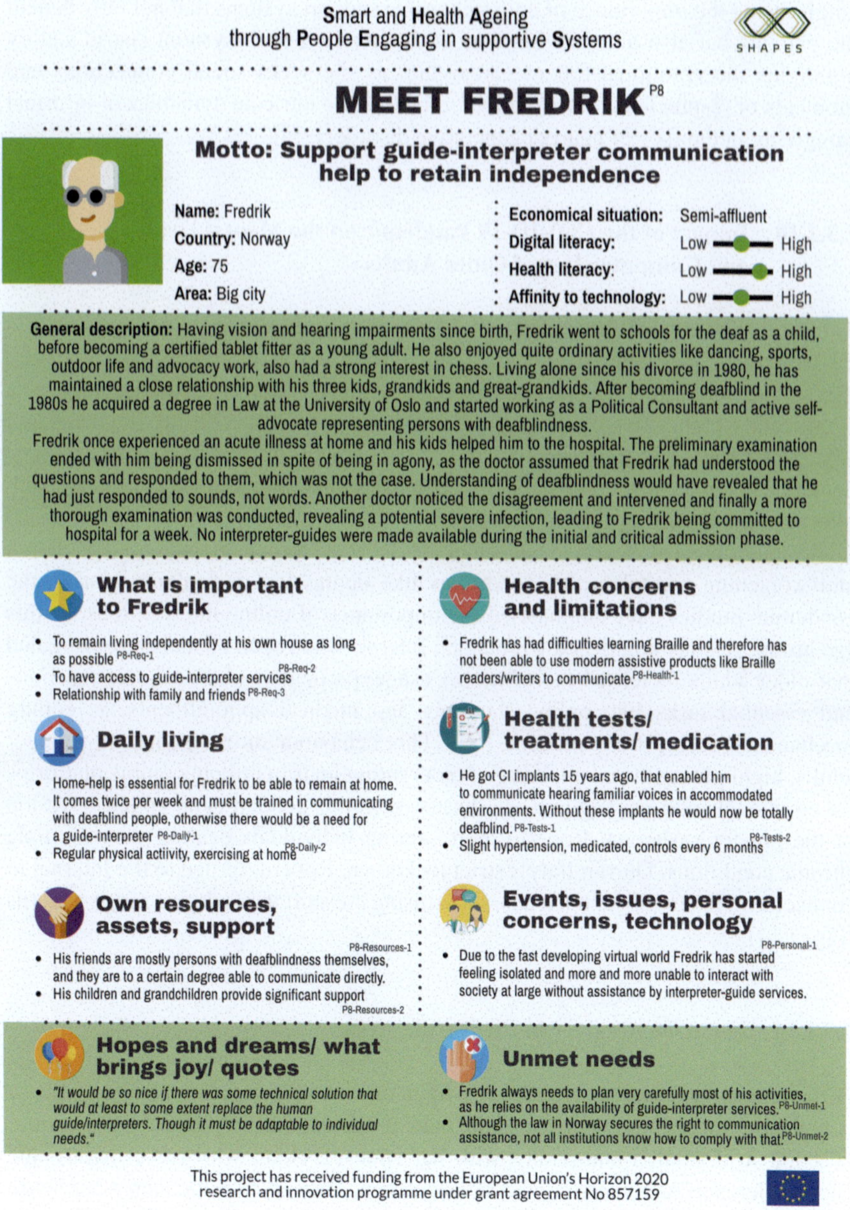

Fig. 7.12 Persona 8: Deafblind older adults (older adults with dual sensory impairment) [83]

often grapple with dilemmas such as preserving relationships, coping with changing behaviours and deciding when to prioritise their own needs, leading to feelings of guilt and frustration. Experts highlight the critical role of informal caregivers, emphasising the importance of comprehensive support systems that not only benefit the patients but also alleviate burdens on the public health system. Astrid's story highlights the emotional toll of caregiving, as she seeks social connections and moments of respite amid her isolation, reflecting the intricate dynamics of informal caregiving in the face of neurodegenerative disorders (Fig. 7.13).

7.3.1.10 Impact of the COVID-19 Pandemic on the Mental Health and Computer Use of Older Adults

The tenth persona, Roberto from Italy, focuses on the impact of the COVID-19 pandemic, particularly on older adults who are at a higher risk of severe illness and mortality. Several studies have indicated that older adults were at a significantly higher risk of increased isolation and loneliness during the pandemic [25], worsening all of the existing mental health conditions like depression, anxiety, dementia and psychosis. The pandemic emphasised the importance of online health interventions to help this age group [92].

Besides physical health risks, older adults were prone to increased isolation and worsening mental health conditions like depression and anxiety during the pandemic. Studies have emphasised the importance of online interventions for this age group. A study conducted with Israeli Internet users aged 60 and above revealed that older adults increased their Internet usage, particularly for social connections and essential tasks like online shopping and medical appointments, as coping mechanisms during the pandemic [62]. This behaviour mirrored that of younger adults, highlighting the adaptability of older individuals in utilising online platforms for emotional support. The persona discussed in this context is an updated version of the previous persona, Roberto, representing individuals dealing with multiple chronic conditions. During Italy's strict lockdown, Roberto turned to the Internet to connect with his family and friends, showcasing the shift in his digital usage patterns (Fig. 7.14).

7.3.1.11 Formal Caregiver in the Nordic Area

Persona number eleven, Anna, sheds light on life in a Nordic suburban area, a perspective not covered in previous qualitative research. At 70 years old, she resides in a flat in a small Finnish city with her spouse Pekka, who has Amyotrophic lateral sclerosis (ALS) and requires constant care. They sold their countryside house 5 years ago due to Pekka's mobility issues. Anna, his formal caretaker for a decade, balances her own health concerns while caring for Pekka, who receives support from the public healthcare system. Their routine involves multiple meals, TV, and audio books, but Anna wishes she could provide Pekka more outdoor time despite her physical limitations. Their lives revolve around each other, and both of them desire more independence for Pekka, highlighting the challenges and hopes within their daily existence (Fig. 7.15).

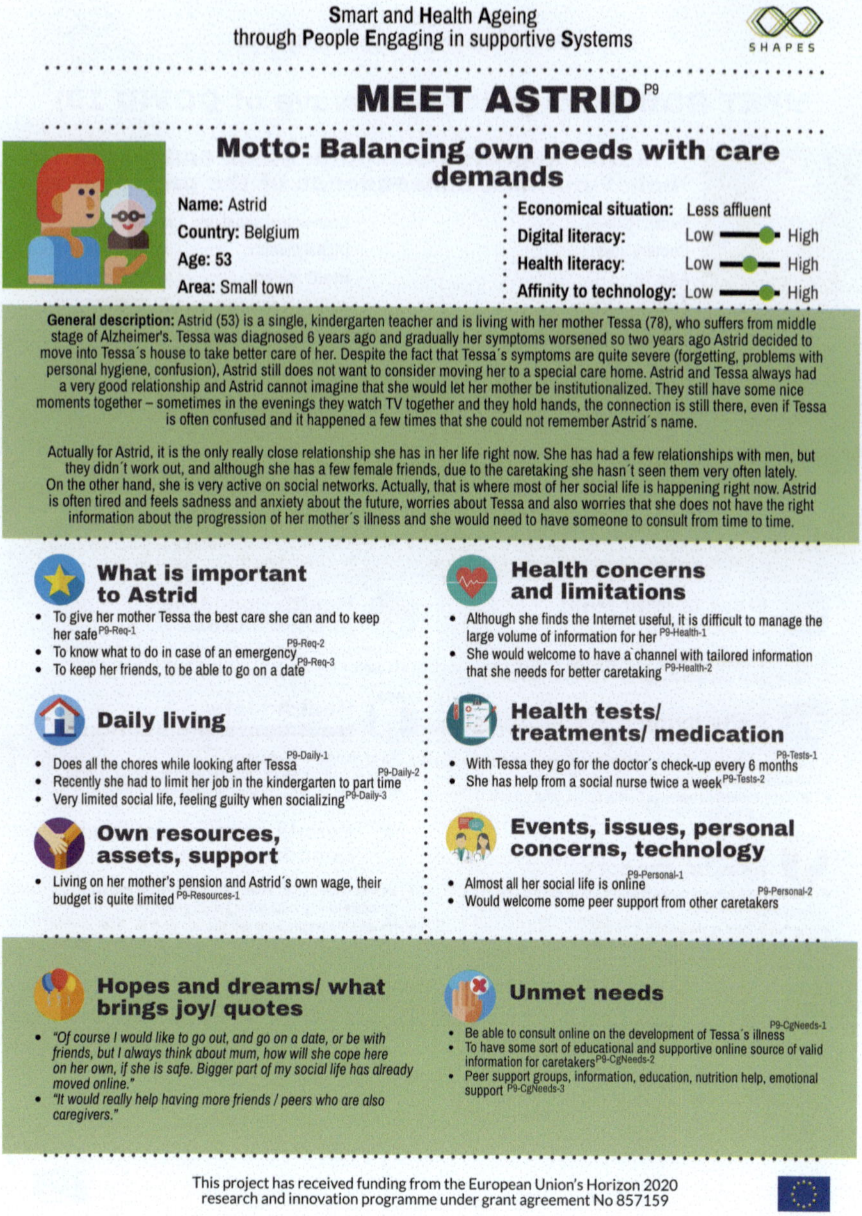

Fig. 7.13 Persona 9: Informal caregivers [83]

Smart and **H**ealth **A**geing
through **P**eople **E**ngaging in supportive **S**ystems

SHAPES

MEET ROBERTO (after first wave of COVID 19)[P10]

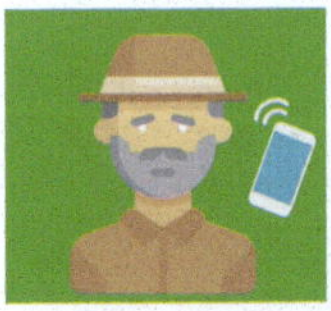

Motto: Improved computer skills and health behaviour as a consequence of the pandemics

Name: Roberto
Country: Italy
Age: 72
Area: Small town

Economical situation: Less affluent
Digital literacy: Low — High
Health literacy: Low — High
Affinity to technology: Low — High

General description: Roberto lives with his wife Bianca in a small Italian town, in a house with a garden. He is the owner of a small shop, which is now run by his nephew. Roberto and Bianca are childless and Bianca was recently diagnosed with Parkinson´s, though she has very mild symptoms so far. Roberto is slightly obese, he has diabetes and hypertension and smokes 20 cigarettes a day. He realizes he has to change his lifestyle.

The COVID19 pandemics has changed lives not only for Roberto, but for all the people in the city. Almost four months it was not possible to go anywhere and people were very afraid of the infection. Roberto knows several people who have been to hospital and unfortunately one of his best friends died of COVID. Roberto was very scared for himself as well as for Bianca´s life and he was anxiously complying with all regulations. Of course he realized that he was in higher danger due to his being overweight, having hypertension and smoking. Some of his friends were also suffering depression. Paradoxically COVID pandemics caused Roberto to take better care of his health. He started to take regular walks around the house and even ride on the exercise bike. Also, as he could not go out, his nephew taught him how to work better with the internet, Roberto started using social networks and evening videocalls with his friends (with an obligatory glass of wine). With their wider family they started seeing each other on Skype.

What is important to Roberto

- To keep a satisfactory social life even amidst pandemics[P10-Req-1]
- Family ties of their brothers, sisters, nieces, and nephews[P10-Req-2]

Daily living

- Still does most of the work around the house and in the garden, but sometimes his nephews come to help[P10-Daily-1]
- Most of the evenings he meets friends online, once a week personally in the town[P10-Daily-2]

Own resources, assets, support

- The business suffered during the pandemics, but it is still functioning[P10-Resources-1]
- Big family, there is always help if needed[P10-Resources-2]
- Also he has many friends and a good local community that he can rely on[P10-Resources-3]

Health concerns and limitations

- To keep some of the good habits that he gained in the first wave of pandemics (training, less drinking, healthier food)[P10-Health-1]

Health tests/ treatments/ medication

- Takes six different medications[P10-Tests-1]
- Visits several specialists (diabetes, heart condition), recently some of the checks were done by videocalls[P10-Tests-2]

Events, issues, personal concerns, technology

- He likes to read about various diagnoses on the internet, considers joining some online patient groups[P10-Personal-1]
- He used to have problems with doctor's visits as he felt ashamed and irritated, but it seems to be much easier with online check-ups[P10-Personal-2]

Hopes and dreams/ what brings joy/ quotes

- *"it is really awful what happened here in the spring with the COVID 19 pandemics. I hope this will never happen again. But surprisingly, thanks to that horrible situation I learned some new tricks with the internet, I never knew it was so easy to videocall or to find friends on social network. I am very enthusiastic about this new technology and all the possibilities."*

Unmet needs

- Online peer support group of patients with hypertension[P10-Unmet-1]
- Online intervention to reduce smoking[P10-Unmet-2]
- Some tools to enhance home training[P10-Unmet-3]

This project has received funding from the European Union's Horizon 2020 research and innovation programme under grant agreement No 857159

Fig. 7.14 Persona 10: Impact of the COVID-19 pandemic on the mental health and computer use of older adults [83]

Smart and Health Ageing
through People Engaging in supportive Systems

SHAPES

MEET ANNA[P14]

Motto: One day at a time, hoping for the good ones

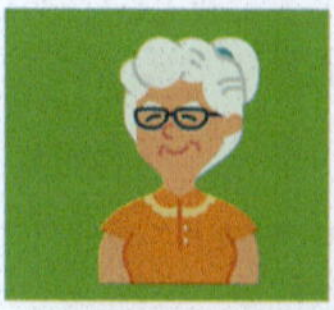

Name: Anna
Country: Finland
Age: 70
Area: Suburb of a small city

Economical situation: Less affluent
Digital literacy: Low —●— High
Health literacy: Low —●— High
Affinity to technology: Low —●— High

General description: Anna has been living with her spouse Pekka for almost 50 years. They live in a block of flats. Pekka has been feeling progressively worse the last couple of years, and Anna, who has already been his formal caretaker for 10 years, does not have time for herself. As a formal caretaker, she receives a monthly payment of 800€ in addition to her pension. Anna is happy that her own symptoms with high blood pressure and cholesterol are mild, and with medication she feels ok most of the time. She just needs to remind herself about her own medication. She also feels pain in her back and joints from time to time, but aims not to pay attention, as she feels that she simply doesn't have time to concentrate on herself, and her health concerns are lesser that Pekka's. In addition to the constant care that Anna provides, the public healthcare system provides Pekka with nurses visiting him two times a day.

What is important to Anna

- Pekka [P14-Req-1]
- Daily routines [P14-Req-2]
- Staying physically capable of acting as the formal caretaker [P14-Req-3]

Daily living

- Nurses visiting two times a day [P14-Daily-1]
- Routines regarding daily cooking and eating together are important [P14-Daily-2]
- Assisting Pekka with all tasks [P14-Daily-3]
- Having TV on and reading digital newspapers [P14-Daily-4]

Own resources, assets, support

- Relies on herself in daily life [P14-Resources-1]
- Calls their private healthcare provider in case needs help for herself or Pekka [P14-Resources-2]
- Daily support from nurses [P14-Resources-3]
- Feelings of isolation and loneliness, and sometimes anxiety [P14-Resources-4]

Health concerns and limitations

- Feeling healthy most of the time, does not experience limitations [P14-Health-1]
- COVID-19 fear [P14-Health-2]
- Concerns for Pekka's deteriorating health [P14-Health-3]
- She need reading glasses (strong nearsightedness) [P14-Health-4]

Health tests/ treatments/ medication

- Takes pills daily to stabilize hood blood pressure [P14-Tests-1]
- Yearly health check-ups [P14-Tests-2]
- Regular dentist visits [P14-Tests-3]

Events, issues, personal concerns, technology

- Digital active, uses smartphone and tablet daily reading, videocalls and occasionally ordering online [P14-Personal-1]
- Concerns about data privacy, does not give consent to third parties [P14-Personal-2]
- Trusts own healthcare service provider [P14-Personal-3]
- Interested, yet highly suspicious about new digital services and data privacy. She is afraid of 5G and its consequences, especially for bees [P14-Personal-4]

Hopes and dreams/ what brings joy/ quotes

- *That everything would stay as it is, and nothing surprising would happen*
- *Having as many good days with Pekka as possible*
- *Being able to contribute to the society somehow*

Unmet needs

- Maintaining individual life and participating actively in society [P14-Unmet-1]
- Feeling guilty for the times being away from Pekka, and not being able to provide him with enough independence and outside activities [P14-Unmet-2]
- Not having time for herself [P14-Unmet-3]

This project has received funding from the European Union's Horizon 2020 research and innovation programme under grant agreement No 857159

Fig. 7.15 Persona 14: Formal caregiver in the Nordic area [83]

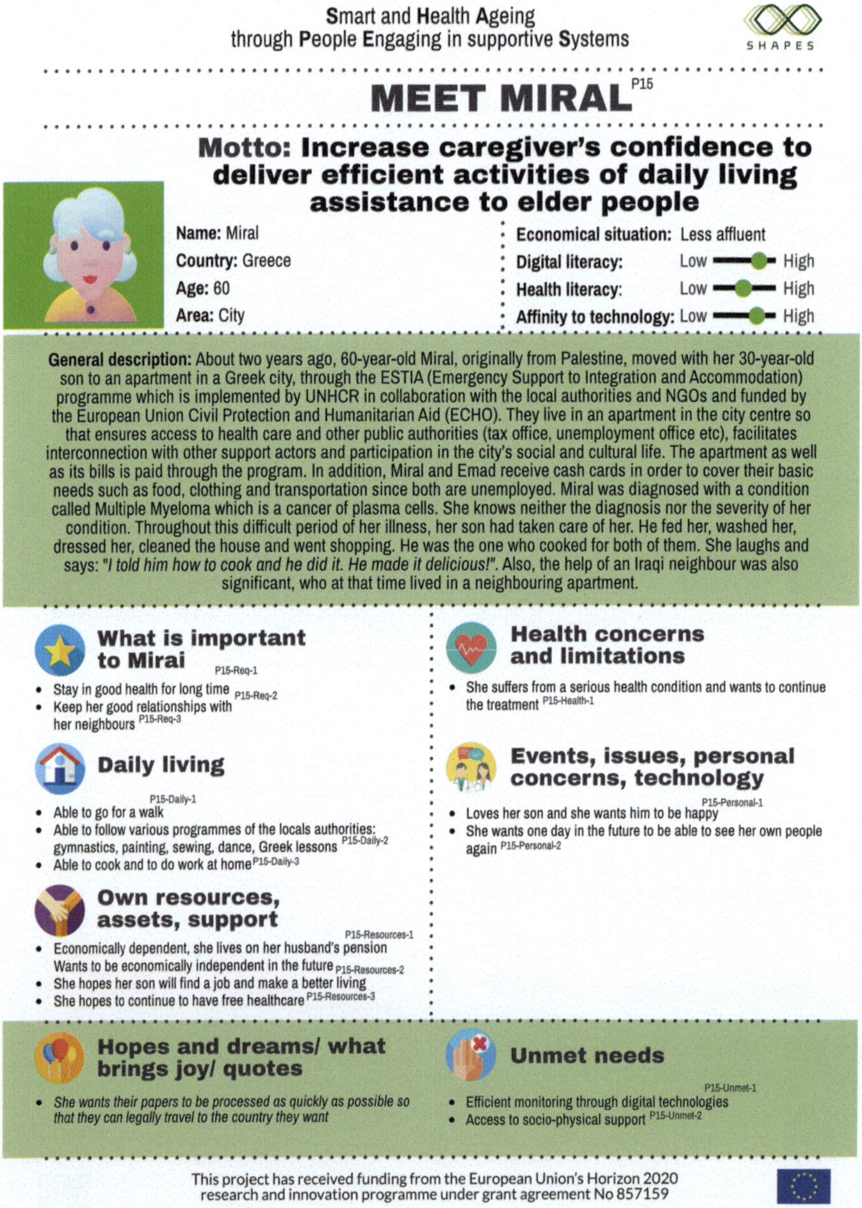

Fig. 7.16 Persona 15: Refugee's perspective [83]

7.3.1.12 Refugee's Perspective

Miral, the final persona, offers a view from a refugee's perspective. Despite not belonging to the older demographic, she represents a vulnerable group that has faced and overcome difficult social conditions that average older European population have not confronted [39]. The life-threatening, stressful experiences of conflict zones are said [9, 88] to take their toll in life expectancy. Originally from Palestine, she moved to a Greek city with her son through the ESTIA programme, a collaboration between UNHCR, local authorities and NGOs funded by the European Union Civil Protection and Humanitarian Aid. Living in a centrally located apartment ensures access to essential services, healthcare and participation in the city's social life. Although supported financially through the programme, Miral has faced considerable health issues, including a cancer diagnosis, which she bravely battles while cherishing her connections with her family and finding solace in her newfound community (Fig. 7.16).

7.4 Conclusion

In examining the varied experiences of ageing, each persona offers a unique perspective on the challenges and successes encountered by older adults and their caregivers. The stories of active, healthy older adults highlight the importance of remaining socially and physically engaged in later years. These individuals not only showcase their physical vitality but also demonstrate mental resilience, enabling them to embrace life's adventures with enthusiasm. Transitioning to older adults with mild yet persistent chronic conditions, we gain insight into the delicate balance they maintain between managing health issues and preserving a sense of normalcy. These individuals embody resilience, adapting to the fluctuations in their health while finding joy in life's simple pleasures.

Shifting our focus to older adults with chronic musculoskeletal disorders, the spotlight is on the determination required to navigate daily tasks despite physical limitations. Their stories underscore the significance of accessibility and adaptation, highlighting the challenges posed by environments not tailored to their specific needs. Our exploration deepens with older adults facing neurodegenerative diseases, where the narratives reveal the profound impact of cognitive decline not only on the individuals but also on their families. We witness the strength displayed by these individuals as they grapple with memory loss and shifting realities, underscoring the vital role of support networks in their lives. Each persona, a unique thread in the fabric of ageing, enhances our comprehension of the diverse human experiences that define this significant life stage.

It should be noted, however, that these personas represent contemporary older people and are valid in a specific time context and depending on the current generation, times and conditions. It should be considered that the generation of older people is evolving. Each generation of older people carries different experiences and perceptions, for example, in the field of information technology. The current generation of older people grew up in an era without mass diffusion of IT technologies, while the current productive generation (future older people) already has experience with IT. However, the evolution towards IT is not only influenced by attitudes but also by other key aspects.

References

1. Aboumatar, H. J., Carson, K. A., Beach, M. C., Roter, D. L., & Cooper, L. A. (2013). The impact of health literacy on desire for participation in healthcare, medical visit communication, and patient reported outcomes among patients with hypertension. *Journal of General Internal Medicine, 28*(11), 1469–1476. https://doi.org/10.1007/s11606-013-2466-5
2. Algren, M. H., Ekholm, O., Nielsen, L., Ersbøll, A. K., Bak, C. K., & Andersen, P. T. (2020). Social isolation, loneliness, socioeconomic status, and health-risk behaviour in deprived neighbourhoods in Denmark: A cross-sectional study. *SSM – Population Health, 10*, 100546. https://doi.org/10.1016/j.ssmph.2020.100546
3. Arnautovska, U., O'Callaghan, F., & Hamilton, K. (2018). Behaviour change techniques to facilitate physical activity in older adults: What and how. *Ageing and Society, 38*(12), 2590–2616. https://doi.org/10.1017/S0144686X17001027
4. Auais, M., French, S., Alvarado, B., Pirkle, C., Belanger, E., & Guralnik, J. (2018). Fear of falling predicts incidence of functional disability 2 years later: A perspective from an International Cohort Study. *The Journals of Gerontology: Series A, 73*(9), 1212–1215. https://doi.org/10.1093/gerona/glx237
5. Baarck, J., d'Hombres, B., & Tintori, G. (2022). Loneliness in Europe before and during the COVID-19 pandemic. *Health Policy, 126*(11), 1124–1129. https://doi.org/10.1016/j.healthpol.2022.09.002
6. Berendonk, C., Blix, B. H., Hoben, M., Clandinin, D. J., Roach, P. M., Compton, R. M., Cave, M. T., & Caine, V. (2020). A narrative care approach for persons living with dementia in institutional care settings. *International Journal of Older People Nursing, 15*(1), e12278. https://doi.org/10.1111/opn.12278
7. Berg-Weger, M., & Morley, J. E. (2020). Loneliness in old age: An unaddressed health problem. *The Journal of Nutrition, Health & Aging, 24*(3), 243–245. https://doi.org/10.1007/s12603-020-1323-6
8. Berlingieri, F., Colagrossi, M., & Mauri, C. (2023). *Loneliness and social connectedness: Insights from a New EU-wide Survey (JRC133351)*. European Commission.
9. Bhatt, J., & Bathija, P. (2018). Ensuring access to quality health care in vulnerable communities. *Academic Medicine, 93*(9), 1271–1275. https://doi.org/10.1097/ACM.0000000000002254
10. Bhattacharyya, O., Mossman, K., Gustafsson, L., & Schneider, E. C. (2019). Using human-centered design to build a digital health advisor for patients with complex needs: Persona and prototype development. *Journal of Medical Internet Research, 21*(5), e10318. https://doi.org/10.2196/10318
11. Bodsworth, S. M., Clare, I. C. H., Simblett, S. K., & Deafblind, U. K. (2011). Deafblindness and mental health: Psychological distress and unmet need among adults with dual sensory impairment. *British Journal of Visual Impairment, 29*(1), 6–26. https://doi.org/10.1177/0264619610387495
12. Bonanno, G. A. (2004). Loss, trauma, and human resilience: Have we underestimated the human capacity to thrive after extremely aversive events? *American Psychologist, 59*(1), 20–28. https://doi.org/10.1037/0003-066X.59.1.20
13. Bronstein, L. R. (2003). A model for interdisciplinary collaboration. *Social Work, 48*(3), 297–306. https://doi.org/10.1093/sw/48.3.297
14. Busse, R., Blümel, M., Scheller-Kreinsen, D., & Zentner, A. (2010). *Tackling chronic disease in Europe: Strategies, interventions and challenges*. World Health Organization. Regional Office for Europe. https://iris.who.int/handle/10665/326484
15. Cacioppo, J. T., & Cacioppo, S. (2018). The growing problem of loneliness. *The Lancet, 391*(10119), 426. https://doi.org/10.1016/S0140-6736(18)30142-9
16. Cacioppo, J. T., Hawkley, L. C., & Berntson, G. G. (2003). The anatomy of loneliness. *Current Directions in Psychological Science, 12*(3), 71–74. https://doi.org/10.1111/1467-8721.01232

17. Cacioppo, J. T., Hughes, M. E., Waite, L. J., Hawkley, L. C., & Thisted, R. A. (2006). Loneliness as a specific risk factor for depressive symptoms: Cross-sectional and longitudinal analyses. *Psychology and Aging, 21*(1), 140–151. https://doi.org/10.1037/0882-7974.21.1.140
18. Cacioppo, J. T., Fowler, J. H., & Christakis, N. A. (2009). Alone in the crowd: The structure and spread of loneliness in a large social network. *Journal of Personality and Social Psychology, 97*(6), 977–991. https://doi.org/10.1037/a0016076
19. Chau, A. K. C., Zhu, C., & So, S. H.-W. (2019). Loneliness and the psychosis continuum: A meta-analysis on positive psychotic experiences and a meta-analysis on negative psychotic experiences. *International Review of Psychiatry, 31*(5–6), 471–490. https://doi.org/10.1080/09540261.2019.1636005
20. Chawla, K., Kunonga, T. P., Stow, D., Barker, R., Craig, D., & Hanratty, B. (2021). Prevalence of loneliness amongst older people in high-income countries: A systematic review and meta-analysis. *PLoS One, 16*(7), e0255088. https://doi.org/10.1371/journal.pone.0255088
21. Choi, N., Marti, C., DiNitto, D., & Choi, B. (2015). Alcohol use as risk factors for older adults' emergency department visits: A latent class analysis. *Western Journal of Emergency Medicine, 16*(7), 1146–1158. https://doi.org/10.5811/westjem.2015.9.27704
22. Clegg, A., Young, J., Iliffe, S., Rikkert, M. O., & Rockwood, K. (2013). Frailty in elderly people. *The Lancet, 381*(9868), 752–762. https://doi.org/10.1016/S0140-6736(12)62167-9
23. Coker, J. F., Martin, M. E., Simpson, R. M., & Lafortune, L. (2019). Frailty: An in-depth qualitative study exploring the views of community care staff. *BMC Geriatrics, 19*(1), 47. https://doi.org/10.1186/s12877-019-1069-3
24. Comeau-Vallée, M., & Langley, A. (2019). The interplay of inter- and intraprofessional boundary work in multidisciplinary teams. *Organization Studies, 41*, 017084061984802. https://doi.org/10.1177/0170840619848020
25. De Jong Gierveld, J., & Van Tilburg, T. (2010). The De Jong Gierveld short scales for emotional and social loneliness: Tested on data from 7 countries in the UN generations and gender surveys. *European Journal of Ageing, 7*(2), 121–130. https://doi.org/10.1007/s10433-010-0144-6
26. Dubovská, E., Chrz, V., Tavel, P., Poláčková Šolcová, I., & Růžička, J. (2017). Narrative construction of resilience: Stories of older Czech adults. *Ageing and Society, 37*(9), 1849–1873. https://doi.org/10.1017/S0144686X16000581
27. Durand, F., & Fleury, M.-J. (2021). A multilevel study of patient-centered care perceptions in mental health teams. *BMC Health Services Research, 21*(1), 44. https://doi.org/10.1186/s12913-020-06054-z
28. Erzen, E., & Çikrikci, Ö. (2018). The effect of loneliness on depression: A meta-analysis. *International Journal of Social Psychiatry, 64*(5), 427–435. https://doi.org/10.1177/0020764018776349
29. Fabbri, E., Zoli, M., Gonzalez-Freire, M., Salive, M. E., Studenski, S. A., & Ferrucci, L. (2015). Aging and multimorbidity: New tasks, priorities, and frontiers for integrated gerontological and clinical research. *Journal of the American Medical Directors Association, 16*(8), 640–647. https://doi.org/10.1016/j.jamda.2015.03.013
30. Fejer, R., & Ruhe, A. (2012). What is the prevalence of musculoskeletal problems in the elderly population in developed countries? A systematic critical literature review. *Chiropractic & Manual Therapies, 20*(1), 31. https://doi.org/10.1186/2045-709X-20-31
31. Fokkema, T., De Jong Gierveld, J., & Dykstra, P. A. (2012). Cross-national differences in older adult loneliness. *The Journal of Psychology, 146*(1–2), 201–228. https://doi.org/10.1080/00223980.2011.631612
32. Franke, T., Tong, C., Ashe, M. C., McKay, H., & Sims-Gould, J. (2013). The secrets of highly active older adults. *Journal of Aging Studies, 27*(4), 398–409. https://doi.org/10.1016/j.jaging.2013.09.003
33. GBD. (2019). *VizHub – GBD compare*. VizHub – GBD Compare. https://vizhub.healthdata.org/gbd-compare/

34. Goodman-Deane, J., Waller, S., Demin, D., González de Heredia, A., Bradley, M., & Clarkson, P. (2018). *Evaluating inclusivity using Quantitative Personas*. https://doi.org/10.21606/drs.2018.400
35. Goodman-Deane, J., Bradley, M., Waller, S., & Clarkson, P. (2021). *Developing personas to help designers to understand digital exclusion*.
36. Granbom, M., Löfqvist, C., Horstmann, V., Haak, M., & Iwarsson, S. (2014). Relocation to ordinary or special housing in very old age: Aspects of housing and health. *European Journal of Ageing, 11*(1), 55–65. https://doi.org/10.1007/s10433-013-0287-3
37. Hajek, A., & König, H.-H. (2021). Asymmetric effects of obesity on loneliness among older Germans. Longitudinal findings from the Survey of Health, Ageing and Retirement in Europe. *Aging & Mental Health, 25*(12), 2293–2297. https://doi.org/10.1080/13607863.2020.1822285
38. Hansen, T., & Slagsvold, B. (2016). Late-life loneliness in 11 European countries: Results from the Generations and Gender Survey. *Social Indicators Research, 129*(1), 445–464. https://doi.org/10.1007/s11205-015-1111-6
39. Hatzidimitriadou, E. (2010). Migration and ageing: Settlement experiences and emerging care needs of older refugees in developed countries. *Hellenic Journal of Psychology, 7*, 1–20.
40. Hawkley, L. C. (2022). Loneliness and health. *Nature Reviews Disease Primers, 8*(1), 1–2. https://doi.org/10.1038/s41572-022-00355-9
41. Hawkley, L. C. (2023). *Loneliness*. https://www.britannica.com/science/loneliness
42. Hawkley, L. C., & Cacioppo, J. T. (2010). Loneliness matters: A theoretical and empirical review of consequences and mechanisms. *Annals of Behavioral Medicine, 40*(2), 218–227. https://doi.org/10.1007/s12160-010-9210-8
43. Hersh, M. (2013). Deafblind people, communication, independence, and isolation. *Journal of Deaf Studies and Deaf Education, 18*(4), 446–463. https://doi.org/10.1093/deafed/ent022
44. Holt-Lunstad, J., Smith, T. B., Baker, M., Harris, T., & Stephenson, D. (2015). Loneliness and social isolation as risk factors for mortality: A meta-analytic review. *Perspectives on Psychological Science, 10*(2), 227–237. https://doi.org/10.1177/1745691614568352
45. Hoogendijk, E. O., Smit, A. P., Van Dam, C., Schuster, N. A., De Breij, S., Holwerda, T. J., Huisman, M., Dent, E., & Andrew, M. K. (2020). Frailty combined with loneliness or social isolation: An elevated risk for mortality in later life. *Journal of the American Geriatrics Society, 68*(11), 2587–2593. https://doi.org/10.1111/jgs.16716
46. Huh, J., Kwon, B. C., Kim, S.-H., Lee, S., Choo, J., Kim, J., Choi, M.-J., & Yi, J. S. (2016). Personas in online health communities. *Journal of Biomedical Informatics, 63*, 212–225. https://doi.org/10.1016/j.jbi.2016.08.019
47. Hunter, D. (2012). In practice: Loneliness: A public health issue. *Perspectives in Public Health, 132*(4), 153–153. https://doi.org/10.1177/1757913912449564
48. Iezzoni, L. (2003). *When walking fails: Mobility problems of adults with chronic conditions* (Vol. 8). University of California Press.
49. Igami, K., Hosozawa, M., Ikeda, A., Bann, D., Shimizu, T., & Iso, H. (2023). Adolescent loneliness in 70 countries across Africa, America, and Asia: A comparison of prevalence and correlates. *Journal of Adolescent Health, 72*(6), 906–913. https://doi.org/10.1016/j.jadohealth.2022.12.029
50. Jones, S. A., Alicea, S. K., & Ortega, J. D. (2020). A self-determination theory approach for exercise motivation in rural dwelling older adults. *Activities, Adaptation & Aging, 44*(1), 24–41. https://doi.org/10.1080/01924788.2019.1581022
51. Kemperman, A., Van Den Berg, P., Weijs-Perrée, M., & Uijtdewillegen, K. (2019). Loneliness of older adults: Social network and the living environment. *International Journal of Environmental Research and Public Health, 16*(3), 406. https://doi.org/10.3390/ijerph16030406
52. Lam, D. (2023). Has the world survived the population bomb? A 10-year update. *Population and Environment, 45*(2), 10. https://doi.org/10.1007/s11111-023-00422-7
53. Luchetti, M., Terracciano, A., Aschwanden, D., Lee, J. H., Stephan, Y., & Sutin, A. R. (2020). Loneliness is associated with risk of cognitive impairment in the Survey of Health, Ageing and Retirement in Europe. *International Journal of Geriatric Psychiatry, 35*(7), 794–801. https://doi.org/10.1002/gps.5304

54. Lykes, V. A., & Kemmelmeier, M. (2014). What predicts loneliness? Cultural difference between individualistic and collectivistic societies in Europe. *Journal of Cross-Cultural Psychology, 45*(3), 468–490. https://doi.org/10.1177/0022022113509881
55. Masten, A. S. (2001). Ordinary magic: Resilience processes in development. *American Psychologist, 56*(3), 227–238. https://doi.org/10.1037/0003-066X.56.3.227
56. Matthews, L. A., Shine, A. L., Currie, L., Chan, C. V., & Kaufman, D. R. (2012). A nurse's eye-view on health literacy in older adults. In *NI 2012: 11th international congress on nursing informatics, June 23–27, 2012, Montreal, Canada* (11th: 2012: Montreal, Quebec) (p. 204). International Congress in Nursing Informatics.
57. McCabe, C., Dinsmore, J., Brady, A. M., Mckee, G., O'Donnell, S., & Prendergast, D. (2014). Using action research and peer perspectives to develop technology that facilitates behavioral change and self-management in COPD. *International Journal of Telemedicine and Applications, 2014*, 1–10. https://doi.org/10.1155/2014/380919
58. McCabe, M., You, E., & Tatangelo, G. (2016). Hearing their voice: A systematic review of dementia family caregivers' needs. *The Gerontologist, 56*(5), e70–e88. https://doi.org/10.1093/geront/gnw078
59. McHugh, J. E., Wherton, J. P., Prendergast, D. K., & Lawlor, B. A. (2012). Teleconferencing as a source of social support for older spousal caregivers: Initial explorations and recommendations for future research. *American Journal of Alzheimer's Disease & Other Dementias®, 27*(6), 381–387. https://doi.org/10.1177/1533317512453491
60. Nicolaisen, M., Pripp, A. H., & Thorsen, K. (2023). Why not lonely? A longitudinal study of factors related to loneliness and non-loneliness in different age groups among people in the second part of life. *The International Journal of Aging and Human Development, 97*(2), 157–187. https://doi.org/10.1177/00914150221112292
61. Nielsen, L. (2019). *Personas – User focused design*. Springer. https://doi.org/10.1007/978-1-4471-7427-1
62. Nimrod, G. (2020). Changes in internet use when coping with stress: Older adults during the COVID-19 pandemic. *The American Journal of Geriatric Psychiatry: Official Journal of the American Association for Geriatric Psychiatry, 28*(10), 1020–1024. https://doi.org/10.1016/j.jagp.2020.07.010
63. O'Mahony, D., Gallagher, P., & Lavan, A. (2016). Methods to reduce prescribing errors in elderly patients with multimorbidity. *Clinical Interventions in Aging*, 857. https://doi.org/10.2147/CIA.S80280
64. OECD. (2023). *Old-age dependency ratio [dataset]*. OECD. https://doi.org/10.1787/e0255c98-en
65. Oswald, F., & Rowles, G. (2006). *Beyond the relocation trauma in old age: New trends in today's elders' residential decisions* (pp. 127–152).
66. Perissinotto, C. M., Stijacic Cenzer, I., & Covinsky, K. E. (2012). Loneliness in older persons: A predictor of functional decline and death. *Archives of Internal Medicine, 172*(14). https://doi.org/10.1001/archinternmed.2012.1993
67. Pinquart, M., & Sorensen, S. (2001). Influences on loneliness in older adults: A meta-analysis. *Basic and Applied Social Psychology, 23*(4), 245–266. https://doi.org/10.1207/S15324834BASP2304_2
68. Prohaska, T., Burholt, V., Burns, A., Golden, J., Hawkley, L., Lawlor, B., Leavey, G., Lubben, J., O'Sullivan, R., Perissinotto, C., Van Tilburg, T., Tully, M., Victor, C., & Fried, L. (2020). Consensus statement: Loneliness in older adults, the 21st century social determinant of health? *BMJ Open, 10*(8), e034967. https://doi.org/10.1136/bmjopen-2019-034967
69. Randall, W. L. (2009). The anthropology of dementia: A narrative perspective. *International Journal of Geriatric Psychiatry, 24*(3), 322–324. https://doi.org/10.1002/gps.2179
70. Richardson, J. C., Grime, J. C., & Ong, B. N. (2014). 'Keeping going': Chronic joint pain in older people who describe their health as good. *Ageing and Society, 34*(8), 1380–1396. https://doi.org/10.1017/S0144686X13000226

71. Ritchie, H., Rodés-Guirao, L., Mathieu, E., Gerber, M., Ortiz-Ospina, E., Hasell, J., & Roser, M. (2023). *Population growth*. Our World in Data. https://ourworldindata.org/population-growth
72. Ryan, R., Patrick, H., Deci, E., & Williams, G. (2007). Facilitating health behavior change and its maintenance: Interventions based on Self-Determination Theory. *European Health Psychology, 10*, 2–5.
73. Salminen, J., Guan, K., Jung, S.-G., Chowdhury, S. A., & Jansen, B. J. (2020). A literature review of quantitative persona creation. In *Proceedings of the 2020 CHI conference on human factors in computing systems* (pp. 1–14). https://doi.org/10.1145/3313831.3376502
74. Salminen, J., Guan, K., Jung, S.-G., & Jansen, J. (2021). A survey of 15 years of data-driven persona development. *International Journal of Human-Computer Interaction, 37*, 1–24. https://doi.org/10.1080/10447318.2021.1908670
75. Schäfer, K., Rasche, P., Bröhl, C., Theis, S., Barton, L., Brandl, C., Wille, M., Nitsch, V., & Mertens, A. (2019). Survey-based personas for a target-group-specific consideration of elderly end users of information and communication systems in the German health-care sector. *International Journal of Medical Informatics, 132*, 103924. https://doi.org/10.1016/j.ijmedinf.2019.07.003
76. Scharf, T., & De Jong Gierveld, J. (2008). Loneliness in urban neighbourhoods: An Anglo-Dutch comparison. *European Journal of Ageing, 5*(2), 103–115. https://doi.org/10.1007/s10433-008-0080-x
77. Scheffer, A. C., Schuurmans, M. J., Van Dijk, N., Van Der Hooft, T., & De Rooij, S. E. (2008). Fear of falling: Measurement strategy, prevalence, risk factors and consequences among older persons. *Age and Ageing, 37*(1), 19–24. https://doi.org/10.1093/ageing/afm169
78. Scheibl, F., Farquhar, M., Buck, J., Barclay, S., Brayne, C., & Fleming, J. (2019). When frail older people relocate in very old age, who makes the decision? *Innovation in Aging, 3*(4), igz030. https://doi.org/10.1093/geroni/igz030
79. Snyder, H. (2019). Literature review as a research methodology: An overview and guidelines. *Journal of Business Research, 104*, 333–339. https://doi.org/10.1016/j.jbusres.2019.07.039
80. Stenner, P., McFarquhar, T., & Bowling, A. (2011). Older people and 'active ageing': Subjective aspects of ageing actively. *Journal of Health Psychology, 16*(3), 467–477. https://doi.org/10.1177/1359105310384298
81. Surkalim, D. L., Luo, M., Eres, R., Gebel, K., Van Buskirk, J., Bauman, A., & Ding, D. (2022). The prevalence of loneliness across 113 countries: Systematic review and meta-analysis. *BMJ*, e067068. https://doi.org/10.1136/bmj-2021-067068
82. Tatzer, V. C. (2019). Narratives-in-action of people with moderate to severe dementia in long-term care: Understanding the link between occupation and identity. *Journal of Occupational Science, 26*(2), 245–257. https://doi.org/10.1080/14427591.2019.1600159
83. Tavel, P., Dubovska, E., Meier, Z., Trnka, R., Pesoutova, M., Cohlova, J., Pinaka, R., Stamatiadis, V., Gioulekas, F., Tzikas, A., Gounaris, K., D'Arino, L., Jensen, R., Roche, P., Sarlio-Siintola, S., Purola, A., Isaris, P., Labor, M., Grigoleit, S., … Gutter, Z. (2021). *Smart and healthy ageing through people engaging in supportive systems, D2.7—SHAPES personas and use cases*. Unpublished document. SHAPES consortium.
84. Torraco, R. J. (2005). Writing integrative literature reviews: Guidelines and examples. *Human Resource Development Review, 4*(3), 356–367. https://doi.org/10.1177/1534484305278283
85. Valtorta, N. K., Kanaan, M., Gilbody, S., Ronzi, S., & Hanratty, B. (2016). Loneliness and social isolation as risk factors for coronary heart disease and stroke: Systematic review and meta-analysis of longitudinal observational studies. *Heart, 102*(13), 1009–1016. https://doi.org/10.1136/heartjnl-2015-308790
86. Wang, Z., Wang, A., Eichi, H., Liebenthal, E., Schutt, R., Ongur, D., Rauch, S., Dixon, L., Onnela, J.-P., Baker, J., & Valeri, L. (2021). Loneliness of schizophrenia and bipolar disorder patients in a multi-year mHealth study. *Biological Psychiatry, 89*, S222. https://doi.org/10.1016/j.biopsych.2021.02.560
87. Whittemore, R., & Knafl, K. (2005). The integrative review: Updated methodology. *Journal of Advanced Nursing, 52*(5), 546–553. https://doi.org/10.1111/j.1365-2648.2005.03621.x

88. WHO. (2019). *Promoting the health of refugees and migrants: Global action plan, 2019–2023*. https://www.who.int/publications-detail-redirect/WHA72-2019-REC-1
89. WHO. (2023a). *Ageing*. https://www.who.int/health-topics/ageing#tab=tab_1
90. WHO. (2023b). *Life expectancy at birth (years)*. World Health Organization (WHO). Life Expectancy at Birth (Years). https://www.who.int/data/gho/data/indicators/indicator-details/GHO/life-expectancy-at-birth-(years)
91. World Federation of the Deafblind. (2018). *WFDB global report 2018 – WFDB*. https://wfdb.eu/wfdb-report-2018/
92. Xie, Y., Wang, Z., Liao, H., Marley, G., Wu, D., & Tang, W. (2020). Epidemiologic, clinical, and laboratory findings of the COVID-19 in the current pandemic: Systematic review and meta-analysis. *BMC Infectious Diseases, 20*(1), 640. https://doi.org/10.1186/s12879-020-05371-2
93. Yang, K., & Victor, C. (2011). Age and loneliness in 25 European nations. *Ageing & Society, 31*(8), 1368–1388. https://doi.org/10.1017/S0144686X1000139X
94. Zeytinoglu, M., Wroblewski, K. E., Vokes, T. J., Huisingh-Scheetz, M., Hawkley, L. C., & Huang, E. S. (2021). Association of loneliness with falls: A study of older US adults using the national social life, health, and aging project. *Gerontology and Geriatric Medicine, 7*, 2333721421989217. https://doi.org/10.1177/2333721421989217
95. Zhong, R., Han, S., & Wang, Z. (2023). Developing personas for live streaming commerce platforms with user survey data. *Universal Access in the Information Society*. https://doi.org/10.1007/s10209-023-00996-x
96. Ziebland, S., & McPherson, A. (2006). Making sense of qualitative data analysis: An introduction with illustrations from DIPEx (personal experiences of health and illness). *Medical Education, 40*(5), 405–414. https://doi.org/10.1111/j.1365-2929.2006.02467.x

Chapter 8
Health Data Analytics: Frameworks, Tools, and Impact on the Administration Efficiency and Performance in Healthcare

Ourania Kitsou, Constandinos X. Mavromoustakis, Evangelos K. Markakis, George Mastorakis, Evangelos Pallis, Athina Bourdena, and Markos Kourgiantakis

8.1 Introduction

New technology has enabled society in having access to more data reaching to a point where this overload of information becomes too large to be processed optimally and is described as too large and unmanageable [14]. Health Data refers to differentiated datasets that have large size which both facilitate and make more complex the extraction and application of knowledge about a situation that can be seen and noted. The ability to be analyzed can create opportunities for innovative

O. Kitsou (✉) · G. Mastorakis
Department of Management Science and Technology, Hellenic Mediterranean University, Agios Nikolaos, Crete, Greece
e-mail: gmastorakis@hmu.gr

C. X. Mavromoustakis
Department of Computer Science, University of Nicosia and University of Nicosia Research Foundation, Nicosia, Cyprus
e-mail: mavromoustakis.c@unic.ac.cy

E. K. Markakis
Department of Electrical and Computer Engineering, Hellenic Mediterranean University, Heraklion, Crete, Greece
e-mail: markakis@pasiphae.eu

E. Pallis
Department of Industrial Design and Production Engineering. School of Engineering. University of West Attica, Athens, Greece
e-mail: epallis@uniwa.gr

A. Bourdena · M. Kourgiantakis
Department of Business Administration & Tourism, Hellenic Mediterranean University, Heraklion, Iraklion, Greece
e-mail: bourdena@hmu.gr; mkourg@hmu.gr

© The Author(s), under exclusive license to Springer Nature Switzerland AG 2024

A. Bourdena et al. (eds.), *Intelligent Technologies for Healthcare Business Applications*, Signals and Communication Technology,
https://doi.org/10.1007/978-3-031-58527-2_8

and practical solutions in the healthcare service so as to become more effective and efficient without excess spending [11–13, 42].

According to [13], Health Data Analytics has developed as a significant field of research and application, showing how important is the utilization of this magnitude of data and management based on this information on giving solutions and taking applicable actions in hospitals and healthcare organizations. In order to meet our social needs of today and tomorrow, we need to find solutions to organize this data which result in applicable and meaningful decisions. Taking into consideration the fact that spending for healthcare is one of the biggest financial challenges worldwide, optimizing it while enhancing the quality of care is of great importance to patients, clinicians, administrators, and governments. Although the literature indicates an increasing interest in Big Data Analytics and their connection with better performance and better administrative solutions, there is still a gap between the practical use of Healthcare Analytics and Health Data in healthcare services as it has not yet presented its potential capabilities in simple and practical shapes.

8.2 Definition of Health Analytics

Health Analytics is considered to be the use of data, technology of information, quantitative analysis, statistical methods, or mathematical models based on computers that help healthcare providers understand the needs of patients and make better and more focused decisions [16]. The forms of Health Data include clinical, administrative, demographic, machine generated data, data based on literature surveys or presentations from social media that refer to health issues. Furthermore, the data may be internal (coming from healthcare organizations and hospitals such as EHR) or external (governments, pharmacies, and insurance organizations) and may also be structured (such as financial reports) or unstructured (such as medical notes or medical prescriptions). Big healthcare data refer to heterogeneous, with different dimensions, not completed, and not well-depicted observations such as diagnosis, therapies, illnesses, injuries, and physical and mental impairments coming from different sources using differentiated sampling [1].

The volume and complexity of Health Data are greater than the human ability to process effectively and find results easily. What is more, the diversity and interdependence of Health Data makes the analytical technology more appropriate.

Despite the fact that the definition for Health Data Analytics is not exact, the characteristics, which are presented by many scientists [14, 24, 25, 26, 38], include the following:

- Volume describes the amount of data that must be analyzed. Data can also vary from terabytes to petabytes or exabytes.
- Veracity is recognized to show the accuracy of data from the processing methods of a system.

- Value is referred to what the user benefit or gain based on the processing outcomes.
- Variety shows the differentiation of data and its separation in structured or unstructured information (emails, audio, images, posts from social media or blogs, files from networks, websites, and mobile applications).
- Velocity describes how quickly the data is created, processed, and evaluated based on health analytics procedures. Also, it shows how fast the data is updated.

New medicine, protocols, advances in technology, new ways of treatment, enhanced communication [2, 3], and science appear daily leading to more complex procedures and decisions. All the new developments, from the personalized genetic therapies to robotics and telemedicine create opportunities for solving challenging situations, but these improvements also confuse patients, health professionals, and governments [10, 46]. Usually, hospitals as healthcare organizations are utilizing descriptive health analytics, which refer to medical data. For implementing Health Analytics it is of high importance the usage of queries, reports and collection of data based on healthcare services. In order to manage and analyze the magnitude and variety of data generated at fast rates, an accessible and readable file format is needed [14]. Nowadays, the big data sources include different types of data coming from different systems. Data Warehouses include differentiated information and with the use of Big Data Analytics Applications can result in dashboards for operational use, records, and effective decisions (Fig. 8.1, Health Data Analytics procedure). However, there are not only advantages but also shortcomings and things to be considered before the implementation or during the process (Fig. 8.2 Thoughts for further investigation).

8.3 Examples of Data Analytics in Healthcare

The use of Electronic Health Records has resulted in many advances in the modern healthcare management [5]. Health professionals have easier access to the medical history of each patient. This history refers to previous examinations, prescriptions, diagnoses, orders, clinical tests, and results from laboratories. The information that is provided can lead to a decrease in unnecessary and additional examinations, lost prescriptions and orders, and better recognition of the patient's situation and treatment. Furthermore, the improved coordination of healthcare providers enables them reduce delays and ambiguities in the billing and claims [14].

Of course, an extremely interesting and up-to-date application of health analytics refers to the COVID-19 results, which enabled governments to develop public health activities and communicate effectively by using proper tools. The utilization of Data Analytics enables governments evaluate the decisions taken and the way current technologies can serve as tools in order to overcome the pandemic crisis of COVID-19 and improve the quality and innovation in the healthcare services in turbulent periods [15].

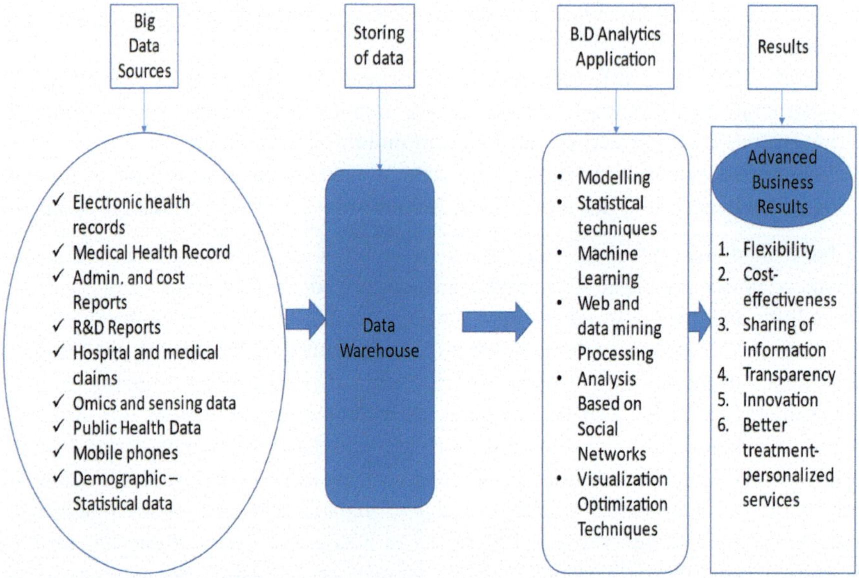

Fig. 8.1 Health Data Analytics procedure. Data taken from data sources are stored in data warehouse. With the Data Analytics application, the organization can become more flexible and efficient

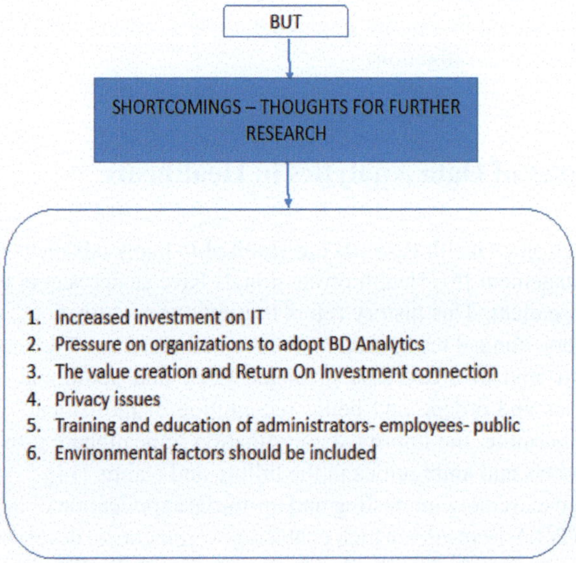

Fig. 8.2 Thoughts for further investigation

On the other hand, when comparing previous studies regarding EHR results on the healthcare service provision efficiency, it can be seen that results may be affected by the size of the organization and the people who participate in the research [9].

In Alameda County as published by KHN organization [6], patients and staff were facing problems in the area of frequent visits in the emergency departments. Many patients had to change emergency room in order to solve their health problems and the staff who served at the different emergency rooms had no idea the patients had already visited other hospitals so they treated them as independent incidents and often patients had to repeat blood or diagnostic tests. This situation led hospitals in Alameda County to coordinate and use the records of patients' health and other information which happened in real time among the departments which were responsible for tackling emergency situations. The different hospitals shared the Pre Manage ED system, and they could track all of their ER patients. This system resulted in treating patients more effectively, faster and without performing unnecessary tests.

Urban Health Plan, which is a patient-focused medical center in South Bronx, New York, is another example of how the power of Health Analytics and especially the strategic use of Electronic Health Records can improve care coordination [35]. More specifically, it introduced a program for low-income patients with chronic psychosocial, behavioral, and mental problems. Based on this action, its community referral department scheduled electronically the appointments with the specialists of the Bronx Lebanon Hospital resulting in better and faster access to proper specialists.

New technology under proper utilization is necessary for giving proper solutions [30, 31, 37, 43, 44, 47].

Great developments in technology, such as Artificial Intelligence and robotics, can promote the service given from the healthcare system [18]. Table 8.1 presents the layers of health data based on the work of Wang L and Cheryl Ann Alexander [18].

Table 8.1 Layers of Health Data

Layers of health data	
Layer 1	Smartphones, internet search, EHR, devices, IoT sensors, services
Layer 2	Demographic, medical, clinical data, which are clustered, saved, and shared to third parties
Layer 3	Companies from private sector gather information from layers 1 and 2 or other sources and sell it in different forms
Layer 4	Governments, public or private organizations process again and sell the data
Layer 5	International actions and governments decisions for the protection of personal health information

Table 8.2 Types of Big Data in healthcare with its typical instances

Big Data's types	Typical instances
Descriptive	Reports of patients' hospitalization or physicians' performance
Predictive	Plan healthcare responses, predict the cost of services
Prescriptive	Personalized health treatment, personalized healthcare services
Discovery	New alternative treatments, new drugs, new medical conditions

8.4 Types of Health Analytics

In recent years, the use of descriptive and analytic methods from healthcare organizations has transformed to predictive and prescriptive analytics procedures as they are more sophisticated and offer the ability to find the proper solutions among available alternatives [13].

The four types of big data as described by many researchers can be divided into (see Table 8.2):

1. Descriptive analytics in the healthcare system is the data referred to past and current data used in order to analyze decisions, quality, and outcomes. One question may answer is what percent of people did use home therapy last week.
2. Predictive analytics is based on past information in order to predict a future outcome. More specifically, it depends on machine learning, creating algorithms so as to extract knowledge based on existing data, combine it and determine future actions [40].
3. Prescriptive analytics is a more complex type which uses more complicated data and includes health and medical information in addition to other data. This type of Health Analytics suggests action in different circumstances. It is strongly connected with optimization techniques in order to find the best solution. The problems, which are solved by prescriptive analytics, can be categorized into four types [40]: (1) Blind Search (all solutions are tested, there is certainty for optimal solution). (2) Local Search (there are given initial solutions based on previous local problems). (3) Population-Based Search (increased diversity, defining new solutions, which are created by combining the attributes related to many search points), (4) Multi-objective Optimization (combining many objectives in an algorithm, creation of the best possible balance).
4. The fourth type is called discovery and uses knowledge that exists in order to discover new knowledge.

8.5 Application Areas of Health Analytics for More Effective Impacts

Based on Burke's option [4], while there are many different areas of healthcare to apply analytics, such as clinical results or financial performance, the healthcare

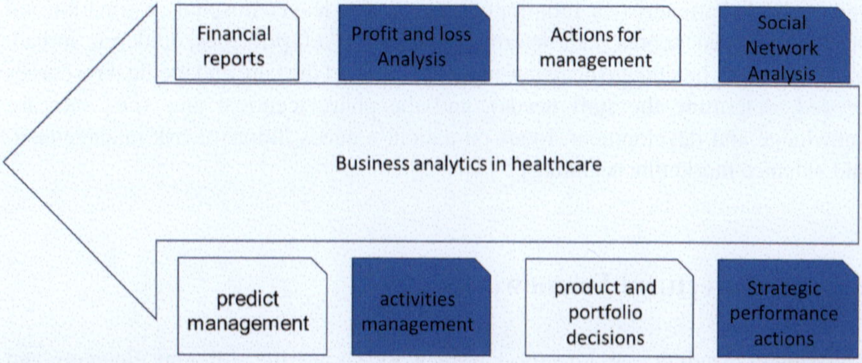

Fig. 8.3 Business analytics in healthcare. (Source: Burke [4]. Gaining the Insights to transform Healthcare, Health Analytics)

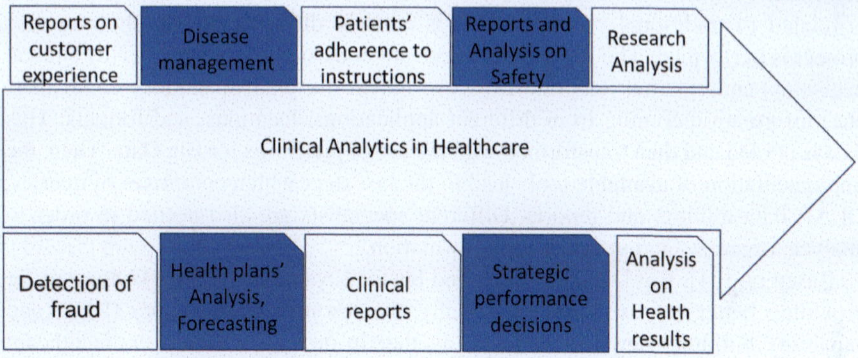

Fig. 8.4 Clinical analytics in healthcare. (Source: Burke [4]. Gaining the Insights to transform Healthcare, Health Analytics)

giver has to choose the area of his interest and focus on the specific subject. Health Analytics applications today are connected with each other and presented to have as edges the business analytics area and the clinical analytics (see Figs. 8.3 and 8.4).

Wirtz [8] also supports the view that the focused service factory strategy can lead to cost-effective service performance in the healthcare.

Venkatraman S et al. [38] proposed a typology for Healthcare Analytics adoption model so as to be more practical. Their study focused on applications for supporting decisions, operations which refer to clinical data, administration, organizational/enterprise, and inter-organizational Health Analytics applications. Their results showed that analytics can be successful when the whole departments of the organization are involved.

Alsunaidi S J et al. [41] revealed four areas for Big Data applications in healthcare in an attempt to control the great and varied amount of data for controlling the global pandemic COVID-19 more effectively. These areas include the following: diagnosis (i.e., detection of COVID-19 pre symptoms, detection of COVID-19 cases and medical characteristics, monitor of patients who leaved hospital), estimation and prediction of risk scores (i.e., determine the care level, priorities, epidemic spread, trace contacts), healthcare decision-making (i.e., find the care and medical resources needed, determine the staff needs), and the pharmaceutical area (i.e., increase knowledge and development, focus on patient's needs, improve risk management, and enhance marketing scanning).

8.6 Architectural Frameworks

The Health Analytics architectural framework shows the different elements and their connection with each other in order to be useful. First, the conceptual design for implementing analytics in the healthcare's decision system is clearly presented by [16], who supported the view that while Big Data Analytics today is related to traditional concepts what is entirely different now is the way this project is performed. The Big Data sources are consisted of internal (EHR, clinical decisions) and external (laboratories, government decisions, insurance companies, etc.) information coming from different applications, locations, and formats. This data is pooled and then transformed with the use of platforms for Big Data. Then, the implementation of available tools lead to the last step, which comprises of queries, OLAP, data mining, and reports. Different specialists are also needed in order to analyze, organize, and visualize the information.

Based on [21], Big Data Analytics and business value models are connected for providing better results. More specifically, the resource-based theory (RBT) and capability building view can be used together in order to develop the healthcare system. This model is called RBT-BV and includes the resource-based theory and capability building view so as to combine the available resources, which can provide competitive advantage and the ways of how specific IT systems can create this advantage and lead the healthcare providers and administrators to better strategic decisions and performance.

Despite the fact that many studies have been conducted based on big data and healthcare system during the last few years, there is a lack in addressing the temporal dimension of big data. The framework which was introduced by [7] called Temporal Big Data Maturity Model was designed to fill this gap. This model can be used by an organization to measure its data sets and enables the effectiveness of available analytical tools in order to adapt properly and plan for the future taking into consideration the time parameter. This framework also includes a self-assessment form, which is used to assess the current Big Data Analytics in order to follow new directions and plan the next steps.

8.7 Tools and Techniques for the Implementation of Big Data Analytics in the Healthcare Service

Information that is available at high speed has to be collected and bundled in order to save time. After that, it is extremely important to update and create proper queries. The last element for the Big Data Analytics process is to properly manage the storage space. Nowadays, computers are also needed, but the analytic processing includes the clustering and scanning of different nodes in order to handle the large and complicated datasets. Some of the most popular tools are Hadoop, Scoop, MapReduce, and HBase Avro [17].

8.7.1 Hadoop

Hadoop is an application tool for handling large and heterogeneous data. The open-source distribution of data is available when we refer to this tool. It also introduces algorithms like map reduce, which enables the processing and combining of certain values in order to promote the machine communication [14]. This tool is widely utilized when we refer to Big Data applications. Bilal et al. [20] with the use of Hadoop Distributed File System investigated how profitable can be the construction of projects and simultaneously used the Resource Description Framework and Network Data Model for storing the data [20].

8.7.2 Machine Learning

Machine learning is useful in cases where the information, which is available, is in different forms (videos, signals, hand writing). Knowledge from the past can be digitized and used for future decisions and actions. For example, Mahout is a program used for creating applications based on past data, which have the ability to correlate and analyze information for predictive purposes [16].

8.7.3 Pig

Pig tool is used for making Hadoop easier and simpler [22]. It is used for cleaning and analyzing large amounts of data sets. Pig also includes PigLatin, which is a language used to show the input of data and the processing in order to produce the final result. PigLatin is simple and makes it easier the connection of structured, semi-structured and unstructured data.

8.7.4 MapReduce

Map Reduce is a model for programming, processing, and analyzing great data sets with the use of distributed clustering.

MapReduce includes the map and reduce capabilities. First, the mapping capability includes the filtering and clustering of data, and the reduction capability includes the summarize of information. This model can solve a problem by divide it into smaller sub-areas or the data inputs are separated into independent clusters, which are processed in a parallel way, and after that follows the combination of data for producing the result [24]. The MapReduce algorithm provides flexibility and fault tolerance in analyzing massive volumes of data.

8.7.5 Data Mining

Data Mining is referred to the procedure of discovering and analyzing great quantities of information with the use of automatic means with no or little human influence. Data Mining includes certain algorithms which under accepted modification can, result in Knowledge and patterns based on large amounts of data. It is primarily used in statistics and computer science [23]. Not only advanced computer technology is required such as parallel architecture but also knowledge of the specific business issue in order to formulate proper questions and interpret the results. Data Mining software is available by some famous enterprises such as SAS Enterprise Miner (www.sas.com/), SPSS Clementine (www.spss.com), XLMiner (www.xlminer.net), and Quadstone (www.quadstone.com).

8.7.6 Trusted Analytics Platform

It is crucial for hospital administrators to predict the number of patients' visits to emergency departments and the admission rates in order to allocate the human resources effectively. Also, the waiting time can be reduced and the staff can offer better service quality to the people. Intel and the Assistance Publique-Hopitaux managed to create a cloud-based application so as to predict the number of patients' visits and admission with the use of the Trusted Analytics Platform or TAP.

TAP is another tool used as an open-source platform, which make the procedure of Big Data Analytics go faster. Data scientists and medical experts based on data from four departments evaluated three approaches with the utilizing of time series analysis, optimization parameters, and the inclusion of the best predictive options. The ARIMAX approach (which included exogenous input) was used, and the Akaike Information Criterion made the model less complex and more accurate [19].

8.8 How Big Data Affect Performance and Administration in the Healthcare Service Sector

8.8.1 *Strategic Planning*

The utilization of descriptive, diagnostic, and prescriptive analytics affects positively the emergency room's performance and enables administrators plan their actions. For example, [13] identified that the classification of patients based on the severity of their situation, the individual treatment, the introduction of a fast track, and an internal waiting area for those with less severe situations could lead to better performance levels and enhance efficiency, effectiveness, and patient-focused treatment.

8.8.2 *Flexibility*

Despite the fact that better service provision is considered to be in conflict with cost-effectiveness, [27] have introduced a model called CESE (Cost-Effective Service Excellence) in order to describe how performance can be promoted with the use of competitive tools, which result in better customer satisfaction and simultaneously better cost allocation. Wirtz J & Zeitham V [27] focused for their research on the healthcare system of Singapore, which is one of the most effective systems worldwide. They highlighted the importance of Health Data Analytics in order to achieve these goals. For example, the use of an Electronic Medical System in the Singapore's Ministry of Health resulted in better access to more accurate information by physicians, clinics, and managers so as to prevent the duplication of asking the same information or testing and also reduced the administrative load.

8.8.3 *Cost-Effectiveness*

Operational waste is one substantial impediment in the healthcare service sector. The duplication of treatment or testing because of the lack of proper communication and coordination, the medical errors, the unnecessary medical equipment, services, and expensive specialists lead to higher cost expenses for healthcare organizations. Healthcare suffers from greater supply expenses for covering the demand of healthcare services contrary to other industries and companies where demand determines the supply [28].

Administrative costs are also a burden for a better healthcare system. Based on [29], about one quarter of medical waste is estimated to be administrative expenses, which is twice the spending on cardiovascular problems and three times above the spending for cancer treatment. Fraud and abuse add to the excess spending.

Berry [28] supported that technology is necessary for innovation in the healthcare system. The application of artificial intelligence, combined with robotics, Big Data, and new technology can increase the service quality and productivity and reduce the costs for healthcare organizations.

8.8.4 Impact on Government Services

New management processes adopted by public services and governments, which utilize Big Data Analytics and include perception, evaluating methods, decision-making process, proper management, and dissemination of information, are essential components of creating a service-targeted and transparent governmental system. Based on [32] a model for governments' big data capabilities can be developed which depends on three parameters: management, system, and human capabilities. The connection and inter-connection of these capabilities can lead to smarter service performance for governments. This research also showed how important is a plan for research and development, the use of new modern platforms, and the importance of training and education of talents in order to result in open, intelligent, personalized, and interactive government services. Governments play a pivotal role in healthcare delivery for the people so their performance can affect healthcare services and can enhance the provision of public services.

8.8.5 Better Decision-Making Ability

Based on the comparative study of [33], who focused on private and public hospitals in Beijing, China, the adoption of Big Data organizational culture can improve the decision-making power. This fact leads to better and more effective decisions not only for hospitals but also for their environmental performance. Another interesting result from this study is the better management of Big Data decision-making ability in the public sector. This fact is also attributed to better infrastructure of this sector, more available funds and government's control on Big Data Application.

Not only tools, hardware, and protocols are needed for the efficient analysis of data, but also experts from different backgrounds such as biologists, mathematicians, information technologists, and managers have to cooperate [39].

8.8.6 Opportunities for Better Staff Positioning

Proper staff positioning is a challenging issue for many countries worldwide. The development of a sustainable health and care workforce will enhance universal health, health security, and the Sustainable Goals for Development, but the current situation in healthcare is urgent. The actions proposed for the alleviation of the problem include funding from governments and oversupply of staff in healthcare [34]. While these options offer a temporal solution to the problem, strategic investment should be targeted in the education of workforce so as to be multi-skilled in order to correspond to present needs. What is more, investing in new analytic tools such as telehealth and mhealth, Electronic Health Records and their analysis could lead in great efficiency gains and provide extra capacity to the health system. Healthcare service systems can implement Health Data Analytics so as to improve accuracy and reduce the time needed for processing and result measurements. What is more, new analytic tools could be used in health systems in order to assess the improvement strategies and enable managers understand what works, why, and how [35]. The creation of proper platforms for regional learning with the use of networks and meetings could promote the dissemination of successful processes and avoid the duplication of failures.

Another interesting application field of Big Data Analytics is the human resource area, which is introduced by organizations that attempt to discover exceptional workers known as knowledge stars or innovative skills and ideas and then identifying programs for the retention and creation of exceptional workers [36].

Staff shortages, dissatisfied healthcare workers, and burnout are burning issues especially for the Greek reality [48]. It is therefore interesting implementing new technology in addressing these problems. Human Resource Information Systems, which include both Human Resource Management and Human Resource Technologies, can collect, store, and report workforce data in an attempt to bring innovations in recruitment, advance the healthcare workforce well-being, and result in better performance management [49]. For example, the Organizational Network Analysis can enhance understanding of workflow exchanges and how they are interconnected at three levels: team level, organizational level, and enterprise level.

8.9 Conclusions and Suggestions for Future Research

Despite the fact that most healthcare organizations utilize real-time data monitors (especially for monitoring Intensive Care Units), however real-time Health Data Analytics procedures are not implemented [45]. This chapter focuses on the presentation of Health Analytics, the frameworks, and tools which are available in the healthcare service provision. Based on previous studies, I tried to connect the computational side of Health Analytics with managerial and administrative opportunities and results. Also, by showing the opportunities offered by the availability of data sources and Health Analytics implementation, I try to explain the ways new technology and transformation can result in improvements and value creation in the healthcare service provision.

Security, privacy, and trust are also issues of great concern for healthcare management [50]. A healthcare system, which is well designed, depends on patients' information in order to achieve advanced health results, healthier people, and cost-effective management [45]. If providing personal information is to benefit, providers and individuals must have confidence in sharing the privacy and security of their personal healthcare experience.

The challenge for healthcare managers and leaders should be the linkage of new analytics strategies with their programs. The questions to be answered should be as follows:

- How organizations can operate and adopt health analytics taking into consideration their own special characteristics and capabilities and also their connection with other organizations, governments, and staff?
- How difficult is the assessment of an organization's analytical capability?
- Which should be the proper actions and decisions for a health organization in order to combine its plan or strategy with the new analytics methods and transform the healthcare activity. Where should leaders focus and what about priorities given?

References

1. Galetsi, P., Katsaliaki, K., & Kumar, S. (2020). Big data analytics in health sector: Theoretical framework, techniques and prospects. *International Journal of Information Management, 50*, 206–216.
2. Ann, A. C., & Lidong, W. (2017). Big data analytics in identification, treatment and cost reduction in hypertension. *American Journal of Hypertension Research, 4*(1), 1–8.
3. Papadokostaki, K., Mastorakis, G., Panagiotakis, S., et al. (2017). *Handling big data in the era of Internet of Things (IoT). Advances in mobile cloud computing and big data in the 5G era* (pp. 3–22). Springer International Publishing.
4. Burke, J. (2013). *Gaining the insights to transform healthcare, health analytics* (pp. 4–58). Wiley & Sons.
5. Yadav, P., Steinbach, M., Kumar, V., & Simon, G. (2018). Mining electronic health records (EHRs): A survey. *ACM Computing Surveys, 50*(6), 85:1–85:40.
6. Gold, G. (2016, June). In Alameda County, a big data effort to prevent frequent ER visits. *KFF Health News*.
7. Olszak, C. M., & Maria, M.-K. (2018) *A conceptual framework for assessing an organization's readiness to adopt big data*. MDPI, Department of business informatics, University of Economics in Katowice.
8. Wirtz, J. (2019). Cost-effective service excellence in healthcare. *Academy of Marketing Science Review, 9*(1–2), 98–104. https://doi.org/10.1007/s13162-019-00139-7
9. Thakkar, M., & Davis, D. C. (2006). Risks, barriers, and benefits of EHR systems: A comparative study based on size of hospital. *Health Information Management, 3*, 5.
10. Cozzoli, N., Salvatore, F. P., Faccilongo, N., & Milone, M. (2022). How can big data analytics be used for healthcare organization management? Literary framework and future research from a systematic review. *BMC Health Services Research, 22*, 809.
11. Batko, K., & Ślęzak, A. (2022). The use of big data analytics in healthcare. *Journal of Big Data, 9*, 3. https://doi.org/10.1186/s40537-021-00553-4
12. Wang, Y., Kung, L. A., & Byrd, T. A. (2018). Big data analytics: Understanding its capabilities and potential benefits for healthcare organizations. *Technological Forecasting and Social Change, 126*, 3–13.

13. Khalifa, M., & Zabani, I. (2016). Utilizing health analytics in improving the performance of healthcare services: A case study on a tertiary care hospital. *Journal of Infection and Public Health, 9*, 757–765.
14. Dash, S., Shakyawar, S. K., Sharma, M., & Kaushik, S. (2019). Big data in healthcare: Management, analysis and future prospects. *Journal of Big Data, 6*, 54. https://doi.org/10.1186/s40537-019-0217-0
15. Andreou, A., Mavromoustakis, C. X., & Mastorakis, G. (2020). Modified Machine Learning Technique for Curve Fitting on Regression Models for COVID-19 projections. In *IEEE Xplore, 2020 IEEE 25th International Workshop on Computer Aided Modeling and Design of Communication Links and Networks (CAMAD), Pisa, Italy, 14–16 September 2020.*
16. Raghupathi, W., & Raghupathi, V. (2014). Big data analytics in healthcare: Promise and potential. *Health Information Science and Systems, 2*, 3. https://doi.org/10.1186/2047-2501-2-3. Retrieved from: http://www.hissjournal.com/content/2/1/3.
17. Kumar, S., & Singh, M. (2019). Big data analytics for healthcare industry: Impact, applications, and tools. *Big Data Mining and Analytics, 2*(1), 48–57. https://doi.org/10.26599/BDMA.2018.9020031
18. Wang, L., & Alexander, C. A. (2019). Big data analytics in healthcare systems. *International Journal of Mathematical, Engineering and Management Sciences, 4*(1), 17–26.
19. Ambert, K., Beaune, S., Chaibi, A., Briard, L., Bhattacharjee, A., Bharadwaj, V., Sumanth, K., & Crowe, K. (2016) *French hospital uses trusted analytics platform to predict emergency department visits and hospital admissions*. Available at: https://www.intel.com/content/dam/www/public/us/en/documents/white-papers/french-hospital-analytics-predict-admissions-paper.pdf. Accessed 03 Aug 2023.
20. Bilal, M., Oyedele, L. O., Kusimo, H. O., et al. (2019). Investigating profitability performance of construction projects using big data: A project analytics approach. *Journal of Building Engineering, 26*, 100850.
21. Wang, Y., & Hajlib. (2016). Exploring the role of big data analytics capabilities in creating business value in healthcare industries: A synthesis of the resource-based theory and capability building view. *Journal of Business Research, 70*, 287. https://doi.org/10.1016/j.jbusres.2016.08.002
22. Pramanik, P. K. D., Pal, S., & Mukhopadhyay, M. (2022) Healthcare big data: A comprehensive overview. In *Intelligent systems for healthcare management and delivery* (Chap. 4, pp. 72–100). https://doi.org/10.4018/978-1-5225-7071-4.ch004
23. Tsui, K.-L., Chen, V. C. P., Wei Jiang, Y., & Aslandogan, A. (2023). Data mining methods and applications. In *Handbook of engineering statistics* (pp. 1–32). Springer.
24. Sarkar, B. K. (2017). Big data for secure healthcare system: A conceptual design. *Complex & Intelligent Systems, 3*, 133–153.
25. Grover, V., Chiang, R. H. L., Liang, T.-P., & Zhang, D. (2018). Creating strategic business value from big data analytics: A research framework. *Journal of Management Information Systems, 35*(2), 388–423.
26. Kopanakis, I., Vassakis, K., & Mastorakis, G. (2016). Big data in data-driven innovation: The impact in enterprises' performance. In *Proceedings of 11th Annual MIBES International Conference, Heraklion, Crete, Greece, 22–24 June 2016* (pp. 257–263).
27. Wirtz, J., & Zeitham, V. (2018). Cost-effective service excellence. *Journal of the Academy of Marketing Science, 46*, 59–80.
28. Berry, L. L. (2019). Service innovation is urgent in healthcare. *Academy of Market Science Review, 9*, 78–92.
29. Cutler, D. M. (2018). What is the health spending problem? *Health Affairs, 37*(3), 493–497.
30. Mastorakis, G., Pallis, E., Mantakas, C., et al. (2006). Exploiting digital switchover for broadband services access in rural areas. *Journal of Communications, 1*(6), 45–50.
31. Sousa, M. J., Pesqueira, A. M., Lemos, C., Sousa, M., & Rocha, Á. (2019). Decision-making based on big data analytics for people Management in Healthcare Organizations, systems – Level quality improvement. *Journal of Medical Systems, 43*, 290.

32. Zhang, A., & Na, L. V. (2021). Research on the impact of big data capabilities on government's smart service performance: Empirical evidence from China. *Special Section of Intelligent Big Data Analytics for Internet of Things, Services and People, IEEE Access, 9*, 50523–50537.
33. Nisar, Q. A., Nasir, N., Jamshed, S., Naz, S., Ali, M., & Ali, S. (2020). Big data management and environmental performance: Role of big data decision-making capabilities and decision-making quality. *Big Data Management and Environmental Performance, 34*(4), 1061–1096.
34. Barbara, M. P., Prarthna, D., Julia, Z., & Williams, G. A. (2023). What steps can improve and promote investment in the health and care workforce? Health systems and policy analysis; World Health Organization. *European Observatory on Health Systems and Policies; Policy Brief, 54*, 1–40.
35. Kruk, E. M., Gage, D. A., Arsenault, C., et al. (2018). High-quality health systems in the sustainable development goals era: Time for a revolution. *The Lancet Global Health Commission on High Quality Health Systems in the SDG Era, 6*(11), e1196–e1252. https://doi.org/10.1016/S2214-109X(18)30386-3
36. Hamilton, R. H., & Sodeman William, A. (2020). The questions we ask: Opportunities and challenges for using big data analytics to strategically manage human capital resources. *Business Horizons, 63*(1), 85–95.
37. Figueras, D. (2012). *Urban health plan in New York uses its HER meaningfully to improve care coordination*. https://www.healthit.gov/case-study/urban-health-plan-new-york-uses-its-ehr-meaningfully-improve-care-coordination.
38. Venkatraman, S., Sundarraj, R. P., & Seethamraju, R. (2015). Healthcare analytics adoption-decision model: A case study. In *PACIS 2015 Proceedings Association for Information Systems AIS Electronic Library (AISeL) Pacific Asia Conference on Information Systems (PACIS)*, Paper 51.
39. Black, N. C. (2023). *How healthcare big data analytics information asymmetry influences organizational design absorptive choices*. Dissertation, Walden University.
40. Agbehadji, I. E., Osita Awuzie, B. O., Ngowi, A. B., & Millham, R. C. (2020). Review of big data analytics, artificial intelligence and nature-inspired computing models towards accurate detection of COVID-19 pandemic cases and contact tracing. *International Journal of Environmental Research and Public Health, 17*(15), 5330. https://doi.org/10.3390/ijerph17155330
41. Alsunaidi, S. J., Almuhaideb Abdullah, M., Ibrahim, N. M., et al. (2021). Applications of big data analytics to control COVID-19 pandemic. *MDPI Sensors, 21*(7), 1–24. https://doi.org/10.3390/s21072282
42. Lopes, J., Guimarães, T., & Santos, M. F. (2020). Predictive and prescriptive analytics in healthcare: A survey. *Procedia Computer Science, 170*, 1029–1034.
43. Mavromoustakis, C. X., Mastorakis, G., & Batalla, J. M. (2016). Internet of Things (IoT) in 5G mobile technologies. In *Modeling and optimization in science and technologies* (Vol. 8). Springer. https://doi.org/10.1007/978-3-319-30913-2
44. Markakis Evangelos, K., Politis, I., Lykourgiotis, A., et al. (2017). Efficient next generation emergency communications over multi-access edge computing. *IEEE Communications Magazine, 55*(11), 92–97.
45. Srivastava, D., Pandey, H., & Agarwal, A. K. (2023). Complex predictive analysis for health care: A comprehensive review. *Bulletin of Electrical Engineering and Informatics, 12*(1), 521–531.
46. Shahbaz, M., Gao, C., Zhai, L., et al. (2019). Investigating the adoption of big data analytics in healthcare: The moderating role of resistance to change. *Journal of Big Data, 6*(6), 1–20. https://doi.org/10.1186/s40537-019-0170-y
47. Mukherjee, M., Kumar, S., Zhang, Q., Matam, R., Mavromoustakis, C. X., Lv, Y., & Mastorakis, G. (2019). Task data offloading and resource allocation in fog computing with multi-task delay guarantee. *IEEE Access, 7*, 152911–152918.
48. Galanis, P., Moisoglou, I., Katsiroumpa, A., et al. (2023). Increased job burnout and reduced job satisfaction for nurses compared to other healthcare workers after the COVID-19 pandemic. *Nursing Reports, 13*(3), 1090–1100. https://doi.org/10.3390/nursrep13030095

49. Tursunbayeva, A. (2019). Human resource technology disruptions and their implications for human resources management in healthcare organizations. *BMC Health Services Research, 19*, 268.
50. Skourletopoulos, G., Mavromoustakis, C. X., Mastorakis, G., et al. (2017). Big data and cloud computing: A survey of the state -of -the -art and research challenges. In *Advances in mobile cloud computing and big data in the 5G era* (pp. 23–41). Springer.

Chapter 9
How to Evaluate Digital Healthcare Applications in a Large-Scale Pilot?

Sonja Grigoleit, Richard Lombard-Vance, Nicola Goodfellow, Glenda Fleming, Michael Scott, Pedro Rocha, Fotios Gioulekas, María José Santofimia Romero, Xavier del Toro García, Alexia Zurkuhlen, and Anna Schüttler

9.1 Introduction

The EU Horizon 2020 project SHAPES (Smart and Healthy Ageing through People Engaging in Supportive Systems, https://shapes2020.eu/, GA No. 857159) posed the question of how to evaluate healthcare solutions in large-scale pilot? SHAPES ran from 2019 to 2023 and had the objective of facilitating long-term healthy and active ageing/and the maintenance of a high-quality standard of life. The Innovation Action built, piloted, and deployed a large-scale, EU-standardised open platform. The digital solutions integrated in the SHAPES platform cover a wide spectrum of areas including Internet of Things (IoT) and Big data Platforms; online

S. Grigoleit (✉)
Fraunhofer Institute for Technological Trend Analysis INT, Euskirchen, Germany
e-mail: sonja.grigoleit@int.fraunhofer.de

R. Lombard-Vance
School of Psychology, Dublin City University, Dublin, Ireland
e-mail: rlv.psych@gmail.com

N. Goodfellow · G. Fleming · M. Scott
Northern Health and Social Care Trust, Medicines Optimisation Innovation Centre, Antrim, UK
e-mail: Nicola.goodfellow@northerntrust.hscni.net; Glenda.Fleming@northerntrust.hscni.net; DrMichael.Scott@northerntrust.hscni.net

P. Rocha
Departamento de Ciências do Comportamento, ICBAS-Instituto de Ciências Biomédicas Abel Salazar, Universidade do Porto, Porto, Portugal
e-mail: parocha@icbas.up.pt

CINTESIS-Centro de Investigação em Tecnologias e Serviços de Saúde, Porto, Portugal
e-mail: parocha@icbas.up.pt

© The Author(s), under exclusive license to Springer Nature Switzerland AG 2024
A. Bourdena et al. (eds.), *Intelligent Technologies for Healthcare Business Applications*, Signals and Communication Technology,
https://doi.org/10.1007/978-3-031-58527-2_9

communication and accessibility tools; cognitive stimulation and rehabilitation; conversational assistants and chatbots; solutions based on robotics, health, and wellbeing platforms; solutions to ensure security as well as solutions in the area of data analytics, such as predictive systems and wellbeing assessment tools. The different digital solutions were combined in 25 use cases —each adapted to a specific target group. Overall, the use cases were categorised in seven pilot themes (PTs) [1]:

- (PT1) Smart Living Environment for Healthy Ageing at Home
- (PT2) Improving In-Home and Community-Based Care
- (PT3) Medicine Control and Optimisation
- (PT4) Psychosocial and Cognitive Stimulation Promoting Wellbeing
- (PT5) Caring for Older Individuals with Neurodegenerative Diseases
- (PT6) Physical Rehabilitation at Home
- (PT7) Cross-Border Health Data Exchange

The 25 use cases were piloted in 43 individual pilot activities at 15 pilot sites across 11 European Countries, including five EIP on AHA[1] Reference Sites.

The main objectives of the SHAPES project involve the evaluation of the SHAPES solutions in two specific areas:

- *The technological evaluation of the digital tools and applications:* This means an evaluation of the pure technological performance—do all technical tools work as they should and without any errors, are the tools interoperable with the local infrastructure, etc.
- *An evaluation of the impact of the SHAPES solution*: How did the SHAPES solutions have an impact on the individual people and society overall in a number of different ways—the health status and the wellbeing of the people, the satisfaction of the user with the SHAPES solution, the effect on the caregiver, organisational aspects for the healthcare community, economic aspects for national health systems as well as socio-cultural aspects for the society in general.

The technical evaluation of the digital health & care solutions was straightforward. Usually the user requirements or system requirements are taken as a basis, so

[1] European Innovation Partnership on Active and Healthy Ageing.

F. Gioulekas
5th Regional Health Authority of Thessaly & Sterea, Larissa, Greece
e-mail: fogi@dypethessaly.gr

M. J. Santofimia Romero · X. del Toro García
Universidad de Castilla-La Mancha, Ciudad Real, Spain
e-mail: mariajose.santofimia@uclm.es; xavier.deltoro@uclm.es

A. Zurkuhlen · A. Schüttler
Gewi-Institut für Gesundheitswirtschaft e.V, Cologne, Germany
e-mail: zurkuhlen@health-region.de

that the number of requirements met represents a good measure to assess the quality of a digital solution from a pure technological perspective.

To measure the impact of a digital solution on the life of the older persons themselves and on their caregiver and the healthcare community at large is more complex.

Several different evaluation methodologies are described in the literature, and each has its advantages and disadvantages and specific perspectives. The World Health Organisation (WHO) has published guidelines for evaluating digital health interventions [2], describing both qualitative and quantitative data capture methods.

The mHealth Assessment and Planning for Scale (MAPS) Toolkit was also published by the WHO as a self-assessment and planning guide designed to improve the capacity of projects to pursue strategies that increase their potential for scaling up [3].

The MAFEIP model (Monitoring and Assessment Framework for the European Innovation Partnership on Active and Healthy Ageing) was developed under the EIP-AHA[2] initiative. It is a web-based tool whose purpose is to estimate the health and economic outcomes of a large variety of ICT-enabled social and health innovations [4].

The non-adoption, abandonment, scale-up, spread, and sustainability (NASSS) framework assesses complexities of health technology projects in various domains to help identify risks of project failures, non-adoption, and challenges to scale-up [5].

The MOMENTUM Blueprint offers critical success factors and performance indicators that help decision-makers to scale up remote monitoring of healthcare services would aid readability and understanding by using more common terminology [6].

The Model for Assessment of Telemedicine (MAST) provides a structure for the assessment of telemedicine applications, including a pre-implementation assessment, followed by multidisciplinary assessment, including description of the patients and the application and assessment of safety, clinical effectiveness, patient perspectives, economic aspects organisational aspects, and socio-cultural, legal, and ethical aspects [7].

9.1.1 How Do Other Health Projects Evaluate Their Solutions?

SHAPES is part of the OPEN DEI (Aligning Reference Architectures, Open Platforms and Large-Scale Pilots in Digitising European Industry) cluster. As part of the Horizon 2020 programme, the OPEN DEI project focuses on 'Platforms and Pilots' to support the implementation of next generation digital platforms in four basic industrial domains, among them the healthcare domain. Currently 14 healthcare projects belong to the OPEN DEI cluster [8].

Most of the healthcare projects in the OPEN DEI framework have published their evaluation method on their respective homepage, and the majority of the OPEN DEI health projects use key performance indicators (KPIs) for their evaluation.

The EU project InteropEHRate used the principles: usability, usefulness (also in healthcare processes), information quality, and interface quality for the evaluation of their solution. In more detail, the questionnaires used were the System Usability Scale (SUS) [9] and Post-Study System Usability Questionnaire—PSSUQ [10, 11]. Smart4Health used qualitative interviews with citizens, healthcare professionals, and researchers [12]. The ACTIVAGE project used key performance indicators (KPIs) on the basis of the MAST domains and the Triple Win strategy for indicators classification[2] [13]. SMART BEAR used KPIs (both clinical KPIs as well as technical KPIs) and also the MAFEIP framework for their evaluation [14]. GATEKEEPER also used KPIs in different categories—clinical, impact assessment, technology, and societal [15]. The evaluation framework of ADLIFE involves an assessment of the effectiveness, implementation, technology acceptance, and socio-economic impact [16]. Finally, HOSMARTAI evaluated the outcome of their project with KPIs in the area of diagnosis revolution, logistic efficiency, treatment improvement, surgical support, and assistive care [17].

9.1.2 How Does SHAPES Evaluate Their Digital Health & Care Solutions?

The SHAPES consortium decided to use a multiple method approach. As pre-evaluation tools, the NASSS and MOMENTUM frameworks were selected to identify difficulties in the use cases and adapt the pilot plan accordingly. Key performance indicators (KPIs) were used to evaluate SHAPES from a project management perspective, and MAST was used to evaluate the impact of the SHAPES solution.

Whilst this multiple method approach had the disadvantage of being more time-consuming than a KPI evaluation alone, the SHAPES evaluation was more detailed and also provides insights into the why and how the impact of a digital health & care solution is other than expected. Another advantage is that this multiple method approach also contains tools to detect risks and challenges early in the use case design (Fig. 9.1).

After the pan-European pilot campaign, interviews were conducted with all pilot sites to evaluate the organisation and management of the pilot activities. One important topic was also the evaluation method used within the SHAPES project.

[2] EIP-AHA triple win strategy refers to (1) more healthy life years, (2) a sustainable health system, and (3) innovation and growth.

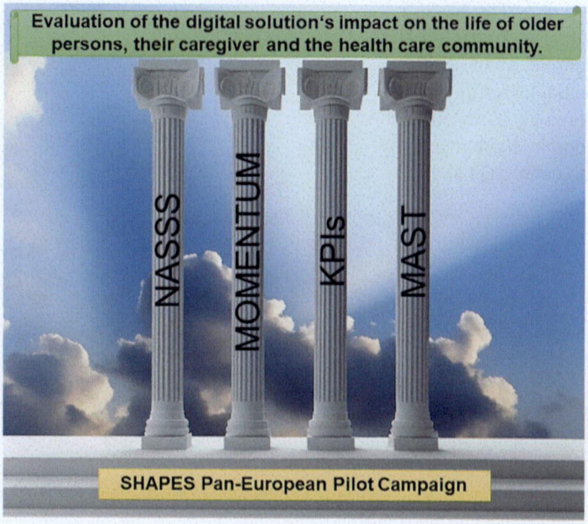

Fig. 9.1 Evaluation methodology of SHAPES digital solutions. (Created by AI)

This chapter contains a description of the four evaluation methods used in SHAPES, the outcomes of the evaluation with the respective method, and also recommendations on the basis of the results of the post-pilot interviews.

9.2 NASSS Framework

9.2.1 Background

It was observed that numerous healthcare projects fail to deliver the expected outcome(s). There are several reasons for this non-adoption of healthcare technologies: lack of user acceptance, reluctance of professionals to use the new technologies, and difficulties integrating the new technology into legacy systems or processes or regulatory frameworks' conditions [5, 18].

Greenhalgh et al. developed the non-adoption, abandonment, scale-up, spread, and sustainability (NASSS) framework, which showed that the failure of the implementation of new health technologies is mainly due to the complexity of the project or because the complexity is not managed optimally. The more complex the (technological) change in healthcare, the less likely it is that the new technology will be implemented into the healthcare system [18, 19].

The NASSS framework consists of seven domains, each of which may be simple (few components, predictable), complicated (many components but still largely predictable), or complex (many components interacting in a dynamic and unpredictable way). The more complexity there is in the system, the less likely the technology is to achieve a sustainable adoption and the more likely it is to be abandoned [19].

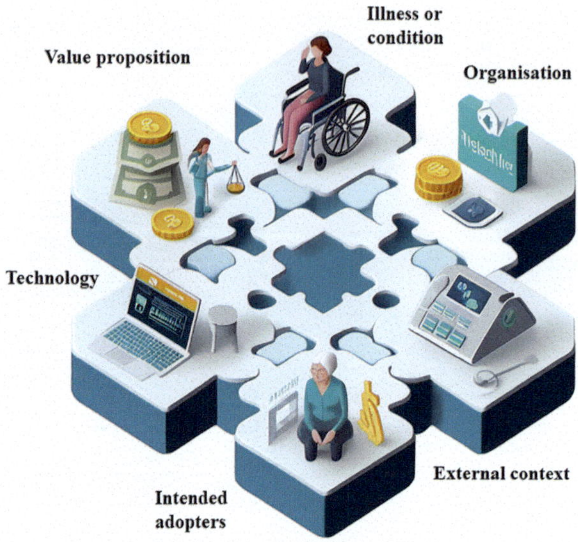

Fig. 9.2 The NASSS framework analyses the complexity of health technologies in various domains. (Created with AI, complexity domains by Greenhalgh et al. [5])

More specifically, these seven domains are as follows [20]:

1. The *illness or condition*
2. The *technology* (e.g. the maturity, reliability, interdependency)
3. The *value proposition* (e.g. the value to the user, the healthcare organisation, and the healthcare system)
4. The *intended adopters* (e.g. user acceptability)
5. The *organisation implementing the technology* (e.g. readiness of the organisation)
6. The *external context* for the innovation (e.g. political, legal, or societal context)
7. *Emergence over time* (e.g. the population with the condition or the technology is likely to change over the next 3–5 years)

Greenhalgh et al. also developed the NASSS-CAT Tools (Complexity Assessment Tools) to analyse the complexity of a planned project and also to identify how complexity could be reduced [18–20] (Fig. 9.2).

9.2.2 Results of the Usage of the NASSS Framework

The NASSS-CAT tools were used at a very early stage of the pilot campaign—at the time of the planning of the different use cases. The aim of this complexity check was to identify potential difficulties in the use cases in order to adapt and mitigate the pilot plan.

Almost all of the use cases identified complexities in the technology domain. Most use cases also identified issues in the domains value proposition and intended adopters, whereas, the illness or condition, the organisation implementing the technology and also the external context were defined as simple for most use cases.

A *complicated or complex condition* was identified, for example, for use cases involving people with reduced mobility, people who required rehabilitation, or people with cognitive impairments. For these cases, the illness described covered a spectrum of different conditions (e.g. mild and severe cognitive impairment), for which different health & care digital solutions are required. As a mitigating measure, the inclusion and exclusion criteria were adapted to be more specific, allowing only people with similar conditions (e.g. only people with mild cognitive impairments or cognitive decline) to participate in the pilot.

In the *technical domain*, the main concerns were about the many interdependencies of the different digital solutions, the data transfer between different health solutions and devices in each use case, and final definition of the SHAPES technological Platform connecting the different health & care solutions, which was still under development at the time of the planning of the use cases. Equally important was that several of the digital health & care solutions did not exist in a robust and definite form at the time of use case planning. This has both advantages and disadvantages for the success of the project. The advantage is that the final adopters could be involved in the development process and have the opportunity to validate mock-ups and prototypes to ensure that the final version of the digital solution reflects the needs of the intended users. The disadvantage is that it is difficult to foresee the number and seriousness of interdependencies and data transfer issues, so that several mitigation measures have to be put in place, such as constant testing, feedback loops, and frequent meetings with all technical partners and pilot sites. It is considered advantageous for the pilot activities to start early with the deployment in order to identify potential problems early in the project.

Other issues identified in the technology domain were the complicated procurement process (stock availability and increasing prices of electronic components during the COVID-19 pandemic) and subsequently an uncertain outcome of the device integration and interoperability, the availability of applications in the local language, a stable network connection at the participants' home, and the number of local IT experts available for the pilot activity.

In the domain *value proposition*, the main uncertainty was that the final combination and integration of digital solutions had not been finalised at the time of the planning of the pilots. As a result, it was not possible to make a realistic assessment of the costs and the effectiveness of the solution before the pilots started.

In the domain *intended adopters*, the main concern was about the digital literacy and the possible low technology acceptance of potential participants. To mitigate this, the participants were involved in the development phase and training was provided on how to use the digital solutions.

Another aspect identified was the continuous engagement of the participants in the pilot activities (e.g. use the devices, take all the necessary measurements, complete the evaluation questionnaires) over a longer period of time. Since the early stages of the project, the pilot sites have been worried about possible drop-outs and less than expected usages of the digital solutions. As a mitigation measure, the potential participants were involved from the beginning of the development process in order to maximise the usability of the digital solutions. For the special case of the use of robots in the participant's home, also the suitability of the home environment was identified as a complexity.

In the domain *organisation*, the general technology readiness of the nursing homes or hospitals was mentioned as well as the initial financial investment. Regarding the *external context*, the main issues mentioned were the regulatory context (e.g. use of robots and artificial intelligence, data protection, and privacy) and the possible impact of the COVID-19 pandemic on the pilot campaign.

9.2.3 Results of Post-Pilot Interviews for NASSS-CAT

During the post-pilot interviews with all pilot sites, the experience of the pilot sites with using the pre-evaluation methods NASSS and MOMENTUM were discussed. Many pilot sites indicated that it was very time-consuming to complete all the questionnaires of the NASSS and MOMENTUM framework. Nevertheless, it was also seen as helpful to double-check their specific use case at the beginning of the pilot campaign.

The complexities identified with the NASSS framework before the beginning of the pilot activity were compared with the real challenges during the pilot campaign. It emerged in the post-pilot interviews with all pilot sites that the main challenges were identified in the technological domain.

Overall, the main issue identified on the basis of the interviews was that the development of the digital health & care technologies and the SHAPES Technology Platform on the one hand and the planning of the pilot on the other hand were running in parallel. As a result, the pilot sites had to deal with several uncertainties during the project such as the interdependencies of the different digital solutions and possible integration issues with the equipment procured.

While most digital solutions were well implemented and ran smoothly during the pilot activities, there were some digital solutions, which were challenging for the pilot sites. The main challenges were as follows:

1. **Voice Assistant** The voice assistant was very popular with the pilot sites, as many use cases only make sense when the application or the robot speaks to the participant (e.g. to remind the person to take their medication, to inform about events or appointments, to engage socially with the participant, or to help the participant during night-time monitoring). In order to ensure that more pilot sites could use the voice assistant, it was decided to include more languages than the originally planned English and Spanish only in the natural language processing (NLP) application.

   However, the programming and training of the chatbot (with typical sentences for the use case) was much more demanding for the pilot sites than expected. During the pilot phase, using the voice assistant was stressful for the participants.

Some participants found the interaction with the voice assistant frustrating and mentioned that the chatbot did not respond reliably to audio commands or that the voice assistant only understood short sentences. In particular, when there were problems with the internet connection, the interaction between the participant and the voice assistant was difficult.

2. **Interoperability Between Different Digital Solutions and (Procured) Devices** In use cases where multiple digital solutions and multiple procured devices had to work together, long testing periods were required. In particular, the time needed to integrate procured devices (e.g. glucometers, blood pressure monitors, pulse oximeters, tablets, and wearables) was underestimated.

   Several pilot sites reported that they had to field test the complete set of digital solutions and devices several times to check for errors and malfunctions. This resulted in a high workload for the pilot sites.

3. **Robots** Apart from the voice assistant, some use cases also reported problems with the robot's trajectories. Sometimes it was not possible to predict how the robot would behave in terms of stops and route, so in one use case the robot was left static in the same place for the whole experimental phase, while in another use case the robot only moved with the participants for a very short distance.

   Another important issue identified with the NASSS-CAT questionnaires were the openness of potential adopters to new technologies in general, the digital literacy, the internet connectivity, and the home environment of potential participants.

   The complex situation of the adopters also turned out as one of the challenges mentioned in the post-pilot interviews with the pilot sites. Although in general the recruitment phase was successful, there were some pilot sites (or some use cases) for which the recruitment was challenging. The main reasons for recruitment difficulties were as follows:

   - The overburdened healthcare sector, which made it difficult to find medical teams with the capacity to co-operate
   - A low level of digital literacy among older people in the region of the pilot site
   - Low internet connectivity
   - Potential participants lacked a laptop or Android device
   - An unsuitable home environment for the usage of a robot
   - Other competing health pilots in the same area

This meant that the use of the NASSS-CAT framework accurately predicted challenges encountered by some use cases. In particular, the complexity due to the large number of different digital solutions and devices and possible interdependencies led to long testing periods and thus also to challenges for the pilot's timetable. It is therefore helpful to invest some time in identifying complexities based on the NASSS framework and to think about possible mitigation actions to minimise risks and challenges in the later stages of the project. It might also be useful to have an independent panel of experts assessing the use case on the basis of the NASSS-CAT.

Recommendation

- Invest the time to go through the NASSS-CAT questionnaire to identify the complexities in a health project.
- Adapt the use case to avoid or reduce complexities.
- Technological complexities (in several cases) can be mitigated by allowing for long testing periods and frequent collaboration between technical partners and pilot sites.
- Complexities on the side of the adopters can be avoided (in several cases) by tailoring the use case to a very specific user group (e.g. specific illness, digital literacy, home environment) or by providing the potential participants with standardised equipment (e.g. internet connectivity, smartphone, tablet).

9.3 MOMENTUM

9.3.1 Background

The MOMEMTUM project released the European telemedicine deployment blueprint to assist 'telemedicine doers' introduce remote healthcare services through the use of information technology [6].

The MOMEMTUM blueprint offers critical success factors and performance indicators that help decision-makers to scale-up of remote monitoring of healthcare services from a distance through information technology. It also delivers a self-assessment toolkit that helps an organisation determine whether it is 'ready' for telemedicine deployment.

The blueprint contains 18 critical success factors (CSF) overall, and each critical success factor is followed in turn by a relevant set of 1–6 performance indicators. These indicators can be used by telemedicine doers to test how important each critical success factor is to their specific deployment circumstances [6].

These indicators are statements which telemedicine doers use to rate their telemedicine deployment initiative on a scale from 1 to 5. The overall scaling indicates the degree of readiness of a telemedicine solution for large-scale deployment [6].

The critical success factors (CSF) defined by MOMENTUM are laid out in four subgroups [6]:

The context

1. Ensure that there is cultural readiness for the telemedicine service.
2. Come to a consensus on the advantages of telemedicine in meeting compelling need(s).

People

3. Ensure leadership through a champion.
4. Involve healthcare professionals and decision-makers.
5. Put the patient at the centre of the service.
6. Ensure that the technology is user-friendly.

Plan

7. Pull together the resources needed for deployment.
8. Address the needs of the primary client(s).
9. Prepare and implement a business plan.
10. Prepare and implement a change management plan.
11. Assess the conditions under which the service is legal.
12. Guarantee that the technology has the potential for scale-up.

Run

13. Identify and apply relevant legal and security guidelines.
14. Involve legal and security experts.
15. Ensure that telemedicine doers and users are privacy aware.
16. Ensure that the appropriate information technology infrastructure and eHealth infrastructure are available.
17. Put in place the technology and processes needed to monitor the service.
18. Establish and maintain good procurement processes (Fig. 9.3).

9.3.2 Results of the Usage of the MOMENTUM Framework

During the planning phase of the project, the use cases were rated on a scale of 1 to 5 for each of the 18 critical success factors in the MOMENTUM framework. Most of the critical success factors were addressed from the beginning of the project—involving the right and committed stakeholders and putting the patient at the centre (PEOPLE); considering the economic, organisational, and legal context (PLAN); and ensuring the right technological infrastructure that meets all security and legal requirements (RUN).

Only a few of the critical success factors were considered challenging in the planning phase of the pilot activities. One of these was cultural readiness for the health & care solution. Particularly for use cases involving very new technologies such as robots, the pilot sites were uncertain whether older people would accept the new tool and find it helpful in their daily lives.

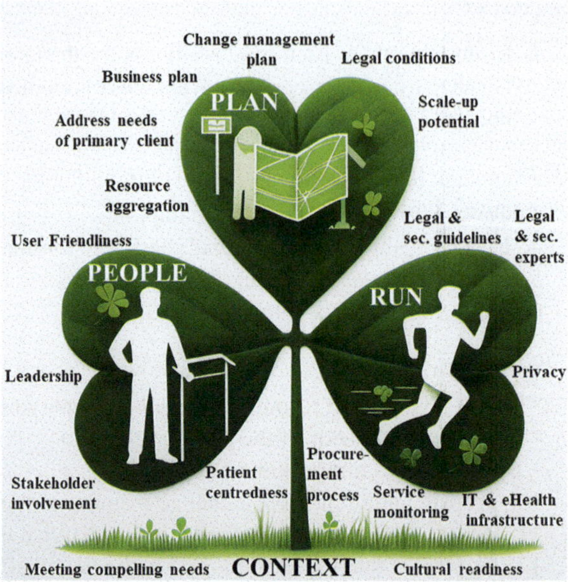

Fig. 9.3 The 18 critical success factors of the MOMENTUM framework [6]. (Created by AI, adaptation of the Shamrock model of the MOMENTUM framework [6])

Another challenge was seen in the involvement of health & care professionals. Particularly in the aftermath of the COVID-19 pandemic, many hospitals and nursing homes were understaffed and, in many cases, overworked. As a result, in several cases, health professionals were not able to devote time to a research project and had to withdraw their involvement. However, it might be a solution to hire full-time staff at the respective organisation dedicated to the project.

One issue that was not fully addressed during the course of the research project was the scaling up of new technologies. Especially for expensive technologies such as robotics, it is difficult to accurately calculate the cost balance for large-scale production.

A further issue was the appropriate information technology infrastructure. The pilot sites had to assess on a case-by-case basis whether the potential participants in the pilots had sufficient internet coverage and a suitable smartphone or tablet.

9.3.3 Results of the Post-Pilot Interviews for MOMENTUM

The MOMENTUM self-assessment tool, with its critical success factors and performance indicators, was generally seen as a useful test to examine whether the different use cases were ready for scale-up in Europe.

However, most of the critical success factors were inherent to the SHAPES project, such as the identification of user needs; the involvement of older people themselves in the development of the solutions to ensure usability; the involvement of health professionals, legal and IT experts, the digital solutions and IT infrastructure; and the consideration of data protection and privacy regulations as well as the preparation of a business and change management plan.

Given that the use of the MOMENTUM self-assessment tool was also considered to be time-consuming, the overall impact of using MOMENTUM during the project was limited.

MOMENTUM would be more helpful at a much earlier stage, namely, during the planning of the SHAPES project itself. This would enable all the necessary aspects of innovation management to be considered and enable an overview of how the new innovation can best be implemented by organisations.

Recommendation

- Use MOMENTUM to plan research and innovation projects in the health area.
- The 18 Critical Success Factors provide a good way to check if the project includes all the necessary aspects for a successful innovation management.

9.4 MAST

9.4.1 Background

The Model for Assessment of Telemedicine (MAST) framework was developed as part of the MethoTelemed Project, a multidisciplinary effort aimed at evaluating the effectiveness of telemedicine interventions.

The use of MAST includes three steps. As a first step, the maturity of the telemedicine technology and the organisation using the service is assessed before the assessment of effectiveness is carried out. If the maturity of the technology needs to be developed further, studies such as usability studies or feasibility studies must be carried out, and, similarly, if MAST is to be used for the development of the organisation using the telemedicine, optimisation studies need to be performed.

Following implementation of the service or pilot, a multidisciplinary assessment of the effectiveness of the technology can be carried out using MAST. These seven domains addressed by MAST include clinical effectiveness, patient experience and satisfaction, economic impact, technical reliability, ethical considerations, legal compliance, and organisational feasibility [7, 21].

Finally, an assessment of the transferability of the results to other locations, regions, or countries should be completed (Fig. 9.4).

MAST provides a comprehensive approach to assess telemedicine programmes across seven key domains. To effectively measure the impact of telemedicine

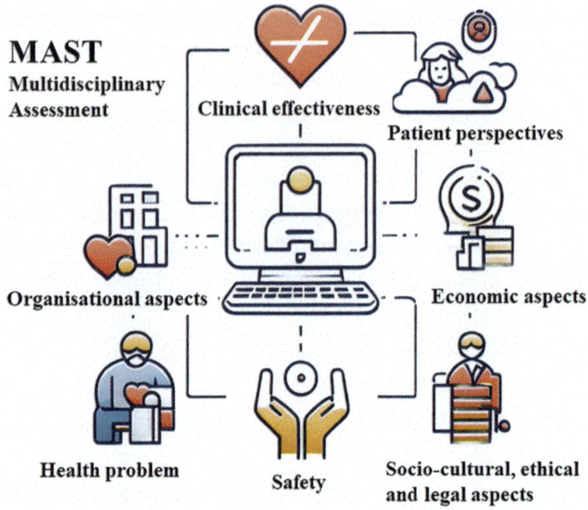

Fig. 9.4 The seven domains of the multidisciplinary assessment of MAST (Model for Assessment of Telemedicine) [22]. (Created by AI)

interventions within each domain, MAST employs a selection of validated questionnaires and surveys. The choice of questionnaires and surveys is driven by the specific objectives of the assessment and the intended outcomes to be measured.

9.4.2 Results of the Usage of the MAST Framework

To apply the MAST framework for the evaluation of the digital health & care solutions, the relevant domains and the questionnaires for each domain have to be selected. Overall, the relevant data for the evaluation of SHAPES was captured with 35 different questionnaires.

An important domain for the evaluation is the clinical effectiveness of the digital health & care solution. For the 25 use cases of the SHAPES project, a broad range of questionnaires to measure the clinical effectiveness were selected depending on the specific health status of the target group. However, nearly all use cases measure the effects on health-related quality of life (HRQOL) by using the WHOQOL-BREF [23] score and the EQ-5D-5L [24] score. The EQ-5D-5L consists of the EQ-5D descriptive system and the EQ visual analogue scale (EQ-VAS) [25]. Additionally, the majority of use cases applied the Oslo Social Support Scale (OSSS-3) [26].

Depending on the specific objective of the use case, other scales are applied within this domain. For the use case dedicated to improve deficiencies in the adherence to medicines and treatments for people with multi-morbidities, additionally the effects on mortality, the usage of health services and behavioural outcomes like the Beliefs about Medicines (BMQ) [27] and the Medication Adherence Report Scale (MARS) [28] were applied.

In the use cases dedicated to cognitive stimulation and training further cognitive health assessments, such as the Trail Making Test [29] and the Montreal Cognitive Assessment (MoCA) [30] were used.

Use cases with a focus on mental health applied the UCLA Loneliness Scale [31] and/or the Scale of Positive and Negative Experience (SPANE) [32].

Psychosocial assessment scales applied were the Beck Anxiety Inventory (BAI) [33], the Geriatric Depression Scale (GDS-15) [34], and the Friendship Scale Assessment [35].

In the patient perspective MAST domain, all use cases applied the System Usability Scale (SUS) [9] and nearly all the General Self-Efficacy Scale (GSE) [36]. To measure the satisfaction and acceptance of the digital health & care solution, most use cases also applied the Technology Acceptance Model (TAM) [37] and the User Experience Questionnaire-Short Version (UEQ-S) [38]. Use cases dedicated to the understanding of information and confidence in treatment also used the 1-item health literacy [39].

In addition to the questionnaires, system data such as the number of logins, video calls, used functions, or visited pages were also used to measure the engagement and self-efficacy of the participants.

In the economic domain, the cost of the medical and other devices, the SHAPES Technological Platform and the staffing were assessed. Additionally, the saved expenses related to patient transport as well as hospitalisation and A&E attendances are analysed. The safety domain was only relevant for the use case with robots to measure possible collisions.

The organisational, socio-cultural, ethical, and legal domains were not used within the SHAPES project. As the pilot ran for several weeks or months (depending on the use case) and the overall number of participants per use case was relatively low, it was not possible to measure any effect on the staff, workflow, or management in nursing homes or hospitals. The same holds true for measuring social or legal aspects. The time span of the pilot was too short to lead to changes in the patients' role in major life areas or a general change in the service model of healthcare. The list of all data captured for the MAST evaluation is compiled in Table 9.1.

9.4.2.1 Holistic Psychosocial Evaluation Via Harmonised Outcome Measurement

The different technologies used in SHAPES, the different pilot sites and languages spoken, and the target groups with very different life situations, such as older adults, people with chronic health conditions, impairments, or disabilities, were the reasons why a total of 35 different questionnaires were selected for the evaluation.

In order to provide a comprehensive evaluation of SHAPES, a longitudinal assessment of psychosocial outcomes (using a harmonised set of outcome measures) was chosen. The range of possible important outcomes is very broad. Psychosocial wellbeing outcomes hold particular importance and meaning for older adults. Therefore, the SHAPES Project focused on the harmonisation of outcomes related to

Table 9.1 Selected domains and specific types of outcomes for the MAST evaluation

MAST domain	MAST topic	Data required
Health problem and description of the application	Health problem	Medical information about patients
		Number of GP contacts, number of nurse contacts, number of out-of-hours contacts, number of ambulance calls
Safety	Technical safety (technical reliability)	Protocol for collisions
Clinical effectiveness	Effects on mortality	Number of deaths
	Physical health	Heart rate, sleep quality, wellbeing: risks of falls; physical status (Senior Fitness Test—Fullerton) [40]; balance (Berg Balance Scale, Tinetti Test) [41]; static balance (Stork Balance test—1 leg) [42]; body mass index (BMI); balance while walking (10 min Walk Test) [43]; short physical status (Short Physical Performance Battery Protocol) [44]; aerobic capacity (6-min walk) [45]; RISC score (risk of hospitalisation) [46]; gait speed test: Eadon Scale [47]
	Mental health	OSSS-3 [26]; SPANE [32]; UCLA [31]; Beck Anxiety Inventory (BAI); Geriatric Depression Scale 15 (GDS-15) [33]; Friendship Scale Assessment
	Cognitive health	Trail Making Test [29]; Montreal Cognitive Assessment (MoCA) [30]; Mini Mental Examination [48]; Digit Symbol Substitution Test (DSST) [49]; Verbal Fluency [50]; STROOP/'Name that colour' test [51]; 6CIT [52]; QMCI [53]

	Effects on health-related quality of life (HRQL)	EQ-5D-5L [24]; WHOQOL-BREF scores [23]
	Behavioural outcomes	BMQ-scores [27]; MARS scores [28]; steps, fluid and nutrition intake, sleep duration; dance score, number of choreographies danced, the ratio of correct steps, time danced, level of difficulty, and type of interaction (continuous or erratic)
	Usage of health services	Number of hospitalisations; number of A&E attendances; number of GP contacts; number of nurse contacts; number of out-of-hours contacts; number of ambulance calls
Patient perspectives	Satisfaction and acceptance	TAM score [37]; UEQ-S score [38]
	Understanding of information; confidence (in treatment);ability to use the application; access & accessibility	SUS [9]; 1-item health literacy [39]; Semi-structured interviews
	Empowerment, self-efficacy	General Self-Efficacy Scale (GSE) [36]; participation questionnaire; activities (e.g. number of logins, video calls, used functionalities, visited pages); interviews
Economic aspects	Amount of resources used when delivering the application and comparators	Cost of (medical) devices; costs per device maintenance (IT support, medical device regular checks, calibration, etc.); cost of using digital solutions and technical platform; cost of staffing; patients travel expenses
	Related changes in use of healthcare	Cost of hospitalisations; cost of A&E attendances; cost and length of rehabilitation process

quality-of-life (QOL), health-related quality-of-life (HRQOL), social participation, and constructs which might intrinsically be considered outcomes, but may also function as moderators or mediators of QOL, HRQOL, and participation: self-efficacy, social support, and health literacy. Additionally, the measurement of the usability and acceptance of measures was harmonised. These constructs were prioritised following a fruitful process of iterative engagement with use case leaders and other stakeholders across the SHAPES Project, ensuring that a broad spectrum of persons could contribute views and ideas in relation to what was measured across all pilots, and with what measure.

Various challenges present for navigation in the design of a harmonised outcome set. First, where possible, existing measures with satisfactory validity and reliability are key to facilitating measurement. Second—Europe is a continent of many languages—the availability of appropriately translated versions of extant, valid, and reliable outcome measures is a central concern. Fortunately, it is possible to source an outcome measure for most constructs in the languages required. SHAPES required English, German, Greek, Italian, Portuguese, Spanish, and Swedish. A third challenge presents in terms of comprehensiveness versus burden. Comprehensive coverage of important psychosocial constructs needs to be balanced with the burden of assessment, both for individual respondents and for assessment administrators. Selecting a brief measure, such as the WHOQOL-BREF instead of the WHOQOL, is likely to provide sufficient, meaningful data in this context. Assessment administration itself can be piloted to refine and reduce the expected duration of administration. For SHAPES, and at the time of assessment design, measures such as the WHOQOL-BREF to measure QOL, EQ-5D-5L to measure HRQOL, General Self-Efficacy Scale to measure self-efficacy, Oslo Social Support Scale-3 to measure social support, system usability scale to measure usability, and technology acceptance model to measure acceptance and intention to use satisfied all criteria. A simple, single-item, English-validated measure was deemed the best option to measure health literacy. We relied upon newly constructed participation items (based on an extant measure) to measure social participation, as we did not have available a reliable, translated measure. Language is not the only construct which varies across Europe. Diversity of education systems, cultures, and income levels, for example, warrants consideration in the design and collection of socio-demographic data alongside psychosocial and socio-technical variables.

Accessibility and inclusion are other key challenges. Are participants enabled to complete assessments across pilots? This is no more or less important than an individual pilot's outcome assessment, but this is always worthy of consideration. Participants with impairments or health challenges have a right to participate in research activity—particularly where research concerns issues which may affect them as a population, or where they have historically been neglected. Participants should be enabled to engage in those activities, for example, via accessibility supports or supported procedures for informed consent [54]. In addition to operationally, inclusion ought to be considered at point of design and analyses.

Heretofore, evaluations may have relied on use case-level or pilot-level outcome data. The small-n nature of the reality of piloting new technologies in complex contexts—not least peri- and post-pandemic—would engender limitations in the scope of analyses. Harmonisation of outcomes enabled cross-project, holistic, quantitative analyses with $N > 300$, which would otherwise simply not have been possible. Harmonised analyses present challenges and limitations regarding research design and analytic interpretation, but these present an additional, data-rich option for the co-evaluation of multiple pilots.

9.4.3 Results of the Post-Pilot Interviews for MAST

The MAST framework was the main evaluation method used for the SHAPES project. All pilot sites agreed to use MAST and recognised the usefulness of the methodology. However, there was some criticism regarding the number of questionnaires to be included in the MAST evaluation.

Within the SHAPES framework, the partner organisations agreed to use 8 'harmonised' questionnaires (6 psychosocial—WHOQOL-BREF, EQ-5D-5L, self-efficacy (GSES), OSSS-3 (social support) & life events, 1-item health literacy, participation questions, and 2 socio-technical—SUS and TAM to be able to compare the results of the 25 use cases and also to complete an overarching evaluation of SHAPES. In addition to these questionnaires, the pilot sites used other more specific questionnaires (e.g. on caregiver burden, gait speed, or loneliness scale).

For this reason, almost all the pilot sites reported that the total number of questionnaires was too much for the participants. They reported that it was 'very demanding' and 'a burden for the participants' (and also for the researcher) as the total interviews lasted more than an hour. It was recommended that interviews should not last longer than 20 min.

It was also mentioned that in several cases the intervention time was too short to see a significant change in health-related quality of life. A larger number of participants and an intervention period of around 12 months would be needed to observe significant changes in participants' health-related quality of life.

Recommendation

- The MAST framework is a good overall evaluation method which covers all important aspects regarding the impact of a digital health & care solution in a real-life situation.
- The number of questionnaires for one or more of the 7 domains of the MAST framework should be limited so that the interviews with the participants do not take longer than 20 min.

(continued)

- To observe significant changes in the health-related quality of life, larger numbers of participants need to be recruited and longer intervention periods should be allowed (e.g., around 12 months).
- Harmonised analyses present an additional, data-rich option for the co-evaluation of multiple pilots.

9.5 Key Performance Indicators

9.5.1 Background

Key performance indicators (KPIs) were defined as a set of measures that focus on the factors that are most critical to an organisation's success and reflect on the efficiency of its operational flow and business processes. KPIs tell management how the organisation is performing on its previous defined critical success factors (CSFs) and, by monitoring them, management can improve performance [55].

CSFs can be understood as 'a limited number (usually between 3 and 8) of characteristics, conditions, or variables that have a direct and serious impact on the effectiveness, efficiency, and viability of an organisation, programme or project' in the case of SHAPES [56]. KPIs measured a performance in critical areas by showing the progress or lack of it towards realising the objectives by monitoring activities [56].

The SMART rule summarises the basic requirements for effective KPIs. The five conditions of the SMART rule are as follows [57, 58]:

- Specific: It must be clearly stated what the parameter measures. This means that the parameter to be measured must be unambiguous.
- Measurable: The parameter must quantify the progress of a capability (e.g. with a quantity, frequency, cost, or time).
- Achievable: The means of measuring a parameter must be realistic.
- Relevant: The parameter must be an indicator that is of key interest to the project and is not already quantified by another indicator.
- Time-bound: The indicator must represent the status at a specific point in time during the pilot campaign.

In addition to the SMART rule, the number of KPIs for a use case should be kept to a minimum. It has been shown that a manageable number of parameters can increase to about 20 variables [59].

In summary, SHAPES defined a manageable set of KPIs for each use case in order to evaluate after the pilot, whether the use case was successful or not. An

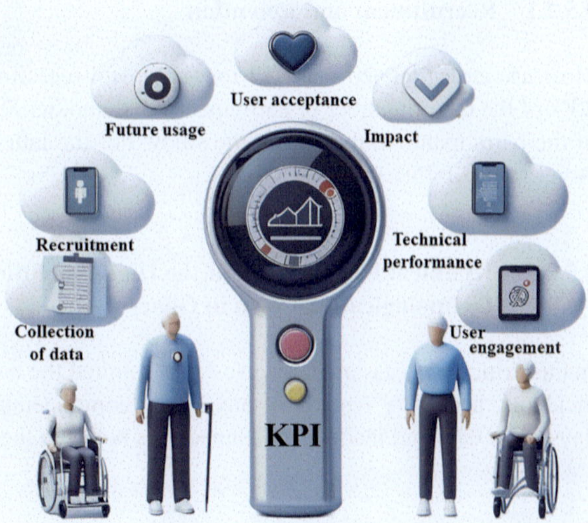

Fig. 9.5 The seven domains of the key performance indicators (KPIs) used within the SHAPES project. (Created by AI)

'unsuccessful use case' meant that major changes needed to be made to the digital solutions, the target group or the overall pilot setting, before scaling-up the use case.

9.5.2 *Results of the Use of KPIs*

To be able to evaluate whether the use case was successful during the pilot or not a manageable number of KPIs were defined for each use case. For each use case, an average number of 6–7 KPIs were defined.

To be able to evaluate the success of the pilot activities, it is necessary to monitor the progress in all areas which are critical to achieving the underlying objectives of the SHAPES project. The following topics were identified as critical success areas:

1. Recruitment and retention
2. Technical performance of the digital solutions/the technological platform in general
3. User engagement
4. Collection of data (via sensors and/or questionnaires)
5. User acceptance
6. (Positive) impact of the pilot activity
7. Intention to use SHAPES in the future (Fig. 9.5)

Depending on the specific objectives and planning of each use case, a set of KPIs were defined and adapted for evaluation.

9.5.2.1 Recruitment and Retention

Most use cases defined one KPI for successful recruitment, with a target value of 80% of the target number of participants, and another KPI for successful enrolment of the participants to the end of the study. For the latter KPI, most use cases set a target value of 75% or 80%.

9.5.2.2 Technical Performance of the Digital Solutions/the SHAPES Technological Platform in General

In this critical success area, the use cases counted the number of (serious) technical incidents, necessary restarts of any of the components (at more than 10% of the days), lost data and inadequate connections between the devices/ solutions.

9.5.2.3 User Engagement

To measure the user engagement, the pilot sites counted the number of participants, who had repeated interaction with the digital solutions (e.g. daily or on 50/60% of the days), or they counted the number of exercises (e.g. 80% of the exercises or twice per week).

9.5.2.4 Collection of Data (Via Sensors and Questionnaires)

The number of questionnaires completed by the participants (e.g. 50/60%) and how many measurements such as blood pressure, oxygen saturation, and heart rate were taken by the participants (e.g. 50% of the days) was counted. In three use cases, whether sufficient data was collected to allow the heart failure decompensation prediction tool to generate a percentage risk of decompensation (for 60% of the participants) was measured.

9.5.2.5 User Acceptance

The results of questionnaires were used to measure user acceptance. In most use cases, the System Usability Scale (SUS) was used (above average rating (>68) for at least 60% of the participants). In many use cases, the User Experience Questionnaire (UEQ-S) was used (the overall experience is to be rated above average). In three use cases, the Technology Acceptance Model (TAM) was used to assess the acceptance of the digital solution (60%).

9.5.2.6 (Positive) Impact of the Pilot Activity

Some use cases assessed the impact of the pilot activity on participants' life. For this assessment, participants completed questionnaires to measure the cognitive and/or physical status, as well as quality of life (WHOQOL-BREF, EQ-5D-5L, GSE, OSSS-3). Typical targets were for 50/70% of the participants to maintain or improve their status, or an average of 5/10% increase in the respective status.

Other indicators to measure the impact of the pilot activity were used, for example, in one case the Eadon scale [47] and in others the cognitive, physical, and social functioning or the perceived anxiety and depression or the quality of gait.

Some use cases also used indicators to measure the impact on the caregivers (burden, mental load, and workload), an eVIP evaluation tool for virtual patients [60], or a general questionnaire for the participants (medical students) to assess, whether they believed that the technology improved the quality of practice.

9.5.2.7 Intention to Use SHAPES in the Future

Some use cases included a projection of the future use of the SHAPES solutions in the evaluation. To measure this the participants were asked, whether they intended to use the digital solution after the test phase (target value is 80% of the participants) and whether it would be useful to develop a specific platform for healthy ageing.

9.5.3 Results of the Post-Pilot Interviews on the Use of KPIs

The KPIs presented a concise way to monitor the progress of the pilot activities towards the objectives of the specific use case. In the interviews, the KPIs were generally accepted as an easy-to-use method of assessing the performance of the use case.

The pilot activity of each of the 25 use cases was evaluated with KPIs. The mean number of KPIs per use case was 7—of these KPIs on average 70% were achieved successfully, 20% have not been achieved, and 10% were not evaluated due to various reasons (e.g. heart disease functions were not used, because there were only patients with diabetes; the usability was not evaluated, because the respective functionality was not used in the pilot).

The main reasons for not achieving KPIs are as follows:

- The participants did not score an above average rating (>68) in the System Usability Scale (SUS)—18 responses.
- The participants did not interact or did not use the digital solution as many times as foreseen—8 responses.
- The overall user experience quality of the digital solution as measured using the User Experience Questionnaire (UEQ-S) was not above average—7 responses.

- The target recruitment number was not achieved—5 responses.
- There were more serious support cases (due to malfunctioning or difficulties with the digital solution) than expected—4 responses.
- The impact on the health-related quality of life of the participants was less than expected—4 responses.
- The impact on healthcare personnel was less positive than expected—2 responses.
- The digital solution had to be restarted various times—2 responses.
- Less than expected number of participants remained enrolled until the end of the intervention period—2 responses.
- The participants did not fill out the questionnaire on a regular basis—2 responses.
- Less than expected number of participants assessed the digital solution to be useful to them according to the Technology Acceptance Model (TAM)—2 responses.
- The participants did not want to use the digital solution after the termination of the pilot activity—1 response.

Although the KPIs provide an easy way to rapidly assess, if a use case is successful, it does not give any information about the underlying problem in the case of unsuccessful pilot activities. For example, a low KPI in the area of user engagement does not give any clues, if the reason lies in a low user friendliness of the digital health & care solution or in problems with the IT infrastructure (e.g. Wi-Fi connection), the health or personal situation, a lack of training with the new technology, or if the digital solution did not match the target group. It was also deduced that the bond of trust established between general practitioner and the associated elder patients is an important factor which bolsters the efficient evaluation of the KPIs.

Overall, KPIs were a helpful tool from a project management perspective, but the MAST evaluation method was more appropriate to describe the impact and possible drawbacks of a new digital health & care solution.

Recommendation

- KPIs were an easy method to assess, if a use case (or pilot activity) was successful or not and also to monitor the progress of the pilot activities towards the objective of the use case.
- However, they should primarily be used as a project management tool. To understand the impact of a digital solution the MAST framework is recommended.

9.6 Conclusion

The NASSS framework was a useful test to check the complexity of a use case at the beginning of the pilot's planning. The MOMENTUM self-assessment tool with its critical success factors and performance indicators was also a useful tool to see if the different use cases were ready for scale-up in Europe. Both pre-evaluation tests are time-consuming. It is recommended to use MOMENTUM during the design of a healthcare project, to make sure that the innovation management of the project is planned in a suitable manner. The NASSS framework is recommended to be used as a check for use cases. Complexities in the use case can be identified so that mitigations can be included in the further planning of the pilot activity.

KPIs were suitable from a project management perspective. They were defined as a set of measures that focus on the factors most critical to the success of the respective use case. They presented a concise way to monitor the progress of the pilot activities towards the objectives of the specific use case. It is recommended to define only a small number of KPIs. Within SHAPES, 6–7 KPIs per use case were defined.

To get a greater insight into the impact of the digital health & care solution on the participants of the pilots and understand which aspects might need to be improved, the more holistic MAST evaluation is better suited.

Thus, the main evaluation tool for SHAPES was the Model for Assessment of Telemedicine (MAST). This method can be easily adapted to the specific objectives of the project or use case. Overall, MAST comprises seven different assessment domains. For SHAPES, the three domains, namely, clinical effectiveness, patient perspectives, and economic aspects were selected.

The data for these domains was captured with 35 different questionnaires. Most use cases used the System Usability Scale (SUS), EQ-5D-5L-VAS, and WHOQOL-BREF to assess the health-related quality of life, General Self-Efficacy-Scale (GSE), Technology Acceptance Model (TAM), Oslo Social Support Scale (OSSS-3), and the User Experience Questionnaire-Short Version (UEQ-S). Depending on the specific objective of the use case, further questionnaires were used. The project clearly showed that is it important to limit the number of questionnaires per use case. The participants should not be overwhelmed with evaluation activities. For the evaluation, it is recommended to limit interview time with the participants to less than 20 min. It is also strongly advised that in case of older individuals, and especially with chronic diseases or with disabilities, the evaluation is performed with the assistance of their general practitioners or the caregivers (formal or informal).

References

1. Seidel, K., Labor, M., Lombard-Vance, R., et al. (2022). Implementation of a pan-European ecosystem and an interoperable platform for Smart and Healthy Ageing in Europe: An innovation action research protocol. *Open Research Europe, 2*, 85. https://doi.org/10.12688/openreseurope.14827.1

2. WHO. (2016). *Monitoring and evaluating digital health interventions: A practical guide to conducting research and assessment*. https://apps.who.int/iris/handle/10665/252183.
3. World Health Organization. (2015). *The MAPS toolkit: mHealth assessment and planning for scale*. WHO Press.
4. Birov, S, Lavin, C., & Stroetmann, V., et al. (2017). *MAFEIP user guide. Version 2.0. Open evidence & empirica*. https://tool.mafeip.eu/assets/files/MAFEIP_User_Guide_v2_Website.pdf
5. Greenhalgh, T., Wherton, J., Papoutsi, C., et al. (2017). Beyond adoption: A new framework for theorizing and evaluating nonadoption, abandonment, and challenges to the scale-up, spread, and sustainability of health and care technologies. *Journal of Medical Internet Research, 19*, e367. https://doi.org/10.2196/jmir.8775
6. MOMENTUM. (2015). *European momentum for mainstreaming telemedicine deployment in daily practice*. https://www.telemedicine-momentum.eu/
7. Kidholm, K., Bowes, A., Dyrehauge, S., et al. (2010). *The MAST manual: MAST – Model for Assessment of Telemedicine*; The manual is part of the results from the MethoTelemed Project. http://www.ouh.dk/dwn154013
8. OPEN DEI. (2023). *OPEN DEI projects*. https://www.opendei.eu/projects/. Accessed 22 Nov 2023.
9. Brooke, J. (1995). *SUS: A quick and dirty usability scale. Usability evaluation in industry* (p. 189). CRC Press.
10. Fruhling, A., & Lee, S. (2005). Assessing the reliability, validity and adaptability of PSSUQ. *AMCIS 2005 Proceedings*, 378.
11. Interopehrate Project. (2021). *D7.1 experimentation scenarios and validation plan*. https://www.interopehrate.eu/wp-content/uploads/2022/09/InteropEHRate-D7.1-Experimentation-scenarios-and-validation-plan.pdf. Accessed 22 Nov 2013.
12. Smart4Health Project. (2023). *WP1: Citizen- and Professional-User participation: User requirements and performance criteria D1.10: Validation Report: D1.7*. https://smart4health.eu/deliverables/. Accessed 22 Nov 2023.
13. Activage Project. (2017) *Consolidated list of KPIs and coordinated methodology for evaluation: D6.1*. http://www.activageproject.eu/docs/downloads/activage_public_deliverables/ACTIVAGE_D6-1_M6_consolidated-KPI-list+evaluation-methodology_v1-0.pdf. Accessed 22 Nov 2013.
14. Smartbear Project. (2022). *SMART BEAR "Smart big data platform to offer evidence-based personalised support for healthy and independent living at home": D53*. https://www.smart-bear.eu/wp-content/uploads/2023/03/D53-D12.2.pdf. Accessed 22 Nov 2013.
15. Gatekeeper Project. (2022). *D7.8 – KPI evolution report (I to VIII)* [M36 updated every 6 months]. https://www.gatekeeper-project.eu/wp-content/uploads/2022/12/GATEKEEPER-WP7-D7.8-DEL-20220930-v1.0.pdf. Accessed 22 Nov 2023.
16. ADLIFE Project. (2023). *D9.1 ADLIFE intermediate progress report*. https://static1.squarespace.com/static/5e6fed256e0cba537c99c528/t/652017b3956c4a1893b5c075/1696602041097/ADLIFE_D9.1_Evaluation_IntermediateProgress+Report_20230630.pdf. Accessed 22 Nov 2023.
17. Hosmartiai Project. (2022). *D1.7 – Report on KPIs definition*. https://www.hosmartai.eu/wp-content/uploads/2022/02/HosmartAI_D1.7-Report-on-KPIs-definition_v1.0_2022-01-31_PhE.pdf. Accessed 22 Nov 2023.
18. Kunze, C. (2020). *(Nicht-)Nutzung, Transfer, Verbreitung und Nachhaltigkeit von Gesundheitstechnologien: Deutsche Version des NASSS-Frameworks*. https://opus.hs-furtwangen.de/frontdoor/index/index/year/2020/docId/6230. Accessed 02 Mar 2023.
19. Greenhalgh, T., & Abimbola, S. (2019). The NASSS framework – A synthesis of multiple theories of technology implementation. *Studies in Health Technology and Informatics, 263*, 193–204. https://doi.org/10.3233/SHTI190123
20. Greenhalgh, T., Maylor, H., Shaw, S., et al. (2020). The NASSS-CAT tools for understanding, guiding, monitoring, and researching technology implementation projects in health and social care: Protocol for an evaluation study in real-world settings. *JMIR Research Protocols, 9*, e16861. https://doi.org/10.2196/16861

21. Kidholm, K., Clemensen, J., Caffery, L. J., et al. (2016). The model for assessment of telemedicine (MAST): A scoping review of empirical studies. *Journal of Telemedicine and Telecare, 23*, 803–813. https://doi.org/10.1177/1357633X17721815
22. Kidholm, K., Jensen, L. S., Kjølhede, T., et al. (2016). Validity of the model for assessment of telemedicine: A Delphi study. Undefined.
23. World Health Organization. (2023). *WHOQOL: Measuring quality of life*. https://www.who.int/tools/whoqol/whoqol-bref. Accessed 19 Jul 2023.
24. EuroQol Research Foundation. (2023). EQ-5D. https://euroqol.org/eq-5d-instruments/. Accessed 19 Jul 2023.
25. EQ-5D. (2023). EQ-5D-5L | About. https://euroqol.org/eq-5d-instruments/eq-5d-5l-about/. Accessed 30 Nov 2023.
26. Kocalevent, R.-D., Berg, L., Beutel, M. E., et al. (2018). Social support in the general population: Standardization of the Oslo social support scale (OSSS-3). *BMC Psychology, 6*, 31. https://doi.org/10.1186/s40359-018-0249-9
27. Thorneloe, R. J., Griffiths, C. E. M., Ashcroft, D. M., et al. (2017). The challenges of assessing patients' medication beliefs: A qualitative study. *BMC Health Services Research, 17*, 119. https://doi.org/10.1186/s12913-017-2020-y
28. Chan, A. H. Y., Horne, R., Hankins, M., et al. (2020). The medication adherence report scale: A measurement tool for eliciting patients' reports of nonadherence. *British Journal of Clinical Pharmacology, 86*, 1281–1288. https://doi.org/10.1111/bcp.14193
29. Reitan, R. M. (1992). *Trail Making Test: Manual for administration and scoring*. Reitan Neuropsychology Laboratory.
30. MoCA Test Inc. (2023). *MoCa cognition*. https://mocacognition.com/. Accessed 19 Jul 2023.
31. Russell, D., Peplau, L. A., & Ferguson, M. L. (1978). Developing a measure of loneliness. *Journal of Personality Assessment, 42*, 290–294. https://doi.org/10.1207/s15327752jpa4203_11
32. Diener, E., Wirtz, D., & Tov, W. (2010). New measures of well-being: Flourishing and positive and negative feelings. *Social Indicators Research, 39*, 247–266.
33. Beck, A. T., Epstein, N., Brown, G., et al. (1988). An inventory for measuring clinical anxiety: Psychometric properties. *Journal of Consulting and Clinical Psychology, 56*, 893–897. https://doi.org/10.1037/0022-006x.56.6.893
34. Yesavage, J. A., & Sheikh, J. I. (1986). 9/geriatric depression scale (GDS). *Clinical Gerontologist, 5*, 165–173. https://doi.org/10.1300/J018v05n01_09
35. Hawthorne, G. (2006). Measuring social isolation in older adults: Development and initial validation of the friendship scale. *Social Indicators Research, 77*, 521–548. https://doi.org/10.1007/s11205-005-7746-y
36. Schwarzer, R., & Jerusalem, M. (1995). Generalized self-efficacy scale. In S. Weinman & M. J. Wright (Eds.), *Measures in health psychology: A user's portfolio causal and control beliefs* (pp. 35–37). NFER-NELSON.
37. Lewis, J. R. (2019). Comparison of four TAM item formats: Effect of response option labels and order. *Journal of User Experience, 14*, 224–236.
38. Schrepp, M., Hinderks, A., & Thomaschewski, J. (2017). Design and evaluation of a short version of the user experience questionnaire (UEQ-S). *IJIMAI, 4*, 103. https://doi.org/10.9781/ijimai.2017.09.001
39. Morris, N. S., MacLean, C. D., Chew, L. D., et al. (2006). The single item literacy screener: Evaluation of a brief instrument to identify limited reading ability. *BMC Family Practice, 7*, 21. https://doi.org/10.1186/1471-2296-7-21
40. Różańska-Kirschke, A. K., Kocur, P., Wilk, M., et al. (2006). Fullerton fitness test as fitness index for the elderly. *Medical Rehabilitation, 10*, 15–19.
41. Miodonska, Z., Stepien, P., Badura, P., et al. (2018). Inertial data-based gait metrics correspondence to Tinetti Test and Berg Balance Scale assessments. *Biomedical Signal Processing and Control, 44*, 38–47. https://doi.org/10.1016/j.bspc.2018.03.012
42. Vellas, B. J., Wayne, S. J., Romero, L., et al. (1997). One-leg balance is an important predictor of injurious falls in older persons. *Journal of the American Geriatrics Society, 45*, 735–738. https://doi.org/10.1111/j.1532-5415.1997.tb01479.x
43. Physiopedia. (2023). *10 Metre Walk Test*. https://www.physio-pedia.com/10_Metre_Walk_Test. Accessed 19 Jul 2023.

44. Guralnik, J. M., Ferrucci, L., Simonsick, E. M., et al. (1995). Lower-extremity function in persons over the age of 70 years as a predictor of subsequent disability. *The New England Journal of Medicine, 332*, 556–561. https://doi.org/10.1056/NEJM199503023320902
45. Casano, H. A. M., & Anjum, F. (2023). *Six-Minute Walk Test.*
46. O'Caoimh, R. (2023). Validation of the Risk Instrument for Screening in the Community (RISC) among older adults in the emergency department. *International Journal of Environmental Research and Public Health, 20*, 3734. https://doi.org/10.3390/ijerph20043734
47. Eadon, H. (2011). Assessing the quality of ward pharmacists' interventions. *International Journal of Pharmacy Practice, 1*, 145–147. https://doi.org/10.1111/j.2042-7174.1992.tb00556.x
48. Arevalo-Rodriguez, I., Smailagic, N., Roqué-Figuls, M., et al. (2021). Mini-Mental State Examination (MMSE) for the early detection of dementia in people with mild cognitive impairment (MCI). *Cochrane Database of Systematic Reviews, 7*, CD010783. https://doi.org/10.1002/14651858.CD010783.pub3
49. Jaeger, J. (2018). Digit Symbol Substitution Test: The case for sensitivity over specificity in neuropsychological testing. *Journal of Clinical Psychopharmacology, 38*, 513–519. https://doi.org/10.1097/JCP.0000000000000941
50. Patterson, J. (2011). Verbal fluency. In J. S. Kreutzer, J. DeLuca, & B. Caplan (Eds.), *Encyclopedia of clinical neuropsychology* (pp. 2603–2606). https://link.springer.com/content/pdf/10.1007/978-0-387-79948-3_1423.pdf
51. Lezak, M. D. (2004). *Neuropsychological assessment.* Oxford University Press.
52. Egton Medical Information Systems Limited. (2023). *Six-item Cognitive Impairment Test (6CIT).* https://patient.info/doctor/six-item-cognitive-impairment-test-6cit. Accessed 19 Jul 2023.
53. O'Caoimh, R., & Molloy, D. W. (2017). The Quick Mild Cognitive Impairment Screen (QMCI), pp. 255–272. https://link.springer.com/content/pdf/10.1007/978-3-319-44775-9_12.pdf
54. Lombard-Vance, R., Soye, E., Ferri, D., et al. (2023). Applying the 'human rights model of disability' to informed consent: Experiences and reflections from the SHAPES Project. *Disabilities, 3*, 28–47. https://doi.org/10.3390/disabilities3010003
55. Parmenter, D. (2015). *Key performance indicators: Developing, implementing, and using winning KPIs* (3rd ed.). Wiley.
56. Business Directory. (2019). *Critical Success Factors (CSF).* http://www.businessdictionary.com/definition/critical-success-factors-CSF.html. Accessed 02 Jul 2019.
57. Doran, G. T. (1981). There's a S.M.A.R.T. way to write management's goals and objectives. *Management Review, 70*, 35–36.
58. Sevilla, R. (2017). *D23.21 – Performance and effectiveness metrics in crisis management experiments: Driving innovation in crisis management for European resilience (DRIVER+).* https://driver-project.eu/wp-content/uploads/2017/11/Performance-and-Effectiveness-Metrics-in-Crisis-Management-Experiments.pdf. Accessed 02 Jul 2019.
59. Kaplan, R. S., & Norton, D. P. (2009). *The balanced scorecard: Translating strategy into action, [Nachdr.].* Harvard Business School Press.
60. eVIP electronic virtual patients. (2023). *Evaluation tool kit.* https://virtualpatients.eu/resources/evaluation-tool-kit/. Accessed 03 Aug 2023.

Chapter 10
Increasing Interoperability by Using Distributed Computation, Machine Learning, and the IoT Ecosystem

Mikhail Tishin, Constandinos X. Mavromoustakis, Athina Bourdena, Evangelos K. Markakis, George Mastorakis, and Evangelos Pallis

10.1 Introduction

10.1.1 Concept

Distributed Computation as a concept in Computer Science is not new and has been a stand-alone topic for research for a couple of decades. The idea of Distributed Computation revolves around the concept of being able to split a large processing load between multiple independent servers/computers in order to solve it. It is fair

M. Tishin (✉) · C. X. Mavromoustakis
Department of Computer Science, University of Nicosia and University of Nicosia Research Foundation, Nicosia, Cyprus
e-mail: tishin.m@live.unic.ac.cy; mavromoustakis.c@unic.ac.cy

A. Bourdena
Department of Business Administration & Tourism, Hellenic Mediterranean University, Heraklion, Iraklion, Greece
e-mail: bourdena@hmu.gr

E. K. Markakis
Department of Electrical and Computer Engineering, Hellenic Mediterranean University, Heraklion, Crete, Greece
e-mail: markakis@pasiphae.eu

G. Mastorakis
Department of Management Science and Technology, Hellenic Mediterranean University, Agios Nikolaos, Crete, Greece
e-mail: gmastorakis@hmu.gr

E. Pallis
Department of Industrial Design and Production Engineering, School of Engineering, University of West Attica, Athens, Greece
e-mail: epallis@uniwa.gr

© The Author(s), under exclusive license to Springer Nature Switzerland AG 2024

A. Bourdena et al. (eds.), *Intelligent Technologies for Healthcare Business Applications*, Signals and Communication Technology,
https://doi.org/10.1007/978-3-031-58527-2_10

to say that with the invention of the LAN and the Internet, this field of Computer Science has been evolving even more rapidly.

Distributed Computation has several major aspects, such as software components and means of inter-process communication, and as it is mentioned in [1, Ch. 2.1, p. 56]; the mixture of both defines certain architectural paradigms/types and their implementation.

10.1.2 Architectural Paradigms

Distributed Computation systems, like many other systems, can be implemented in several ways to achieve different objectives. The well-established and widely used implementations are discussed below.

The architecture types are as follows:

- Layered architecture—essentially represents several independent layers, which are often, for the most part, consist of software components on top of the hardware and OS. Those components are layered on top of each other and process all the incoming tasks in the top-down fashion [1, pp. 57–61, 2, Sec. 2.3.2, pp. 51–52].
- Object-based—in this approach, the interaction between computers/machines is represented by objects and their interfaces. The key feature of this method is one of the object-oriented programming paradigms—encapsulation [1, 2].
- Publisher and Subscriber—it is an event-based approach, which means that servers interact between each other using events and messages [1, pp. 67–71, 2, Sec. 6.3, pp. 242–244]. A common implementation of such an approach includes, but not limited to, a message queuing mechanism, such as RabbitMQ, AWS Simple Queue Service or Kafka, with publisher and subscriber roles.
- Resource-based/Web Services—another commonly used implementation of the Distributed Computation concept and probably the most commonly used on the Internet. In a nutshell, it allows computers/machines to communicate between each other via HTTP/HTTPS calls using either SOAP or REST approach, which are well covered in [1, 2].
- Peer-to-Peer—in this case it is direct communication between two or more machines, where each of them can be both a server and a client [2, 3]. The key idea of this approach is to allow computers/machines, which execute common task, for those processes to communicate in a quick and reliable manner.

Of course, as usual, each of the implementations should consider certain challenges, common for distributed systems; synchronization, security, and fault tolerance are just some of them.

The Healthcare domain is no different from any other data-rich and process-intense computations; therefore, by default, it requires robust hardware to process large workloads. For example, let us imagine a hospital with many patients. The hospital will need to process such images as MRIs, X-Ray, and CT scans, to analyze genomics data or to aggregate large amounts of patient's information to derive insights. These are the most common cases; however, the list can go on, depending on a specific need. Of course, if a hospital uses a Cloud provider, this task becomes simpler, since Cloud providers already have a wide range of solutions to accommodate bulky computations and eliminating the need to host server hardware of premises. For instance, AWS alone has set of solutions:

- https://aws.amazon.com/hpc/
- https://aws.amazon.com/batch/
- https://aws.amazon.com/hpc/parallelcluster/

In any way, even using a Cloud provider, it still requires a certain level of expertise to configure the system properly. Cloud providers simplify Distributed Computation, but only to some extent.

10.2 Machine Learning

10.2.1 Concept

Machine learning is one of the most dynamic and vibrant fields in Computer Science today. Generalizing, its main purpose is to enable computer programs, as much as possible, to adjust their behavior/response to new data considering previous experience (previously input data), hence, to learn. Machine learning as a Computer Science field is relatively new, yet the concepts in which it is based on are fairly old. These concepts belong to the different fields of mathematics starting from simple linear algebra, including calculus and inferential with descriptive statistics methods.

10.2.2 Learning Types and Algorithms

Machine Learning is separated into several major learning types, which go hand in hand with algorithms they use to solve specific tasks. The algorithms in their turn are also separated into several groups by the type of problem they solve and the type of data, categorical or/and continuous, they work with.

Below are discussed major learning types and some of their algorithms:

Supervised—uses labeled data to create a model. Essentially, it uses provided data to identify the relation between features and labels, against which new data is compared. The result of such comparison is often data classification.

KNN—Is one of the base algorithms used to classify new input X against existing Y (trained model). It does so by measuring distances between feature values of X and Y in vector space. There are several frequently used distance measuring techniques, such as Euclidean, Manhattan, Minkowski, Chebyshev [4, pp. 10–

11], and Cosine similarity, which are preferred one over another for the specific nature of data. Euclidean distance takes square root out of the sum of squared differences between features of X and Y, essentially measuring the direct distance between two points. After the final value is found, X is attached to a certain category. Manhattan distance uses sum of the absolute values of differences between X and Y, which on 2D graph can be described as the sum of run and rise between two points. Minkowski distance is somewhat of generalized version of the previous two metrics. It uses exponent as a variable to adjust measurement and is capable of producing results identical to Euclidean and Minkowski metrics, as well as anything in between with correct exponent value. Chebyshev distance, or else known as Chessboard distance, is determined by the maximum, absolute value, between X and Y distances of given points. Cosine similarity is different from the above all, instead of measuring the distance, it finds the angle size to identify proximity.

Regressions—there are two types of regressions Linear and Logistics, which address completely different issues. The current example discusses Linear Regression. This approach comes directly from statistical analysis and is designed to find a regression line on X, Y vector space. In simple terms, LR employs slope intercept formula $y = mx + b$ to build the line and then estimates the distance of other points from it. The values for the formula are derived from X and Y columns, through a series of not complicated calculations [5, Sec. 3.2, pp. 44–45, 6, p. 289]. After the regression line is ready, it is time to compare new data by measuring how far or close its values from the regression line, by finding a standard error of estimate.

Unsupervised—unlike its supervised counterpart, this type of ML does not need labeled data, instead its algorithms are designed to cluster and/or find relations inside of unlabeled data. There is a wide range of all sorts of algorithms, not only to cluster data but to perform clustering related tasks, such as cluster dimensionality reduction using SVD [6, p. 119], PCA, FA, or MDS, which are well covered in [7, pp. 113–125]. The list of algorithms and their complexity is fairly large to be properly addressed in this chapter, though one of them that is worth mentioning is K-means.

- K-Means—one of the most widely used unsupervised learning clustering algorithms. It clusters data around centroids, in which the number is provided by a user. $K =$ number of clusters we want to find, spreading centroids at random locations. The algorithm runs over dataset, compares distances between points to the nearest centroid, and assigns points to the closest centroid (cluster). Every iteration, it assigns a new centroid, which is an average of all points assigned to the cluster in the previous step. After a new centroid has been assigned, points may change their cluster. The algorithm runs until points stop changing belonging cluster [5, Sec. 13.2.1, p. 460, 7, Sec. 7.3, p. 145–149].

Reinforcement—unlike supervised and unsupervised, this type of learning does not have a clear-cut set of algorithms, instead it uses a mixed approach. One of them is the State-Action-Reward model, which helps robotic systems to navigate and perform/adjust their actions based on the incoming data from sensors [7, 8].

Artificial Neural Networks—this sector of Machine Learning uses Artificial Neural Networks to solve both supervised and unsupervised types of tasks, with the best results shown under supervised learning. However, instead of using a specific algorithm for a specific problem, it uses Artificial Neural Networks. Despite having different designs, which basically differ in the number of nodes layers and their connectivity, the core structure is the same—the input layer (nodes), the middle layer (nodes), and the output layer (nodes). The input layer passes its original values multiplied by weights to the middle layer nodes, which sum up the incoming values, add bias value to them, and compare against a threshold. In case of success, the data from the middle layers goes to the output layer, otherwise through backpropagation, the process repeats until the network generates suitable weights. Hence, the updated computation results of weights, values, and bias overcome a threshold [8, p. 81, 5, Sec. 11.3, p. 392].

Let us have a detailed look into some of the above-introduced algorithms and their plain implementation. It is important to mention that Machine Learning algorithms are almost always used alongside other code, which fetches, prepares, and normalizes data. These steps are very important in the Machine Learning workflow, especially data preparation and normalization steps, since they directly influence the quality of analysis outcomes.

The first algorithm to be discussed is KNN with Euclidean distance. For sake of examples, to illustrate some of the basic Machine Learning concepts, the following dataset is used:

The data in Table 10.1 represents a list of [X, Y] points for 2D space and belong to a certain category. In fact, the data can have additional features, since Euclidean distance allows to work with higher than 2D dimensionality. Thus, the features, if needed could be [X, Y, Z] or [X, Y, Z, W]. The visualized version of the table data is provided in Fig. 10.1.

Table 10.1 Test data points

ID	X	Y	Category
1	6.1	6.2	B
2	9.3	9.1	C
3	8.1	8.3	C
4	6.2	5.1	B
5	1.1	2.2	A
6	2.3	3.1	A
7	6.3	5.8	B
8	6.5	6.4	B
9	9.1	9.3	C
10	8.7	8.5	C
11	2.5	3.8	A
12	2.1	2.9	A

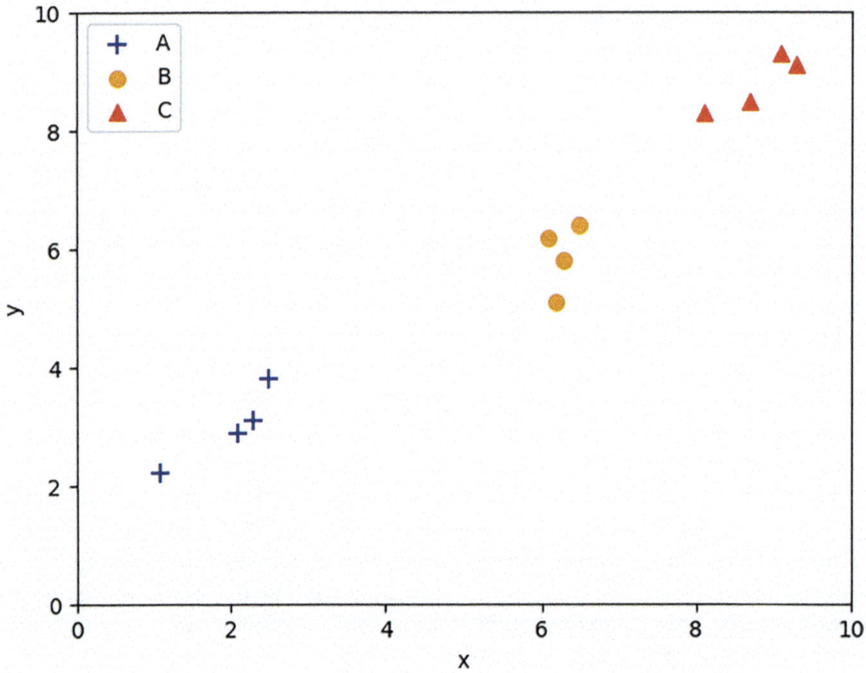

Fig. 10.1 Visualized example data

Having introduced the data, the next step is to classify a new point [5.3, 4.3] by measuring its distance between the existing ones.

$$\text{Distance 1} \quad : \text{sqrt}\left((5.3 - 6.1)^2 + (4.3 - 6.2)^2\right) = 2.062$$

In order to find the rest of the distances, we need to iterate over all the points and compare their distances against the given pair.

$$\text{Distance 2} : [5.3, 4.3] \; [9.3, 9.1] = 6.248$$

$$\text{Distance 3} : [5.3, 4.3] \; [8.1, 8.3] = 4.883$$

$$\text{Distance 4} : [5.3, 4.3] \; [6.2, 5.1] = 1.204$$

$$\text{Distance 5} : [5.3, 4.3] \; [1.1, 2.2] = 4.696$$

$$\text{Distance 6} : [5.3, 4.3] \; [2.3, 3.1] = 3.231$$

$$\text{Distance 7} : [5.3, 4.3] \; [6.3, 5.8] = 1.803$$

$$\text{Distance 8} : [5.3, 4.3] \; [6.5, 6.4] = 2.419$$

$$\text{Distance 9} : [5.3, 4.3]\ [9.1, 9.3] = 6.280$$

$$\text{Distance 10} : [5.3, 4.3]\ [8.7, 8.5] = 5.404$$

$$\text{Distance 11} : [5.3, 4.3]\ [2.5, 3.8] = 2.844$$

$$\text{Distance 12} : [5.3, 4.3]\ [2.1, 2.9] = 3.493$$

Thus, after computing the distances, we can see that there are several points under ID 1, 4, 7, and 8, which seem to be close to the input. However, to classify our new point, we need the closest one, under ID 4. After having identified the closest point, we check its category and assign it to the new point. The positioning of the new point is in Fig. 10.2, where it is marked as a star symbol.

Linear Regression is another popular supervised learning algorithm. It works well with continuous values. It is commonly used to infer future data and to identify if there is a correlation between X and Y; in other words, if changes in either X or Y affect one another. Let us use the previous dataset and plot its regression line as in Fig. 10.3.

Let us see how exactly the line was calculated. Linear Regression is centered around slope intercept formula $y = mx + b$. To plot the line, all the necessary variables must be found.

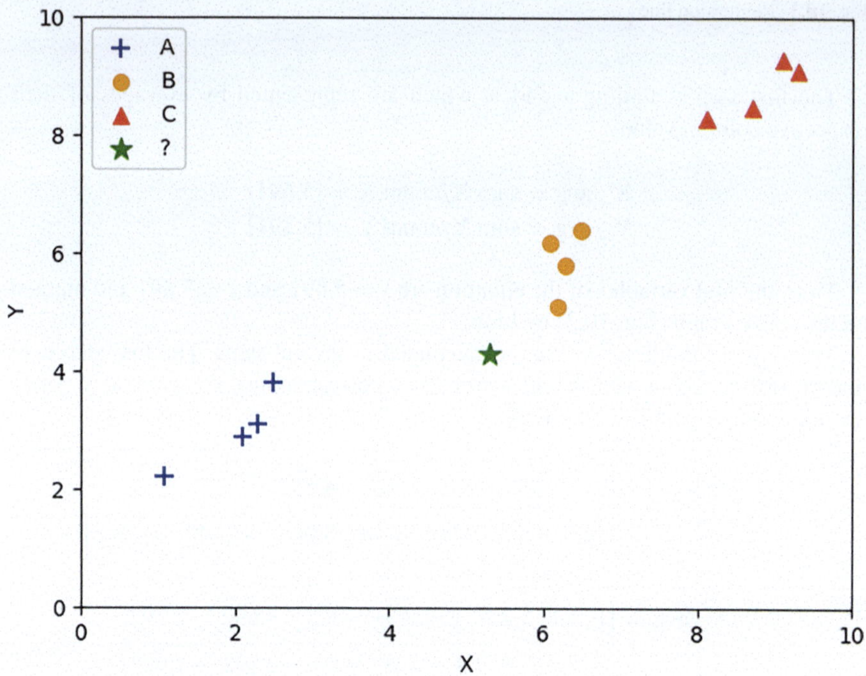

Fig. 10.2 Visualized example data with the new point

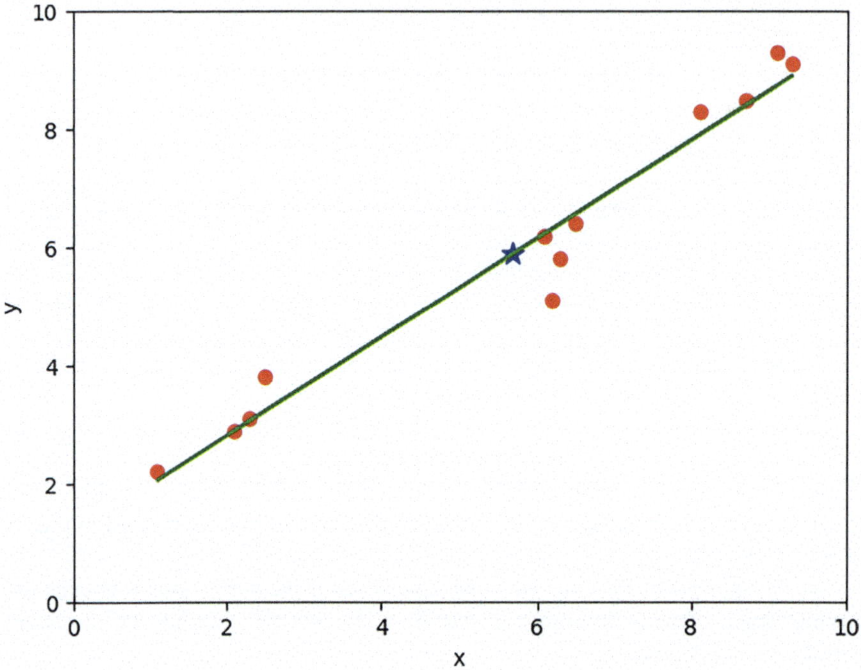

Fig. 10.3 Regression line

The first step is finding x and y, which are represented by averages of their respective column values:

$$X\_avg = \text{sum } X/\text{count } X = [5.691]$$
$$Y\_avg = \text{sum } Y/\text{count } Y = [5.891]$$

Thus, the first variables of the equation are $x = 5.691$ and $y = 5.891$ and marked on the above graph (Fig. 10.3) by blue.

The slope of the line "m" can be calculated in several steps. The first step is to find the difference for each X and Y from their corresponding X _ avg and Y _ avg, i.e., (X – X _ avg), (Y – Y _ avg).

$$\text{X–X\_avg} = [0.408, 3.608, 2.408, 0.508, -4.592, -3.392, 0.608, 0.808, 3.408, 3.008, -3.192, -3.592]$$

$$\text{Y–Y\_avg} = [0.308, 3.208, 2.408, -0.792, -3.692, -2.792, -0.092, 0.508, 3.408, 2.608, -2.092, -2.992]$$

The next step is to find the dot product of (X – X _ avg) $_*$ (Y – Y _ avg) and squared (X – X _ avg) ^{2}.

$$(X–X\_avg) * (Y–Y\_avg) = \big[0.126, 11.577, 5.800, -0.402, 16.951, 9.468, - 0.056, 0.411, 11.617, 7.847, 6.676, 10.745\big]$$

$$(X - X\_avg)^2 = \big[0.167, 13.020, 5.800, 0.258, 21.083, 11.503, 0.370, 0.653, 11.617, 9.050, 10.187, 12.900\big]$$

Having found all the required components, "*m*" = sum((X – X _ avg) $_*$ (Y – Y _ avg))/sum((X – X _ avg) ^{2}) = 80.759/96.609 = 0.836.

So far, there have been found all of the variables, except "*b*", which can be found by solving the equation for "*b*"; $b = y - m_* x$.

$$"b" = 5.891 - 0.836 * 5.691 = 1.134$$

Now Y can be found by using "*m*" = 0.836, "*b*" = 1.134 and X column values.

$$Y = 0.836^*6.1 + 1.134 = 6.233$$

$$Y = 0.836^*9.3 + 1.134 = 8.908$$

$$Y = 0.836^*8.1 + 1.134 = 7.906$$

$$Y = 0.836^*6.2 + 1.134 = 6.317$$

$$Y = 0.836^*1.1 + 1.134 = 2.053$$

$$Y = 0.836^*2.3 + 1.134 = 3.057$$

$$Y = 0.836^*6.3 + 1.134 = 6.400$$

$$Y = 0.836^*6.5 + 1.134 = 6.568$$

$$Y = 0.836^*9.1 + 1.134 = 8.741$$

$$Y = 0.836^*8.7 + 1.134 = 8.407$$

$$Y = 0.836^*2.5 + 1.134 = 3.224$$

$$Y = 0.836^*2.1 + 1.134 = 2.889$$

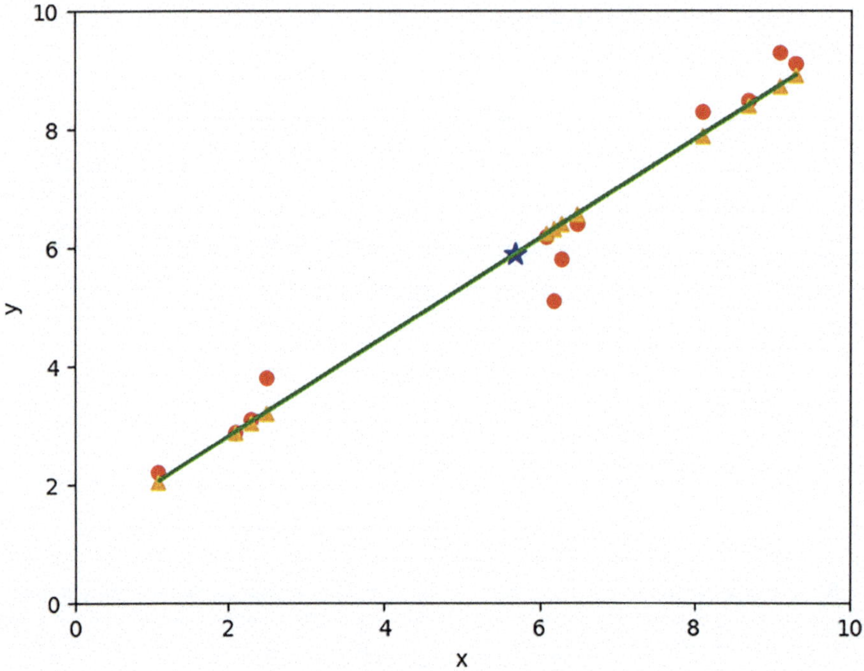

Fig. 10.4 Regression line points

If to plot the [X, Y] points, they should look as on the graph (Fig. 10.4) marked as triangles.

From the graph, it is clear that all of the derived points lie on the regression line, in other words, finding these points allows to draw the line.

In context of Healthcare, Machine Learning has multiple implementation scenarios, from classification of patients by body mass index, clustering their analysis results to identify patterns on medical images and scans, or to infer future state of a patient based on previous cases. The results of the computations can be used by doctors or as instructions to a device. The key idea is to use Machine Learning to allow computers in some cases to recognize health problems on their own and to provide additional advice to a doctor. Essentially, Machine Learning should have no problem diagnosing issues which have clear mathematical definitions. The problem comes when there is a need to diagnose based on symptoms, which can manifest due to a wide range of issues, and it is not always easy to quantify them. In this case, ultimately a doctor is the one to identify potential reasons and prescribe treatments, while Machine Learning can assist in providing insights. Healthcare is rather a delicate matter; therefore, using analyzed data either for instructing devices or for advising doctors must have strict oversight. Even if Machine Learning diagnosed insights are virtually identical to ones a doctor has, a doctor must provide the final decision.

10.3 Distributed Computation and Machine Learning

10.3.1 Concept

In recent years, Machine Learning has become very popular and is being used almost everywhere, from Education and Healthcare to Trading and Science and almost any other industry in between. Their decision-making process includes model training and analysis of big data. The complication arises because of the amount of data is being used, i.e., in the order of hundreds of gigabytes to terabytes and more, which in its turn makes almost impossible to execute Machine Learning tasks in a reasonable amount of time [9, Ch. 1, pp. 1–2].

Distributed Computation and Machine Learning is a field in Computer Science, which explores how ML tasks, i.e., data transfer, algorithms, and model training can be used in context of Distributed Computation to improve performance [10, Ch. 1, pp. 1, 11, Ch. 1, pp. 1].

10.3.2 Ways to Scale Up Machine Learning Computations

In general, any computational system can be scaled either vertically or horizontally. In the case of scaling up Machine Learning computation, both methods are used. Vertical scaling is represented by using GPUs and dedicated for Machine Learning CPUs [9, pp. 2–3], while horizontal scaling is referred to Distributed Computation and federated learning.

Distributed Computation—this idea is tightly coupled with the Distributed Computation from the previous chapter. The whole idea is to have multiple computation nodes connected between each other and each being able to process its own workload. The key aspect is how the load is partitioned, since there are two major approaches—data parallelism and model parallelism, which are well described in [9, 12]. Model parallelism is a more complicated method out of those two.

Federated Learning—this approach was originally developed by Google. It has a centralized model and, unlike the Distributed Computation, where the common source is used either by sharing or its partitioning, it has decentralized data (locally stored). Here is the overall workflow—centralized model is initially downloaded on a device, which trains it on a locally stored data, and, after the training process is finished, the updated model parameters are being sent back to the centralized server [13, pp. 4, 35, 14]. This workflow allows to avoid usage of centralized large amounts of data, thereby avoiding all the complications related to transferring and processing big data.

Also, it is worth mentioning that there are already some tools and frameworks [9, pp. 16–23] out on the market which either assist or fully perform distributed Machine Learning computations. Some of the notable and available are as follows:

- Horovod—https://learn.microsoft.com/en-us/azure/databricks/machine-learning/train-model/distributed-training/horovod-runner
- TensorFlow—https://www.tensorflow.org/guide/distributed_training
- PyTorch—https://pytorch.org/tutorials/beginner/dist_overview.html

and several others.

It is important to note that alongside the already developed and proven methods to optimize Machine Learning performance, there are future possible optimization using Quantum Computers. The notion of Quantum Computers is not new, has been around for decades, and has many publications on how they operate and can be implemented across various Computer Science fields. Machine Learning is one of such field, where adjusting algorithms to work on Quantum Computers has a promise to drastically improve processing speed [15].

Distributed Computation and Machine Learning have their own challenges. Some of them are as follows: Distributed nodes communication and Fault tolerance, Performance optimization and Privacy and several others, which are all mentioned in [9, pp. 24–25, Sec. 1.2, p. 2]. Each of them alone or combined are topics of ongoing research in search of the best possible solution with the least possible computational cost. In other words, it is the cost versus efficiency balance problem.

10.4 IoT Ecosystem

10.4.1 Concept

IoT is a relatively new, evolving field, which encompasses a whole spectrum of different industries from hardware manufacturers, which make all sorts of devices and sensors capable of computation, to software engineers who program them and network architects who make it possible for those devices to communicate. In simple terms, IoT is a constellation of devices, which are interconnected via different networks and able to exchange data, between each other and remote servers. The list of IoT devices can virtually include everything, starting from a kettle or a fridge with the internet connection, to very sophisticated ones with considerable processing capacity, such as smartphones, drones, self-driving cars, and many others.

The core idea is that IoT devices, while operating, generate data either through sensors or direct interaction and either process it locally or send it to a remote server to analyze it. The analyzed data can be used as an insight into the device's performance or to generate and send back a new set of instructions. This approach allows the device to actuate or calibrate their behavior to the changing circumstances in which they are placed. The use cases of IoT are paramount and depend on the scale of the particular IoT ecosystem, the types of devices, and their purpose. Some of the ideas for IoT implementation include manufacturing, smart city, healthcare, logistics, agriculture, and many others.

10.4.2 IoT Key Components

The typical IoT infrastructure definition varies across different literature sources; however, it shares same base components—devices with some sort of sensors, layered network, server for data storage and analysis, and security.

The scope of IoT devices can virtually include everything, starting from a kettle or a fridge with the internet connection, to very sophisticated ones with considerable processing capacity, such as smartphones, drones, self-driving cars, and many others. The core idea is that IoT devices, while operating, generate data either through sensors or through direct client input. The data is either being processed locally or sent to a remote server for aggregation and analysis. The analyzed data can be used for all sorts of insights including the device's performance or to generate and send back a new set of instructions for devices. The IoT setup is very agile and can be extended by adding new devices. The degree to which devices can be "smart" and adjust their behavior depends on software, from very rudimentary embedded code to turn a device on/off and to very complex based on use of Machine Learning. The complexity of the software depends on the device hardware configuration, such as CPU, RAM, and energy source. Basically, the processing capacity of the hardware elements depends on the energy source that powers them. Devices with low hardware parameters have simpler software and are fully reliant on the server side computation.

Network connectivity is essential for the whole IoT concept to work. This is the component in IoT architecture that enables devices to communicate between each other and the server. For that purpose, there are certain commonly used application-level protocols, including HTTP/S, CoAP, AMQP, XMPP, and MQTT. All of them work over TCP or UDP transport layers [16, 17]. There are significant differences between them that should be considered during designing an IoT architecture. For example, CoAP better fits as request response for devices with low hardware capacity [18, 19]. AMQP and MQTT despite sharing some similar characteristics as publisher and subscriber model, asynchronous messaging, scalability, and being secure, yet differ in messages routing, size, and delivery. MQTT was originally designed for monitoring remote devices accounting for their limited hardware and network resources [16, p. 305, 18, p. 136], while AMQP designed with no such considerations and prioritized maximum reliability and wide range of configurations [16, 18].

Other important aspects of the IoT networking are Wireless and potential use of Content-Centric Network. Wireless is used for both inter device and device server communications and represented by the whole range of different technologies [18, pp. 102–108], including the ideas of using 5G [20, pp. 25–33]. In fact, it is possible to argue that Wireless Communication is vital for the robust and agile IoT ecosystem [21], simply for mobile types of devices to be connected between themselves and Cloud servers. Talking about Content-Centric Network, it is a good alternative to IP/Host-based architecture for devices to communicate by making easier and faster access to data [20, pp. 8–16]. Faster access to data comes in part due to request/response optimization, by skipping the so-called request acknowledgment step, used in IP/Host model.

Data storage and analysis is the "brain" part of IoT ecosystem. It is meant to be scalable and to work with immense amounts of data, therefore requiring extensive computational resources. Depending on the IoT architecture, its initial purpose and use case, such computational resources can be on premise or on Cloud. It is clear that the on-premise option requires purchase and installation of sophisticated hardware and necessary software to facilitate data storage and analysis. On top of that, the whole infrastructure must be kept up to date, i.e., repair, update, and replacement of equipment. On the other hand, modern Cloud providers provide services to address those needs [19, Sec. 1.5.1, p. 13].

Security is an important part of the IoT ecosystem [22]. Both devices and network must be protected from the inside and outside cyberattacks. There is a wide range of attacks such as DDOS, Bruteforce Credentials, Network packets interception, and various others [16, 23]. All these measures, including strict policies on device access, strong passwords and their rotation, honey pots, and properly configured firewalls and SSL certificates, should be implemented to address a variety of cyberattacks. The security can go, as far as, to use Artificial Neural Network to monitor and prevent cyberattacks on the IoT devices. One of such detailed examples is well described in the context of an industrial IoT [24, Sec. C, p. 23194]. The concept of such an approach very well can be applied in other industries, including Agriculture and Healthcare.

10.4.3 Combined Use of Distributed Computation, Machine Learning, and the IoT Ecosystem

This section discusses the use and purpose of Machine Learning and Distributed Computation in the IoT ecosystem. One needs to keep in mind that not all of the IoT ecosystem types require explicit use of Machine Learning and Distributed Computation at the same time. It is all case specific to the IoT ecosystem and its purpose. This chapter covers only those specific cases.

Before diving into examples, let us discuss if the IoT concept is something completely new or a natural evolution of pre-existed concepts. In the next paragraph, I will discuss a smart farm (IoT ecosystem) and its components. However, before that let us ask some questions: Does it really need those components to be smart? Are there any predecessors to smart farms? Let us start answering from the last—there have been farms with certain degree of automation for decades, which is the direct result of replacing human labor with automation. Some of the activities that have been replaced include manual watering with irrigation systems, harvesters instead of handpicking, and thorough environment (heat, humidity, and sunlight) analysis in place of human guessing. The transition from human labor to automation still required significant human involvement to maintain the infrastructure's key parts. The ongoing digital transformation has brought new available technologies, which allowed to cut human interaction even more, by providing synchronization between the key parts, increasing farming efficiency, and delegating some decision-making to computers that control the key parts [25]. Thus, innovation in computing gave prospect to smart farms and reduced human involvement. This brings us to the second question—does a smart farm need those components? Yes, it does, if we want to reduce human labor, increase efficiency, and interoperability between farm infrastructure key parts. This example is not limited to farms; the IoT concept can be implemented to most of the industries. Despite having its unique features, IoT is a natural evolution of automation and human's desire to enable machines to take certain decisions on the spot, in other words—being able to adjust their behavior according to the changing environment.

Let us imagine such IoT devices composition as in Fig. 10.5, which would allow enhancing crop cultivation. Such composition should include sensors to measure heat, air and soil humidity, and an irrigation system to water crops (either in-ground pipes or flying/on-ground drones) and a server in the nearby farming complex. Sensors collect data in real time and pass it over to the server, which after processing data can decide further course of actions. Let us imagine, during the last days the incoming data from the sensors has been indicating favorable weather conditions, thus the irrigation system has been instructed from the server to use 100 liters of water and to water crops two times per day. However, on the next day, during the night the server starts to receive data that the soil and air are getting too dry, and the server instructs the irrigation system to increase watering frequency from 2 to 4 times and water usage from 100 to 200 liters. This example looks quite simple; however, if we decompose it to its primitive components, we find that it consists not only of smart devices but includes Distributed Computation and Machine Learning.

The above composition sounds somewhat rudimentary, a couple of sensors here and there, an irrigation system, and water supply regulation. What can be complicated there? However, in practice, it is not as simple as it might look. The role of the devices is fairly obvious, to collect and send data to the server, and to irrigate the crops. What roles do Machine Learning and Distributed Computation play here? As it was mentioned earlier, the sensors send data about each minor change in the environment to the server in real time, thus generating large amounts of data over the time, including passing seasons/months. The server has to store this data, thus, to have a sophisticated database schema, represented by a Data Warehouse and its additional components to accommodate the ETL process. Essentially, it is a whole software infrastructure pipeline, which receives data from the sensors, transforms it to the format suitable for storage, and provides some sort of admin panel for humans to inspect the storage and the data inside it. To organize such a pipeline alone requires expertise in the domain of Database Management and Big Data. Some of the challenges of managing Big Data in context of IoT are well described here [26, 27]. The next step for the system is to process the accumulated data, in order to provide meaningful instructions for the irrigation system. In order to process the data, Machine Learning algorithms can be used, to derive patterns and relations from the data. For example, the simplest can be Linear Regression to see the relation

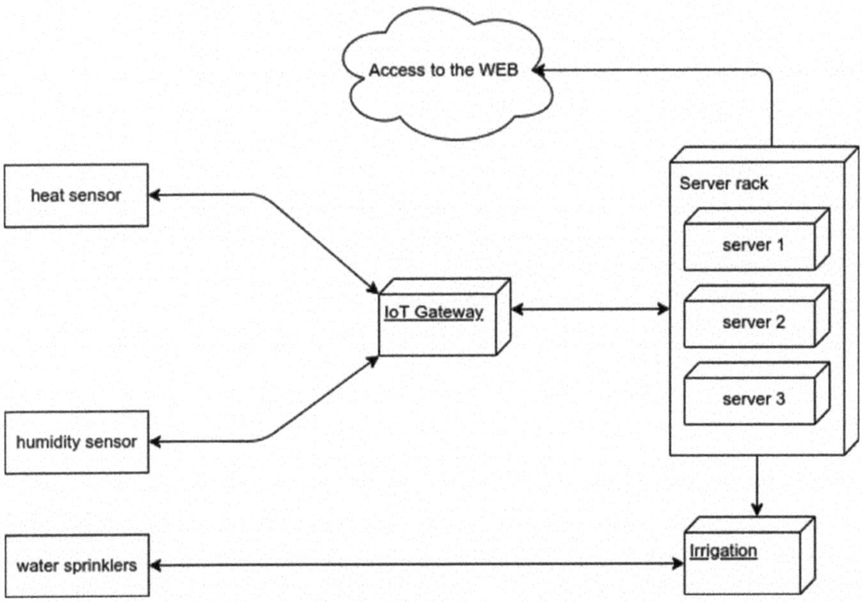

Fig. 10.5 Smart farm

between the heat and levels of humidity, or to run clustering to identify heat and humidity distribution across the fields. From the first view, it looks simple to run Linear Regression or to Cluster data to discover patterns. However, considering the sheer size of data and the need to instruct the irrigation system in reasonable amount of time, Machine Learning has to be done on multiple machines, thus, to incorporate Distributed Computation.

Moreover, talking about Distributed Computation on premises includes installation of a server room to host server rack/racks, which is a typical industrial solution. The servers can be represented by different types with different hardware configurations: some to analyze data and execute Machine Learning computations; others to perform regular activities, such as use of desktop and web applications and work with office files. Those that perform Machine Learning must have certain hardware configuration, somewhat similar to the following:

- RAM—32–128 GB—can support massive datasets.
- Disk—1–2 TB SSD—quick read and write operations.
- Video—NVIDIA Tesla V100—optimized for running Artificial Neural Networks, due to GPU parallelism.
- CPU—Intel Xeon W or D series—versatile for all sorts of work, including AI and data processing.

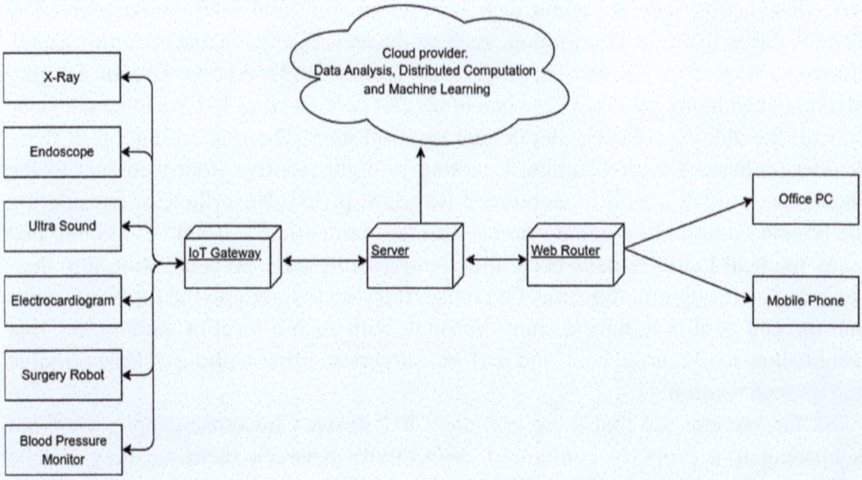

Fig. 10.6 Smart hospital

Servers for regular activities can have the following:

- RAM—8 GB
- Disk—100–200 GB HDD
- Video—Built-in video adapter, such as Matrox G200eW3 Graphics Controller or a cheap alternative from NVIDIA or AMD
- CPU—Intel Xeon Silver

To squeeze maximum performance and compatibility requires servers' proper configuration and maintenance, which is not an easy task, considering the wide range of hardware available on the market, including emerging cutting-edge prototypes.

The next case to be discussed is related to the Healthcare domain and hospitals in particular. However, before describing possible ecosystem configuration, it is good to lay out certain base assumptions:

- The whole system must be practical in use, to ease and improve the day-to-day work of the hospital.
- The system has to be robust, easy to extend, and fault tolerant.
- The system must be secure.

The base system architecture can have, but not to be limited to, peripheral IoT devices, means to be connected and communicate, and a server to process and instruct humans and the devices, as shown in Fig. 10.6.

The ecosystem for the smart hospital could include an array of up-to-date medical machines, which can be outright classified as IoT devices. Most of the modern hospital equipment has undergone digital transformation and always comes equipped, either with built-in or externally connected computers. The very fact that these machines are being controlled/used via computer interface suggests they were designed to have a certain degree of automation and inter-connectivity. The devices range from fairly common, such as devices, X-ray, endoscope, ultrasound, electrocardiogram to the most sophisticated as Surgeon Operating Robotic Surgery Machine, and many others. These machines can be viewed as IoT peripherals, since they all are able to collect/generate and transmit data. The transformation of these devices, enhanced with Machine Learning brought positive improvements to the Healthcare industry, as it is mentioned here [28, p. 13]. Nevertheless, considering the ongoing automation update across different industries, it is safe to assume that many medical facilities have been integrating cutting-edge AI innovation into their work cycle, throughout this time. Of course, if trying to look into the future, it seems that the end goal is to have a smart hospital, with such a level of automation, that would allow to diagnose, heal, and perform surgeries, either without or least possible human intervention.

So far, we can see that there are many IoT devices for our example, yet what is missing is a properly configured connectivity between them, so they can be orchestrated and perhaps even to take some decisions on their own. To address the missing components, we have to factor in AI/ML, network equipment, and computational resources (server). Unlike IoT devices and the network equipment, which hospital has to purchase on its own, AI/ML and computational server require a hospital to consider several options:

- To rely on their own resources, therefore, to mount and configure these parts, which is a serious challenge.
- To delegate it elsewhere, such as AWS https://aws.amazon.com/iot/ https://aws.amazon.com/healthimaging/ https://aws.amazon.com/health/ or IBM https://www.ibm.com/industries/healthcare https://www.ibm.com/cloud/internet-of-things.
- To have a mixed version of both approaches.

Each of the options offers its own benefits and drawbacks. For example, having the whole ecosystem on premises can provide a hospital with full control over the system, direct access at any time to every single part of it, which may be completely not possible with a Cloud provider. The downside, as from the previously discussed examples, in order to implement Distributed Computation and Machine Learning architecture a hospital has to heavily invest in server room equipment, software development, and to have IT personal to maintain the system. On top of that, it should be able to scale up or down the hardware components. None of the issues mentioned above are real problems when using a cloud provider. The mixed approach may look quite appealing due to its flexibility and that it allows us to reduce dependency on certain services from Cloud providers. For example, a hospital IT team can connect and orchestrate all the devices on premises instead of using AWS events or developing their own machine learning models to work with certain types of data or storing the most sensitive data locally, however, to perform all the bulky computations on the Cloud.

Let us talk about devices connectivity. The industrial grade of equipment, such as CISCO or Leonton, is preferred over the regular ones. The devices can be interconnected inside a local network via IoT Gateway, without having direct access to the internet. The gateway itself can be connected to the main server where it streams data from the devices in real time. In fact, employing industrial-level equipment may very well lead to using a very sophisticated industrial-grade network with such attributes as high level of security, access management, and fault tolerance. One of the potential examples is well described here https://www.cisco.com/c/dam/global/en_uk/solutions/industries/pdfs/healthcare-secure-infrastructure.pdf. Although, using proper equipment can increase network security, it is important to remember that there are additional methods to increase security, for example, such as the one described in here [29, 30].

The server and its processing capacity is directly correlated to many factors, among which are whether a hospital uses a Cloud provider or does everything on premises, the number of devices, amount and type of incoming data generated by them, and applications used in day-to-day work by the personnel. For example, if IoT devices involve real-time video processing, then it is better to process it on the local server, which must be specifically designed for that, and later upload it on the Cloud, for further analysis. However, if the devices generate data, which is not crucial in real time, then the server has to be good enough to reliably send those data to the Cloud server and receive it back analyzed.

Nowadays, a large part of medical equipment, despite being digitized, still functions as tools in the hands of doctors, unable to take actions on their own and requiring human operation. The tools can be "smart," connected to a network, and emit data; however, many remain single purpose, cannot take any effective actions nor change their behavior. Instead, they just monitor, measure, and report results. There are certain exceptions, such as life support units, anesthesia machines, robotic surgery machines, and some others, which can be instructed to behave in a crtain way and take actions based on a patient's real-time condition.

Another example is inter-drone communication and navigation while performing certain tasks. Let us imagine an object inside a certain area, and we need to find it. Let the current scenario include the following components: an area that splits into sectors, two average drones (perhaps even Arduino or Raspberry Pi robots), distance and video sensors, a server, and a test object. The baseline objective is to make two drones cooperate and find the test object as represented in Fig. 10.7. In order for this scenario to be successful, the drones should be able to navigate in a given area and to be able to notify each other after searching a sector to avoid double search sectors after each other and to identify the object of the search. Thus, the current scenario has several major questions: communication, navigation, and object identification.

From the search mission objectives and the hardware components given, we already can understand that it will require to use some communication mechanism, route optimization, and image recognition. While the communication part can be fairly simple to implement and utilizes very little computational resources, the other two tasks can be very heavy. Usually, most of the average drones have very limited processing power and storage capacity; thus, they individually cannot perform those two tasks on their own. In order to optimize them, they must be executed in a distributed way. From the previous chapter, we can see that there are several ways for Machine Learning to be used in a distributed fashion, i.e., data parallelism and

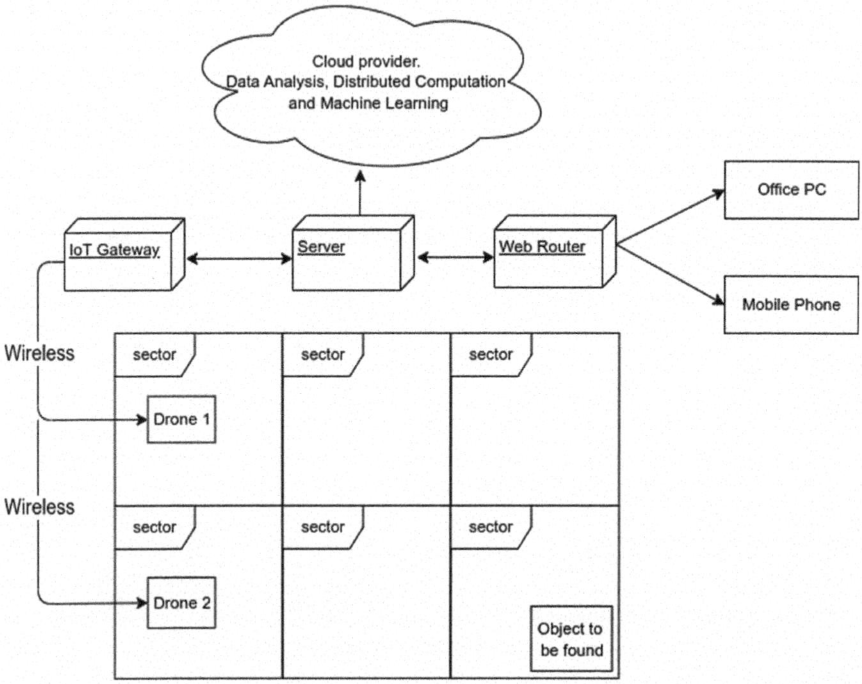

Fig. 10.7 Drones' cooperation

model parallelism, federated learning. Both of the methods are applicable in the current situation. In case of using federated learning, each of the drones should train their own model, which is based on its limited, drone-specific data. After preliminary local processing, the outcomes must be sent to the server, which will aggregate and generate a final result. In case of the regular Distributed Computation, all visual data from the drones has to be streamed back to the server in real time and the server should do data processing, model training, produce final results, and to return instructions to the drones. As for the route optimization, despite drones being able to navigate using sensors, they are constrained by the distance sensors can cover and environment in a given sector. In order for the drones to be able to navigate between sectors, their navigation can be provided either by integrating drones into the already existing systems, which have been used for decades in aerospace and naval industries or by creating a localized version to this particular IoT ecosystem. In either case, navigation in general and for drones in particular, some of its steps include problems similar to A star algorithm [31] or the Traveling Salesman Problem or the Find Shortest Path. These types of problems and the execution time they take are extremely sensitive to the input size. Their Big O in naive implementation starts from $n!$ for the Traveling Salesman Problem and n^2 for the Find Shortest Path. Even after optimization, these algorithms remain fairly computation expensive. In fact, the drones must be able to use Distributed

Computation on demand—access to the server computational resources, even if their complexity is just Big $O(n)$. Let us imagine counting from 0 to N using a loop, which has linear complexity, if the N is large enough the counting can take 2, 5, 10, or even 20 min and more. The counting code execution time fully depends on the input size. Considering that the instructions exchange between the drones and the server must happen quickly, the drones can respond to changes in environment dynamically. Therefore, the computation process must be fast. Thus, Distributed Computation is one of the possible solutions to solve these problems.

From the provided examples, we can see that the introduced IoT ecosystems comprised multiple components: the physical devices are as acting parts, the brain and decision-making are based on Machine Learning, and the speed of the decision-making is Distributed Computation. In fact, Machine Learning and its advanced representation as Artificial Intelligence is the exact component, which makes both of the IoT ecosystems smart, without this component, it is just a network of connected devices and a conventional automation chain.

References

1. van Steen, M., & Tanenbaum, A. S. (2017). *Distributed Systems* (3rd ed.). Pearson Educación.
2. Coulouris, G. F. (2012). *Distributed systems: Concepts and design* (5th ed.). Addison-Wesley.
3. Kshemkalyani, A. D., & Singhal, M. (2011). *Distributed computing: Principles, algorithms, and systems*. Cambridge University Press.
4. Prasath, V. B. S., et al. (2017). Distance and similarity measures effect on the performance of K-nearest neighbor classifier – A review. *Big Data*, no page.
5. Hastie, T., Friedman, J., & Tisbshirani, R. (2017). *The elements of statistical Learning: Data mining, inference, and prediction* (2nd ed.). Springer.
6. Deisenroth, M. P., Faisal, A. A., & Ong, C. S. (2020). *Mathematics for machine learning* (1st ed.). Cambridge University Press.
7. Alpaydin, E. (2014). *Introduction to machine learning* (2nd ed.). MIT Press.
8. Mitchell, T. M. (1997). *Machine learning*. MacGraw-Hill.
9. Verbraeken, J., Wolting, M., Katzy, J., Kloppenburg, J., Verbelen, T., & Rellermeyer, J. S. (2020, March). A survey on distributed machine learning. *ACM Computing Surveys, 53*(2), Article 30, 33 pages. https://doi.org/10.1145/3377454.
10. Galakatos, A., Crotty, A., & Kraska, T. (2017). Distributed machine learning. In L. Liu & M. Özsu (Eds.), *Encyclopedia of database systems*. Springer. https://doi.org/10.1007/978-1-4899-7993-3_80647-1
11. Li, M., et al. (2014). Scaling distributed machine learning with the parameter server. In *11th USENIX Symposium on Operating Systems Design and Implementation*.
12. Rtanase. *What is distributed training? – Azure Machine Learning | Microsoft Learn*. http://learn.microsoft.com/en-us/azure/machine-learning/concept-distributed-training?view=azureml-api-2. Accessed 28 May 2023.
13. Chen, H. (2022). *Reliable and efficient distributed machine learning*. Kungliga Tekniska Högskolan.
14. Collaboration Machine Learning On-Device Learning Optimization. (2017). Federated learning: Collaborative machine learning without centralized training data. *Google AI Blog*, Thursday, April 06. http://ai.googleblog.com/2017/04/federated-learning-collaborative.html. Accessed 28 May 2023.

15. Zeguendry, A., et al. (2023, February). Quantum machine learning: A review and case studies. *Entropy, 25*(2), 287. https://doi.org/10.3390/e25020287
16. Lea, P. (2018a). *Internet of Things for architects*. Packt Publishing.
17. Rayes, A., & Salam, S. (2019). *Internet of Things from hype to reality: The road to digitization*. Springer.
18. Gilchrist, A. (2016). *Industry 4.0: The industrial Internet of Things*. Apress.
19. Buyya, R., & Dastjerdi, A. V. (2016). *Internet of Things: Principles and paradigms*. Morgan Kaufmann.
20. Mavromoustakis, C. X., Mastorakis, G., & Batalla, J. M. (2016). *Internet of Things (IOT) in 5G mobile technologies* (Vol. 8). Springer.
21. Batalla, J. M., Mastorakis, G., Mavromoustakis, C. X., & Zurek, J. (2016, October). On cohabitating networking technologies with common wireless access for home automation system purposes. *IEEE Wireless Communications, 23*(5), 76–83. https://doi.org/10.1109/MWC.2016.7721745
22. Mukherjee, M., Matam, R., Mavromoustakis, C. X., Jiang, H., Mastorakis, G., & Guo, M. (2020, September). Intelligent edge computing: Security and privacy challenges. *IEEE Communications Magazine, 58*(9), 26–31. https://doi.org/10.1109/MCOM.001.2000297
23. Waher, P. (2015). *Learning internet of things: Explore and learn about internet of things with the help of engaging and enlightening tutorials designed for Raspberry Pi*. Packt Publishing.
24. Tran, M.-Q., et al. (2022). Reliable deep learning and IOT-based monitoring system for secure computer numerical control machines against cyber-attacks with experimental verification. *IEEE Access, 10*, 23186–23197. https://doi.org/10.1109/access.2022.3153471
25. Manogaran, G., Hsu, C.-H., Rawal, B. S., Muthu, B., Mavromoustakis, C. X., & Mastorakis, G. (2021, March 1). ISOF: Information scheduling and optimization framework for improving the performance of agriculture systems aided by industry 4.0. *IEEE Internet of Things Journal, 8*(5), 3120–3122. https://doi.org/10.1109/JIOT.2020.3045479
26. Papadokostaki, K., Mastorakis, G., Panagiotakis, S., Mavromoustakis, C. X., Dobre, C., & Batalla, J. M. (2017). Handling big data in the era of Internet of Things (IoT). In C. Mavromoustakis, G. Mastorakis, & C. Dobre (Eds.), *Advances in mobile cloud computing and big data in the 5G era. Studies in big data* (Vol. 22). Springer. https://doi.org/10.1007/978-3-319-45145-9_1
27. Karolewicz, K., Beben, A., Batalla, J., Mastorakis, G., & Mavromoustakis, C. (2016). On efficient data storage service for IoT. *International Journal of Network Management., 27*(3), e1932. https://doi.org/10.1002/nem.1932. Online publication date: 1-May-2017. https://onlinelibrary.wiley.com/doi/10.1002/nem.1932.
28. Bzai, J., et al. (2022). Machine learning-enabled Internet of Things (IoT): Data, applications, and industry perspective. *Electronics, 11*(17), 2676. https://doi.org/10.3390/electronics11172676.
29. Andreas, A., et al. (2021). Robust encryption to enhance IoT confidentiality for healthcare ecosystems. In *2021 IEEE 26th International Workshop on Computer Aided Modeling and Design of Communication Links and Networks (CAMAD), Porto, Portugal* (pp. 1–6). https://doi.org/10.1109/CAMAD52502.2021.9617795
30. Andreas, A., Mavromoustakis, C. X., Mastorakis, G., et al. (2021). Towards an optimized security approach to IoT devices with confidential healthcare data exchange. *Multimedia Tools and Applications, 80*, 31435–31449. https://doi.org/10.1007/s11042-021-10827-x
31. Andreou, A., Mavromoustakis, C. X., Batalla, J. M., Markakis, E. K., Mastorakis, G., & Mumtaz, S. (2023). UAV trajectory optimisation in smart cities using modified A* algorithm combined with haversine and vincenty formulas. *IEEE Transactions on Vehicular Technology, 72*(8), 9757–9769. https://doi.org/10.1109/TVT.2023.3254604

Index

© The Editor(s) (if applicable) and The Author(s), under exclusive license to Springer Nature Switzerland AG 2024
A. Bourdena et al. (eds.), *Intelligent Technologies for Healthcare Business Applications*, Signals and Communication Technology,
https://doi.org/10.1007/978-3-031-58527-2

SPRINGER NATURE

GPSR Compliance

The European Union's (EU) General Product Safety Regulation (GPSR) is a set of rules that requires consumer products to be safe and our obligations to ensure this.

If you have any concerns about our products, you can contact us on ProductSafety@springernature.com

In case Publisher is established outside the EU, the EU authorized representative is:

Springer Nature Customer Service Center GmbH
Europaplatz 3
69115 Heidelberg, Germany

The manufacturer's authorised representative in the EU is Springer Nature Customer Service Centre GmbH, Europaplatz 3, 69115 Heidelberg, Germany. If you have any concerns regarding our products, please contact ProductSafety@springernature.com

Printed and bound by CPI Group (UK) Ltd, Croydon, CR0 4YY
05/10/2026
02227724-0001